A Man's Guide

to

Coping with Disability

Resources for Rehabilitation
Lexington, Massachusetts

Resources for Rehabilitation
33 Bedford Street, Suite 19A
Lexington, Massachusetts 02420
(781) 862-6455 FAX (781) 861-7517
e-mail: info@rfr.org http://www.rfr.org

A Man's Guide to Coping with Disability 2nd edition

Copyright 1999 by Resources for Rehabilitation, Inc.

ISBN 0-929718-23-2

Resources for Rehabilitation is a nonprofit organization dedicated to providing training and information to professionals and the public about the needs of individuals with disabilities and the resources available to meet those needs.

Library of Congress Cataloging-in-Publication Data

A Man's Guide to Coping with Disability -- 2nd ed.
   p.   cm.
       Includes bibliographical references and index
       ISBN 0-929718-23-2 (alk. paper)
1. Physically handicapped men--Medical care. 2. Physically handicapped men--
Rehabilitation 3.Physically handicapped men--Services for
I. Resources for Rehabilitation (Organization)
RC108.M356 1999   98-55559
362.4'081--dc21   CIP

This book is printed on acid-free paper.

For a complete listing of publications available from Resources for Rehabilitation, see pages 285-288

TABLE OF CONTENTS

INTRODUCTION

Although medical research and previous volumes addressing the needs of individuals with disabilities have been the subject of criticism for failing to address the special needs of women, these works have almost universally failed to address the special needs of men. Instead, they have addressed the "generic" human. In fact, a review of the literature reveals that there are no publications that deal specifically with the needs of men with disabilities, while recent years have witnessed the publication of several works for women.

A Man's Guide to Coping with Disability provides the essential information that men need in order to pursue their rights and obtain the services that enable them to be independent. In addition to providing information that is applicable to men with any physical disability or chronic condition, this book covers conditions that are most prevalent in men and those that are likely to affect men's special roles in society or their sexual functioning. Family members and service providers will also find the book to be extremely useful in their search for appropriate services. Because men have different lifestyles, needs, and degrees of impairment, the book is organized so that each man may select the resources that are most appropriate to his own specific needs.

Each chapter includes an introductory narrative, information about national organizations that provide services to men, and information about relevant publications and tapes. Chapters 1, 2, and 3, "Men and Disability," "Coping with Daily Activities," and "Laws That Affect Men with Disabilities" provide information that is useful no matter what disability or condition the reader is interested in.

Beginning with Chapter 4, each chapter has introductory material describing causes and effects of the condition or impairment; sexual functioning; psychological aspects; information on professional service providers and where to find services; assistive devices (when applicable); major service organizations; and publications and tapes. Descriptions of organizations, publications and tapes, and assistive devices are alphabetical within sections. Although many of the publications described are available in libraries or bookstores, for those who wish to purchase the books by mail or phone, the addresses and phone numbers of publishers and distributors are included. Only directories that have timely information and those that are updated regularly are included. Publications that are out of print may be located at libraries or bookstores that specialize in locating out of print books.

Developments in computer technology have greatly increased access to information for the general population as well as people with disabilities and chronic conditions. E-mail and Internet addresses are provided for organizations when available.

The use of "TT" in the listings indicates a text telephone, a special telephone system for individuals who are deaf, have hearing impairments, or have speech impairments (formerly known as TDD, telecommunication device for the deaf). The use of "V/TT" indicates that the same telephone number is used for both voice and text telephone. Toll-free numbers may begin with "800," "888," or "877."

All of the material in this book is up-to-date, and prices were accurate at the time of publication. However, it is always advisable to contact publishers and manufacturers to inquire about availability and current prices.

Chapter 1

MEN AND DISABILITY

The number of individuals who live with a disability or chronic condition constitutes a significant proportion of the population. A recent survey estimates that in 1991 to 1992, 48.9 million Americans, or 19.4% of the population, lived with a disability that limits their functional or socially defined activities; this figure does not include those Americans who live in institutions (McNeil: 1993). Nearly 23 million men were members of this population, representing a disability rate of 18.7%. Not surprisingly, older men had higher rates of disability than younger men; over half of men age 65 years or older (50.9%) had some type of disability (McNeil: 1993).

A wide variety of services exists for this population in both the private and the public sectors. Federal legislation has mandated a variety of programs that provide rehabilitation services and independent living programs. Such programs exist at the regional, state, and local levels. Special programs and services are available at hospitals, libraries, senior centers, independent living centers, and in educational institutions at all levels, from preschool through postsecondary education.

Although the services that exist are both numerous and varied, it is commonplace to discover that people who need these services have not received information about them or about the implications of their own condition. A negative attitude on the part of some physicians and inadequate information about rehabilitation leave men with disabilities and chronic conditions in a position where they are marginal to both the fields of medicine and rehabilitation. Physicians, who are more attuned to acute conditions than chronic conditions or disabilities, in essence often write off many of these people. Rehabilitation professionals are not aware of these individuals and therefore are unable to provide services to them. In many instances, individuals never receive rehabilitation services or else years elapse before they do.

MALE VALUES, HEALTH, AND DISABILITY

Although men make up 48.7% of the population in the United States (McNeil: 1993), they account for only 40.1% of all office visits to physicians who are not employed by the federal government (Schappert: 1996). Men's lower rate of office visits was found in every age category except under 15 years (an age at which their parents are likely to make their medical decisions). Males in the age category 15 to 24 years had the lowest rate of office visits, with each succeeding age category having higher rates than the preceding age group. Rates of office visits made by those in the youngest age group (under 15) and the two oldest age groups (65 to 74 and 75 and over) were not significantly different from women's rates. While some of the difference in physician office visits by gender may be explained by women's needs for medical attention to their reproductive system and pregnancy (Waldron: 1983), dominant male values such as independence and physical strength are likely contributors to less frequent use of the health care system. To many men, the need to visit a physician is an indication of weakness and a devaluation of their masculinity. These values often lead men to deny the symptoms of illness and therefore not to seek out medical attention. Even with severe disabilities, men who place great value on their independence may refuse assistance in their everyday activities and reject rehabilitation services. The masculine value of independence is learned so early in life that a teenager with a severe mobility impairment commented:

> If I ever have to ask someone for help, it really makes me feel like less of a man. I don't like asking for help at all. You know, like even if I could use some, I'll usually not ask just because I can't, I just hate asking... (Gerschick and Miller: 1995, 193).

A study of disability and psychological distress indicates that men are less able to psychologically cope with a disability at a younger age, when their feelings of invulnerability may be stronger (Altman and Smith: 1992). As men age, they place greater value on interpersonal relations and intimacy (Moreland: 1989), and their sense of invulnerability may decrease.

As Hahn (1989) has noted, men who have disabilities are subjected to conflict. While their male values stress strength, society views disability as weakness. The devaluation of men with disabilities often results in rejection in the workplace and in romantic relationships. Attempts to deny their disabilities have prevented many men from participating in the disability rights movement.

Values obviously affect men's use of the health care system and their responses to disabilities and chronic conditions. However, poor health and disability may also affect men's values. For example, men with diabetes who had been "workaholics" prior to developing their disease realized the importance of spending more time with their families instead of working all their waking hours. They also changed their values regarding the importance of income, placing family first. Some comments from men with diabetes interviewed by Peyrot et al. (1988) indicate these changing values:

> ...I'm closer to my family than I was. Prior to this [onset of diabetes] I was working 80 hours a week. I spend many more hours at home than I did.

> I think we're closer together. For one reason we found out we could make it on half the income we were making before. We found out even if we have to really tighten up, we're still a family. We changed our whole life around (p. 372).

A male psychologist with a progressive illness wrote that his disease resulted in the ability to express his concerns openly and to attach more significance to family relationships, although these positive changes followed a period in which he was extremely self-centered:

> During the early period following my diagnosis, I became totally self-absorbed. I had no interest in other people's lives, not even those closest to me. This, however, changed as time passed.

Relationships with members of my family took on new significance. For one thing, I wanted them to know me more than I had before. So I more openly expressed my thoughts and feelings about whatever concerned me....Because of this new way of being with others, I developed a greater capacity for kindness and intimacy than I have had (Flapan: 1996, 2).

Disabilities and chronic conditions compel men to change their lifestyles and their definitions of masculinity and in the process to change their definitions of self. Thus, while physical strength, sexuality, competitiveness, and toughness may have been the accepted male values prior to the onset of disability or disease, men find new ways to define their masculinity after the onset of these conditions. For some men, this search for a new identity may take years; ultimately, however, they may come to view their conditions as positive experiences (Charmaz: 1995). For men who never held the traditional male values or for those whose condition developed at a later stage in life when the dominant male values are not as strong, adjustment may be somewhat easier. The response of significant others, who also face an adjustment process, may prove to be either supportive or disruptive in this redefinition process.

SEXUALITY AND DISABILITY

Although sexuality has been referred to as "the forgotten ADL" [activity of daily living] (Breske: 1996), the effects of disability on sexual interactions can be major and should be addressed by every rehabilitation program. Even when the disability does not directly affect the organs responsible for sexual pleasure, loss of self-esteem and revised perceptions of body image may interfere with sexual desire and performance. Anxiety over the disability or condition and what the future will bring may cause interest in sexual activity to decrease dramatically. Fear on the part of both partners that sexual activity may cause additional health problems also may contribute to a decrease in sexual activity. Sometimes the man withdraws from physical relations with his partner for fear that he will be unable to complete the sexual act; the partner, in turn, interprets this as rejection (Rustad: 1984).

Men who experience disabilities while in an established relationship may avoid resuming sexual activity for fear of failure. Both the man and his partner may have grave concerns over the new character of their relationship. Mobility impairment, loss of sensation, spasticity, and bowel and bladder incontinence may all seem insurmountable problems at first. Learning new positions for intercourse, additional means of stimulation, and ways to avoid embarrassing leakage problems due to incontinence will relieve the sexual partners of these fears. Sexual counseling, as a couple or in group sessions, can provide invaluable information on these topics. To a great extent, the couple's success at restructuring their sexual relationship depends upon the quality of their relationship prior to the disability; those who had good communications are more likely to be able to discuss their fears and needs openly (Lemon: 1993).

Men who were not in an established sexual relationship may experience different problems. Lack of mobility may result in social isolation and the inability to meet potential sexual partners. Overcoming embarrassment and fear of rejection may be intensified in a new relationship. Society's attitudes toward individuals with disabilities may prevent men from initiating a social relationship. Men who are homosexual may find that they face two types of stigma. Society's view that individuals with disabilities are asexual applies to homosexuals as well as heterosexuals. Awareness of this stereotype may cause gay men with disabilities to have trepidations over initiating contact with potential partners. When they do establish a stable relationship, rehabilitation professionals are likely to ignore their partners as legitimate participants in the rehabilitation process or as caregivers.

When men experience a disability, they are often required to modify not only the physical activities that formerly were their source of sexual satisfaction, but there is often the need for a role reversal with their sexual partner. When men have limited or no mobility or are spastic, they must rely upon their partner to initiate the sexual activity or prepare them physically. For men who value their role as the dominant partner in a sexual relationship, such a role reversal may be difficult, causing psychological distress and possibly avoidance of sexual activity. The role reversal may be equally difficult for the partner.

For men with severe disabilities that require drastic changes in their patterns of sexual activity, a concomitant change in values may occur. These men may place stronger emphasis on the emotional aspects of their romantic relationships and on pleasing their partner. A man who frequented bars, rode a motorcycle, and had an active sex life prior to his spinal cord injury said the following about his sex life after his injury:

> I've found a whole different side to having sex with a partner and looking at satisfying the partner rather than satisfying myself, and that has taken the focus off of satisfying myself and being the big manly stud and concentrating more on my partner and that has become just as satisfying (Gerschick and Miller: 1995, 190).

Men are often reluctant to raise the subject of erectile dysfunction with their health care providers, so it is imperative that the professional inquire about it (Sandowski: 1989). In some instances, it is difficult to determine whether physical or psychological factors have caused the failure to achieve erection or orgasm. Even when the primary cause of sexual dysfunction is organic, psychological reactions to the situation may contribute to the dysfunction and should be treated (Tieffer: 1987).

Since men have erections while they are asleep, one possibility is to determine whether this normal process is taking place. Simple tests carried out at home or in the hospital provide an answer to this question; if the man is having erections while asleep but is unable to achieve them during attempts at sexual intercourse, it is likely that the failure to achieve erection is psychological. Depression, which is a common and normal response to disability, may cause a lack of desire for sexual relations and the inability to achieve an erection. According to Sandowski (1989), performance anxiety may result in the failure to have an erection; the next time sexual activity is initiated, the fear increases, based on the previous experience. In time, the man completely avoids attempts at sex because the fear becomes so great. In some instances, men who have had a stroke or a heart attack and their partners may fear that sexual intercourse will cause a recurrence; usually this fear is unfounded.

Physical conditions that affect the ability to have an erection include those that interfere with the blood flow to the penis, such as high blood pressure and hardening of the arteries, and those that cause problems in the nervous system, such as diabetes, spinal cord injury, and multiple sclerosis. Urologists may perform tests to assess the blood supply to the penis and the adequacy of the nerve function (Sandowski: 1989).

Treatments for erectile dysfunction include oral medication, injections into the penis, external vacuum pump devices, and penile implants. In March, 1998, the Food and Drug Administration (FDA) approved sildenafil citrate (Viagra), an oral medication which enables many men to produce an erection in response to sexual arousal. In clinical trials, men with mild erectile dysfunction had better results with Viagra than those with more severe cases. Side effects included headache, transient visual disturbances, flushing, and gastrointestinal discomfort. Men who use nitroglycerin should not use the drug, since it may cause a dangerous drop in blood pressure (D'Arrigo: 1998). Although Viagra attracted immediate attention from the media and the public, shortly after its introduction, there were reports of cardiovascular problems in a small number of men who used the drug. The Food and Drug Administration (FDA) has issued warnings to be placed on the drug's label for men with heart conditions or high or low blood pressure. It is unknown if the reported occurrences of heart attacks, hypertension, stroke, or even death were caused by the drug, sexual activity, or previous health conditions.

Injections, vacuum pump devices, and inflatable implants require manual dexterity; those men with limited mobility in their hands may be able to utilize these prostheses only if their partner operates them. Injections directly into the base of the penis have resulted in satisfactory erections that last from one to two hours and enable men to have intercourse. The drugs traditionally used for this purpose include papaverine, prostaglandin E1, and phentolamine, often used in combination. In July, 1995, the FDA approved alprostadil (Caverject), a synthetic prostaglandin E1, to treat erectile dysfunction; this is the first drug the FDA approved specifically for this purpose (Church: 1996). A possible side effect of penile injections is prolonged erection, which may last from four to six hours (priapism). Although this condition is relatively rare, it may damage the spongy tissue of the penis if not treated promptly; immediate treatment at an emergency room is required, where epinephrine is usually injected (Andersson: 1994). In addition, scarring may occur in the penis, preventing the possibility of surgery for penile implants. A recent study of alprostadil found that the main side effect was mild penile pain, occurring after 11% of the injections (Linet and Ogrinc: 1996).

Vacuum pump devices create a partial vacuum around the penis, drawing blood into the penis and causing an erection. The device consists of a plastic cylinder placed over the penis; a pump which draws air out of the cylinder; and an elastic band placed at the base of the penis to maintain the erection. The vacuum works satisfactorily in most cases and does not have any serious side effects (Nadig: 1994).

Penile implants should be considered only when other treatments have failed. Penile implants may be semi-rigid or inflatable. Possible complications include infection and mechanical malfunction, requiring replacement. If penile implants must be removed (due to recurrent infection), the man loses the ability to have an erection permanently. Prior to scheduling surgery for a penile implant, a man should undergo a psychological evaluation to determine whether the cause of his erectile dysfunction is organic or psychological and to ensure that his expectations of a penile implant are realistic. Penile implants do not result in normal erections, and the man should be aware of this prior to undergoing the surgery. His partner should be included in these counseling sessions, and both partners should learn about the advantages and disadvantages of each type of implant.

Men who are unable to ejaculate due to diabetes, multiple sclerosis, spinal cord injury, or other conditions may still father children by undergoing electroejaculation. In this procedure, an electric probe is inserted in the rectum, stimulating the prostate and enabling the collection of semen for artificial insemination into the woman. For men who retain sensation in this area, the procedure is done under anesthesia; those who have lost sensation due to spinal cord injury do not need anesthesia as they cannot feel the pain. Electroejaculation and artificial insemination do not always result in successful pregnancy. Couples should be aware that the process may need to be repeated several times and that success is by no means guaranteed. In addition, the process is very expensive and may be emotionally draining.

Sexual counseling may prove beneficial to couples. When the illness is in the crisis stage, it may be difficult for the man and his partner to engage in sexual activity. Pain, fatigue, and the effects of medication may interfere with participation in counseling (Schover and Jensen: 1988). Lemon (1993) suggests that the first step in the counseling process be the opportunity to grieve. Exploring the couple's patterns of communication and the role sex played in their relationship prior to the disability may prove useful in adapting to the new situation. The ability to communicate fears and expectations to a sexual partner in order to devise alternative sexual positions and activities may contribute to a satisfying sexual relationship. Those who engage in these alternatives report deriving much satisfaction from them. Sensate focus exercises, developed by the well known sex therapists William Masters and Virginia Johnson, may be used to help the couple identify parts of their bodies that retain the ability to respond to stimulation. These exercises involve the couple's exploration of each other's bodies and the communication of their responses to each other.

PSYCHOLOGICAL RESPONSES

The diagnosis of a disability or chronic condition changes a man's life dramatically. To many members of society, people with physical impairments bear a stigma; their social status has decreased, and they become the objects of others' curiosity. People with disabilities are aware of the way in which society views them. As a result, men who hold the traditional male values of independence and physical strength may deny their physical disability. They may reject the assistance of service providers who try to help them adjust to their new situation and assistive devices such as canes, which are visible symbols of their disability. Men with diseases that cause disabilities, such as diabetes, may deny their disease while they are asymptomatic, refusing to change their lifestyles. They perceive such changes as a threat to their masculinity.

When a disability or chronic condition has a sudden onset, the individual may be in a state of shock. Depression, the most common response to loss, often follows shock. Both shock and depression are normal precedents to emotional recovery. Depression is not always recognized, because it may be masked by weakness, apathy, irritability, and passivity

14

(Hollander: 1982). Denial of the presence of the disability is also a common reaction. Service providers and family members must not encourage the belief that the condition will be reversed. Individuals must fully accept their condition before emotional recovery can occur. Individuals who deny their conditions should be referred for counseling; otherwise, it is unlikely that rehabilitation will be effective.

Not surprisingly, research has shown a significant relationship between disability and depression. A large community based study of individuals with chronic disabilities (Turner and Wood: 1985) found that over a third of the respondents (34.9%) had high scores on a scale that measured depression, indicating that they were clinically depressed. In comparison, studies of the general population have found that about 18 to 19% of the population is depressed. Twice as many men with disabilities were depressed (28.9%) as men in the general population (14%). Higher proportions of men who were separated or divorced were depressed (40%) than those who were married (27.4%). The same study indicates that psychological adaptation to the disability occurs over time, with those whose disabilities had been present the longest least likely to be depressed. Thus, there is empirical evidence that individuals who become disabled go through different psychological stages, usually resulting in acceptance and adaptation.

The psychological impact of a disability may have different effects at different stages of a man's life. When disabilities are congenital, those affected have never experienced life as able-bodied. Nonetheless, their conditions may cause extreme stress within the family and may result in parents spending a great deal of time with the child who is disabled, to the neglect of other children and the parents' own relationship. In cases where the parents' relationship is not strong enough to withstand this stress and divorce results, the child may always feel guilty about the situation.

Disabilities that occur in the teenage years or early adulthood may prove especially difficult to deal with, as peer pressure emphasizes body image and physical prowess, both in athletics and sexual activity. At the age when their peers are starting to date, young men with disabilities may not feel comfortable initiating social contacts for fear of rejection. Obviously, such rejection can be psychologically devastating. Many health care and rehabilitation professionals fail to deal with romantic and sexual aspects of disability. In fact, many individuals with disabilities feel that others view them as asexual. A man with a spinal cord injury described the sexual rejection he felt in his late adolescence:

> A very important measure of somebody's personhood--manhood--
> was their sexual ability... What bothers me more than anything else
> is the stereotypes and even more so, in terms of sexual desirability.
> Because I had a disability, I was less desirable than able-bodied
> people. And that I found very frustrating (Gerschick and Miller:
> 1995, 189).

As young men begin to choose and prepare for their occupational careers, disabilities and chronic conditions may have a major influence. Low self-esteem, in part due to societal reactions that embody negative stereotypes, may prevent them from achieving their true aspirations.

When disability occurs at mid-life, men who are established in their careers and who have families face a different set of stressors. Fear that the disability or condition may result in loss of employment and income places enormous strain on a man who has taken responsibility as the breadwinner for the family. The possibility that his partner may have to obtain employment, while at the same time her caretaker burdens have increased, may make the man feel extremely guilty. In cases where the wife was dependent upon the husband prior to the disability, adapting to this new role may be difficult, especially when there are small children to raise; in some cases, however, the woman who was previously dependent finds the situation an opportunity to take control and pursue her own career (Rustad: 1984).

Men who are part of well adjusted marriages and families are likely to cope better with their newly diagnosed conditions than men in strained relationships. Just as individual coping patterns are developed over a lifetime of experience, family responses to crises are similar to those that they have exhibited in the past. Individuals with supportive spouses find their marriages to be a source of strength, while individuals in weaker relationships may tend to use their condition as an excuse for the strain in their marriages (Rodgers and Calder: 1990).

Role changes, financial hardships, and time constraints place additional burdens upon family members. In some instances, however, family bonds grow stronger and members become more cohesive. For example, Peyrot et al. (1988) found that after a period of disruption and readjustment, families where a member had diabetes became more cohesive. Changes in family relationships may make the wife of a man with diabetes feel more needed.

Advances in medical technology have enabled the population to live longer; however, an increase in the prevalence of disabilities and chronic conditions has accompanied this increased longevity. As noted above, more than 50% of men age 65 and over have at least one disability, the highest rate of disability for men in any age group. Although in most age groups, men have lower rates of limitations in activity due to disability than women, at age 75 and over, men have a higher number of restricted activity days per year (Trupin and Rice: 1995). One study of older men found that those whose health problems imposed physical limitations felt "cut down;" they felt that it was important not to appear weak or emotional (Rubinstein: 1986). Despite their high rate of disability, older men with disabilities are viewed as a minority, and their special needs are often ignored by social service agencies.

If they are widowers, older men who live alone may have difficulties taking care of a household and preparing meals; in the past, many depended upon their wives to tend to these daily activities. Coping with one or more disabilities may contribute greatly to the problem of household management, yet the traditional male value of independence may prevent men from seeking help from informal or formal networks. Utilization of home health services enables individuals with disabilities to reside in the community. Men age 65 and over are less likely to utilize home health services than women in the same age category; men represent only 34% of those using these services (Hing: 1994). The differential use by gender increases with age; women age 65 to 74 use home health services at a rate 36% higher than men. At age 85 and over, women's utilization of these services increases to 65% more than men's (Dey: 1995).

Men with disabilities who are gay may face extreme isolation. In some instances, family may have rejected them because of their sexual orientation. Add to this the status of "disabled," and these men may feel extremely isolated and rejected by both groups of gays and groups of individuals with disabilities who are seeking equality. The advent of HIV/AIDS has resulted in a strong support network for gay men with this condition; similar groups for gay men with other disabling conditions are rare.

Knowledge of the man's reactions to previous stressful situations may provide insight into his responses to a disability or chronic condition. It is common to rely on coping mechanisms that have been developed over a course of a lifetime. Religious faith, family, and friends may help some individuals to face disability and cope with it in a positive manner. A man's reactions may be shaped by the severity of the disability or condition and whether it occurs suddenly or gradually. When the onset of disability is gradual and early intervention measures are taken, men may be motivated to learn new ways of accomplishing ordinary tasks. In addition, men may be better able to handle depression; retain a positive self-image; and strive to be independent. Both men and family members have time to plan for necessary changes, although anxiety over the future course of the condition may be severe.

It is especially difficult to cope with those chronic conditions that fluctuate in their severity and impact. Conditions such as multiple sclerosis and diabetes can leave people relatively free of symptoms for a period of time and then cause devastating problems, such as loss of vision. Adjusting to the current situation is difficult enough; add to this the fear that the condition may worsen and it is easy to understand why people in these circumstances have great emotional burdens.

Brooks and Matson (1987) have described the broad array of coping mechanisms and skills that individuals with multiple sclerosis must develop in order to feel that they have a sense of control over their condition and their lives. They must make decisions about medications and treatment; search for information about their disease; adapt their environment to accommodate their current situation; and take measures to relieve anxiety. All of these factors affect employment, family life, and relationships outside the family.

The knowledge that there are services available to help cope with what may at first seem overwhelming can make the difference in maintaining the ability to continue functioning independently. Learning about new technology that enables people with disabilities and chronic conditions to function in their everyday activities may prove to be the factor that enables these individuals to come to grips with the new dimension of their lives.

The roles of professional service providers may be crucial in shaping individuals' responses to a disability or a chronic condition. Professionals can help people with disabilities to continue functioning in socially productive roles and to avoid the feeling that they need to "pass" or cover up their condition. Combating negative attitudes among professionals toward people with disabilities is an essential first step in serving this growing population.

Accepting the limitations of a disability or chronic condition is not only psychologically liberating, but also makes daily living easier. Zola (1991) discovered that when he finally accepted the label "disabled," he was able to accept the types of assistance he needed in order to make living less of a challenge to his ego. Thus, when he went to airports, he no longer had to prove that he could walk long distances with his crutches but was willing to accept a wheelchair that made his travel easier and enabled him to use his energy for the purpose of his trip. For men with disabilities whose masculinity is threatened by accepting assistance from others, reaching this point may be difficult and take time. The acceptance of realistic limitations and abilities may result in the restoration of self-esteem, the sense of control over life, and pride in achievements for men in all stages of life.

WHERE TO FIND LOCAL SERVICES

A good place to start the search for services is the information and referral office of the local United Way. Other sources of information are local directories of service agencies available in the reference collection of many public libraries. Libraries often have their own special programs for people with disabilities, and some have special needs centers or special reading equipment for people with visual impairments.

State and municipal offices established to serve people with disabilities are other sources of referrals. A study of major cities in the United States (Groch: 1991) found that over half had established special offices to deal with disability issues. The remainder had designated an individual to deal with these issues, and the overwhelming majority (86%) had appointed a person to coordinate the requirements of Section 504 of the Rehabilitation Act (see Chapter 3, "Laws that Affect Men with Disabilities" for a discussion of this section). It is likely that these cities have now appointed individuals to coordinate their efforts to meet the requirements of the Americans with Disabilities Act, which was passed about one and a half years after the survey was completed. At the time of the survey, the cities responded that they provided a wide variety of services, including accessible housing, transportation, public education about disability, job placement, referrals, and special recreational activities.

Rehabilitation agencies, described below, are a major source of assistance for people with disabilities and chronic conditions. Some departments of rehabilitation, human or health services, aging, and education may provide respite care to families of individuals with disabilities. Respite care is temporary help designed to relieve caretakers of the need to be "on call" for 24 hours a day. It relieves the caretaker's emotional burden and allows time to tend to personal needs.

Veterans are eligible for special benefits and rehabilitation services. In the United States, the Department of Veterans Affairs (VA) has established a number of special services, including the provision of prosthetics for veterans with service related disabilities. Visual Impairment Services Teams (VIST) help veterans with vision problems. The VA will specially adapt the homes of veterans with disabilities. A booklet describing all of the benefits and rights of veterans, "Federal Benefits for Veterans and Dependents," is available for $3.75 from the Consumer Information Center, PO Box 100, Pueblo, CO 81002.

REHABILITATION

Rehabilitation agencies provide services that teach new skills that enable individuals with disabilities to live independently and continue working. Rehabilitation services may include any or all of the following:
- rehabilitation counseling
- job placement
- provision of adaptive equipment, prostheses, and medical supplies
- vocational training to remain in one's current position or to learn a new skill

- adapting the home or work environment
- training in activities of daily living and homemaking
- transportation services

Rehabilitation services are provided by both public and private agencies. In the United States, each state is required by law to have a public agency that is responsible for providing vocational rehabilitation services. In about half of the states, there are separate agencies to serve people who are visually impaired or blind. In the remaining states, services for people who are visually impaired or blind are provided within the general vocational rehabilitation agency. Many states offer special rehabilitation services for children and elders. The federal government provides financial support for rehabilitation services and sets standards for service delivery, as required by the Rehabilitation Act of 1973 and its amendments (see Chapter 3, "Laws that Affect Men with Disabilities") and administered by the Rehabilitation Services Administration, U.S. Department of Education.

Some rehabilitation professionals provide services independently on a fee-for-service basis. (Rehabilitation counselors are certified by the Commission on Rehabilitation Counselor Certification, listed in "ORGANIZATIONS" section below.) Rehabilitation services are offered in group settings, in residential settings, or at home.

There is no one rehabilitation plan that will work for all individuals. Individuals must work jointly with rehabilitation counselors to set their goals and establish an appropriate rehabilitation plan to meet those goals. The federal government requires that individuals sign an Individual Written Rehabilitation Program that indicates they approve of the rehabilitation strategy developed jointly with counselors in state rehabilitation agencies. It is also important to involve family members in the rehabilitation process so that they will support, not undermine, the person's attempts to remain independent.

The Client Assistance Program is a federally mandated program that requires states to provide information to all clients and potential clients about the benefits available under the Rehabilitation Act (see Chapter 3, "Laws that Affect Men with Disabilities") and to assist clients in obtaining these benefits.

Individuals with severe disabilities often require assistance with personal care, transportation, and special equipment. Independent living programs enable people with disabilities to continue functioning within the community with a minimal amount of assistance. A crucial element of the independent living movement is that consumers have control over the types of services provided. For some, this means living at home, with or without attendant care, and maintaining employment. Attendants assist people with disabilities in activities such as bathing, grooming, dressing, food preparation, and household tasks. Provisions of both Social Security and Medicaid laws have been used to finance the services of attendants. People with disabilities or chronic conditions may opt to live in group residences, where individuals live under supervision but maintain a degree of responsibility for their own care and maintenance. Independent living programs or centers are sometimes administered by state vocational rehabilitation agencies and sometimes are free-standing organizations administered by individuals with disabilities themselves.

Ideally, the approach to medical treatment and rehabilitation planning should be carried out jointly by health professionals and rehabilitation professionals. Because the medical profession is largely oriented toward cure rather than rehabilitation, such a collaborative approach is often a difficult goal to attain.

SELF-HELP GROUPS FOR MEN WITH DISABILITIES

Self-help groups enable individuals with similar problems or conditions to discuss their problems and offer mutual assistance. Self-help groups offer a number of benefits to participants, including learning to develop coping strategies; acquiring a sense of control over life; combating isolation and alienation; and developing information networks. In addition, members of self-help groups often express a sense of increased self-esteem, because they have offered help to other members of the group.

The traditional roles that men have played and the dominant male values of independence and self-reliance may lead them to believe that self-help groups will detract from their masculinity. Male friendships have a different quality than female friendships; they usually involve socializing and having a good time, but men are unlikely to view their close friends as confidantes and to discuss their intimate problems with them (Sherrod: 1987). Although participants at self-help groups are not usually friends, at least at the outset, it would seem logical that men's traditional bonds with other men would deter them from discussing their problems with their male peers.

A study of male participation in self-help groups for caregivers (Jacobs: 1989) found a number of reasons that men participate in self-help groups at lower rates than women. These include lack of familiarity with self-help groups, fear of appearing that they cannot handle the situation, a lack of other men in the groups, reluctance to reveal their personal feelings, and the need to be strong and independent.

Older men, who often lack experience in group environments, may be hesitant to attend self-help meetings and to express their feelings. They may view attendance at these groups as a sign of weakness and a threat to their sense of independence and masculinity. These feelings may be especially strong regarding mixed gender self-help groups, where there are likely to be more women than men. One solution to this problem is to create groups especially for men. Jacobs (1989) has suggested that mixed gender self-help groups have at least one male and one female leader for the members to identify with. In instances where a disease affects only men, such as prostate conditions, some self-help groups have special meetings for their partners to attend but maintain all male groups for most of their meetings.

Professional service providers are ideally suited to identify and bring together individuals with common problems, and they often are able to offer a site where meetings may be held. However, professionals must understand the new role that they play in helping to create a self-help group. Madara (no date) recommends that professionals assume the role of consultants, providing advice and counsel but not assuming any responsibility for leadership, decision-making, or group tasks. A professional who is the catalyst for the formation of a group must disengage from this initial role to allow the group to develop autonomously. Since professionals often tend to encourage dependent client relationships, they must guard against this type of relationship if a group is to offer true mutual support.

Identifying a group facilitator or coordinator is the first step in developing self-help groups for individuals with disabilities and chronic conditions, their spouses or partners, their parents, or their siblings. One method is to identify someone who has had group experience. Former patients or clients who have had experience in coping with disabilities are likely candidates for starting a group. Another method is to identify an organized, articulate person who has experienced a disability and has some background in a club or other organization. Announcements in publications, at meetings, and on hospital and agency bulletin boards are also good recruitment techniques. Once the group is established, it is up to the members to decide how frequently to meet; the types of discussions or programs to have; and how to recruit members.

It is sometimes necessary to be creative in establishing self-help groups for people with disabilities. Individuals who have difficulty traveling because of mobility impairments may have difficulty arranging for transportation to the meeting site. One solution to this problem is to hold meetings by having telephone conference calls (Romness et al.: 1992). While this system may have the disadvantage of not providing face-to-face contact, it does provide the participants with the opportunity to discuss common problems with peers and may eliminate some of the feelings of isolation.

The most recent form of self-help group has evolved as a result of the technological advances in personal computing. Individuals with a computer and modem may now join a usenet group, where they may exchange information with others who experience the same disabilities or conditions. Individuals have the opportunity to discuss their insights, offer advice, and ask questions; other individuals respond to their questions and comments.

While exchanging information over computer lines is significantly different in character from meeting face-to-face with a group, it provides information and helps to combat social isolation for those in rural areas and those who are unable to leave their homes. It may also serve as a first step in meeting someone with a similar experience who lives in the same geographical area. Notations throughout this book indicate organizations that have web sites for individuals who have disabilities or chronic conditions.

COMPUTERS AND DISABILITIES

Personal computers (PCs) have opened up a wide variety of opportunities for people who have disabilities or chronic conditions. Used alone, adapted computers enable individuals to perform tasks that would be otherwise inaccessible to them; retaining a job is just one major opportunity that computers offer to people with disabilities. Using computers with online subscription services and the Internet, it is possible to communicate with people all over the world. This instant communication provides up-to-the-minute information about new developments and the opportunity to "chat" with individuals in similar situations. Many of these services are free, with the exception of telephone charges or subscription fees for online services.

The reference section of most libraries contains indexes and directories of resources available on the Internet. Look up topics such as disabilities, health, and specific conditions or disabilities. Since new resources become available all the time, sometimes it is necessary to browse various services to obtain up-to-date information. World wide web sites provide access to information from service agencies, educational institutions, and commercial organizations. One web site that provides links to information on health and disability is http://www.yahoo.com. The University of Maryland (http://www.umd.edu) is one source of disability related Internet resources; click on "Information Resources," then "Disability Directory," then "Internet Resources." Other sites listed throughout this book provide links to a wide variety of disability resources.

A variety of formats is available to receive and exchange information. When you join a usenet group, you may read messages and respond to them as well as submit your own information and questions. In order to join a usenet group, your host computer must provide access. When you subscribe to a usenet group, you will automatically receive all new messages whenever you log on. If you decide to exchange messages with just one member, you may send mail directly to that individual's e-mail address.

Listserv enables you to receive information by sending a message to an e-mail address stating you would like to subscribe. You may add your own messages which may in turn generate responses from other members of a group. Protocol requires that you then summarize your responses and mail them to all other members of the listserv group.

CONCLUSION

Men who have accepted their disabilities or chronic conditions often have adopted a new set of values that replace the dominant male values in society. This process may take a good deal of time, depending upon the man's special circumstances, personality, and social situation. A variety of options enables men with disabilities to feel productive and fulfilled. Rehabilitation services, self-help groups, accommodations in the workplace and at home, and the support of family and friends can all contribute to an increased sense of self-esteem and independence for men with disabilities.

References

Altman, Barbara and Richard T. Smith
1992   "Impact of Rehabilitation on Psychological Distress: Gender Differences" International Journal of Rehabilitation Research 15:75-81
Andersson, Karl-Erik
1994   "Pharmacology and Erection: Agents Which Initiate and Terminate Erection" Sexuality and Disability 12:1:53-79
Breske, Sharon
1996   "The Forgotten ADL" Advance/Rehabilitation 5:1(January):43-48
Brooks, Nancy A. and Ronald R. Matson
1987   "Managing Multiple Sclerosis" Volume 6, pp. 73-106 in Julius A. Roth and Peter Conrad (eds.) Research in the Sociology of Health Care Greenwich, CT: JAI Press Inc.
Charmaz, Kathy
1995   "Identity Dilemmas of Chronically Ill Men" pp. 266-291 in Donald Sabo and David Frederick Gordon (eds.) Men's Health and Illness: Gender, Power, and the Body Newbury Park, CA: Sage Publications
Church, Paul
1996   "Impotence: No Need to Suffer in Secret" Harvard Health Letter 21:4(May):4-6

D'Arrigo, Terri
1998 "First Pill to Treat Impotence Hits Market" <u>Diabetes Forecast</u> 51:7(July):35-36-

Dey, A. N.
1995 "Characteristics of Elderly Men and Women Discharged from Home Health Care Services 1991-92" <u>Advance Data from Vital and Health Statistics</u> No. 259 Hyattsville, MD: National Center for Health Statistics

Flapan, Mark
1996 "A Personal Story" cited in <u>The Moisture Seekers Newsletter</u> 14:5(Summer):2

Gerschick, Thomas J. and Adam S. Miller
1995 "Coming to Terms: Masculinity and Physical Disability" pp. 183-204 in Donald Sabo and David Frederick Gordon (eds.) <u>Men's Health and Illness: Gender, Power, and the Body</u> Newbury Park, CA: Sage Publications

Groch, Sharon
1991 "Public Services Available to Persons with Disabilities in Major U.S. Cities" <u>Journal of Rehabilitation</u> July/August/September 23-26

Hahn, Harlan
1989 "Disability and Masculinity" <u>Disability Studies Quarterly</u> 9:2(Summer):54-56

Hing, Esther
1994 "Characteristics of Elderly Home Health Care Patients: Preliminary Data from the 1992 National Home and Hospice Care Survey" <u>Advance Data from Vital and Health Statistics</u> No. 247 Hyattsville, MD: National Center for Health Statistics

Hollander, Laura-Lee
1982 "Normal Aging" pp. 1-39 in Martha Logigian (ed.) <u>Adult Rehabilitation: A Team Approach for Therapists</u> Boston, MA: Little Brown & Co.

Jacobs, Geraldine
1989 <u>Involving Men in Caregiver Support Groups: A Practical Guidebook</u> Bryn Mawr, PA: Graduate School of Social Work and Social Research, Bryn Mawr College

Lemon, Marilyn
1993 "Sexual Counseling and Spinal Cord Injury" <u>Sexuality and Disability</u> 11:1:73-97

Linet, Otto I. and Francis G. Ogrinc
1996 "Efficacy and Safety of Intracavernosal Alprostadil in Men with Erectile Dysfunction" <u>New England Journal of Medicine</u> 334:14(April 4):873-877

Madara, Edward
no   <u>Developing Self-Help Groups - General Steps and Guidelines for Professionals</u>
date   Denville, NJ: New Jersey Self-Help Clearinghouse

McNeil, John M.
1993 <u>Americans With Disabilities 1991-1992</u>, Washington, DC: U.S. Bureau of the Census Current Population Reports P70-33

Moreland, John
1989 "Age and Change in the Adult Male Role" pp. 115-124 in Michael S. Kimmel and Michael A. Messner (eds.) <u>Men's Lives</u> New York, NY: Macmillan Publishing Company

Nadig, Perry W.

1994 "Vacuum Constriction Devices in Patients with Neurogenic Impotence" <u>Sexuality and Disability</u> 12:1:99-105

Peyrot, Mark, James F. McMurry, Jr. and Richard Hedges

1988 "Marital Adjustment to Adult Diabetes: Interpersonal Congruence and Spouse Satisfaction" <u>Journal of Marriage and the Family</u> 50(May):363-376

Rodgers, Jennifer and Peter Calder

1990 "Marital Adjustment: A Valuable Resource for the Emotional Health of Individuals with Multiple Sclerosis" <u>Rehabilitation Counseling Bulletin</u> 34(September)1:24-32

Romness, Sharon, Vicki Bruce, and Catherine Smith-Wilson

1992 "Multiple Sclerosis Telephone Self-Help Support Groups" pp. 220-223 in Alfred H. Katz et al. (eds.) <u>Self-Help: Concepts and Applications</u> Philadelphia, PA: The Charles Press, Publishers

Rubinstein, Robert L.

1986 <u>Singular Paths: Old Men Living Alone</u> New York, NY: Columbia University Press

Rustad, Lynne C.

1984 "Family Adjustment to Chronic Illness and Disability in Mid-Life" pp. 222-242 in Myron G. Eisenberg, LaFaye C. Sutkin, and Mary A. Jansen (eds.) <u>Chronic Illness and Disability through the Life Span</u> New York, NY: Springer Publishing Company

Sandowski, Carol L.

1989 <u>Sexual Concerns When Illness or Disability Strikes</u> Springfield, IL: Charles C. Thomas Publishers

Schappert, Susan M.

1996 "National Ambulatory Medical Care Survey: 1994 Summary" <u>Advance Data</u> Number 273, April 10 Hyattsville, MD: National Center for Health Statistics

Schover, Leslie and Soren Buus Jensen

1988 <u>Sexuality and Chronic Illness: A Comprehensive Approach</u> New York, NY: Guilford Press

Sherrod, Drury

1987 "The Bonds of Men: Problems and Possibilities in Close Male Relationships" pp. 213-239 in Harry Brod (ed.) <u>The Making of Masculinities: The New Men's Studies</u> Boston, MA: Unwin and Hyman

Tieffer, Leonore

1987 "In Pursuit of the Perfect Penis: The Medicalization of Male Sexuality" pp. 165-184 in Michael S. Kimmel (ed.) <u>Changing Men: New Directions in Research on Men and Masculinity</u> Newbury Park, CA: Sage Publications

Trupin, Laura and Dorothy P. Rice

1995 "Health Status, Medical Care Use, and Number of Disabling Conditions in the United States" <u>Disability Statistics Abstract</u> 9, June

Turner, R. Jay and D. William Wood

1985 "Depression and Disability: The Stress Process in a Chronically Strained Population" <u>Research in Community and Mental Health</u> 5:77-109

Waldron, Ingrid
1983   "Sex Differences in Illness Incidence, Prognosis and Mortality: Issues and Evidence" <u>Social Science and Medicine</u> 17:16:1107-1123
Zola, Irving Kenneth
1991   "Bringing Our Bodies and Ourselves Back In: Reflections on a Past, Present, and Future 'Medical Sociology'" <u>Journal of Health and Social Behavior</u> 32(March):1-16

Alliance of Genetic Support Groups
4301 Connecticut Avenue, NW, Suite 404
Washington, DC 20008
(800) 336-4363   (202) 966-5557   FAX (202) 966-8553
e-mail: info@geneticalliance.org   http://www.geneticalliance.org

Provides education and services to families and individuals affected by genetic disorders. Membership, individuals, $25.00; organizations, $50.00; includes monthly newsletter, "ALLIANCE ALERT."

American Association of Sex Educators, Counselors and Therapists (AASECT)
PO Box 238
Mount Vernon, IA 52314-0238
(319) 895-8407   FAX (319) 895-6203
e-mail: aasect@worldnet.att.net   http://www.aasect.org

A membership organization for professionals who counsel individuals with sexual dysfunctions. Membership, individuals, $145.00; organizations, $315.00; includes monthly newsletter, "Contemporary Sexuality." Newsletter only, individuals, $42.00; organizations, $65.00. AASECT will provide lists of its members in a local geographical area upon receipt of a self-addressed, stamped, business size envelope.

American Disabled for Attendant Programs Today (ADAPT)
PO Box 9598
Denver, CO 80209
(303) 333-6698

or

ADAPT\Incitement
1319 Lamar SE Drive, Suite 101
Austin, TX 78704
(512) 442-0252   FAX (512) 442-0522
e-mail: adapt@adapt.org   http://www.adapt.org

An organization dedicated to changing the structure of long term care and helping people with disabilities live in the community with supports instead of being sent to nursing homes and other institutions. Publishes "INCITEMENT,"m a newsletter describing ADAPT activities, three or four times a year (available in standard print and on audiocassette), free. ADAPT has supported federal legislation, the Community Attendant Services Act (CASA), to provide personal attendants to individuals with disabilities. No membership fees, but a willingness to participate in ADAPT's activities is required.

American Foundation for Urologic Disease (AFUD)
300 West Pratt Street, Suite 401
Baltimore, MD 21201
(800) 242-2383   (410) 727-2908   FAX (410) 528-0550
e-mail: admin@afud.org

Sponsors research, education, and patient support services. Provides information about urological diseases, including prostate conditions, incontinence, and male sexual function. Membership, $35.00, includes subscription to quarterly newsletter, "Family Urology."

American Self-Help Clearinghouse
Northwest Covenant Medical Center
Pocono Road
Denville, NJ 07834
(973) 625-9565   (973) 625-9053 (TT)   FAX (973) 625-8848
In NJ, (800) 367-6274   http://www.cmhc.com/selfhelp

Provides information and contacts for national self-help groups, information on model groups and individuals who are starting new networks, and state or local self-help clearinghouses.

Combined Health Information Database (CHID)
Ovid Technologies, Attn: CHID Database
333 7th Avenue
New York, NY 10001
(800) 950-2035   (212) 563-3006
e-mail: chid@aerie.com   http://chid.nih.gov

A federally sponsored database that includes bibliographic citations and abstracts from journals, reports, books, and patient education brochures.

Commission on Accreditation of Rehabilitation Facilities (CARF)
4891 East Grant Road
Tucson, AZ 85712
(520) 325-1044 (V/TT)   FAX (520) 318-1129   http://www.carf.org

Conducts site evaluations and accredits organizations that provide rehabilitation. Publishes the "Directory of Accredited Organizations." $60.00 plus $7.00 shipping and handling

Commission on Rehabilitation Counselor Certification
1835 Rohlwing Road, Suite E
Rolling Meadows, IL 60008
(847) 394-2104

Provides certification to rehabilitation counselors.

Department of Veterans Affairs (VA)
(800) 827-1000   http://www.va.gov

This nationwide toll-free number connects veterans with the VA regional office in their vicinity.

Impotence Information Center
PO Box 9
Minneapolis, MN 55440
(800) 843-4315   http://www.ammedsys.com

Sponsored by American Medical Systems, Inc., a subsidiary of Pfizer, Inc., this center provides free information and physician referrals. Pfizer is the manufacturer of Viagra.

Impotence World Institute (IWI)
PO Box 410
Bowie, MD 20718-0410
(800) 669-1603   (301) 262-2400   FAX (301) 262-6825
e-mail: IWABOWIE@aol.com   http://www.impotenceworld.org

A membership organization with support groups throughout the country, including Impotents Anonymous (IA) and I-ANON (for partners) . Produces a variety of fact sheets, books, videotapes, and audiotapes that address the various causes and treatments for impotence. Operates a help line and makes referrals to physicians. Membership, $25.00, includes quarterly newsletter, "Impotence Worldwide."

MedWatch
Food and Drug Administration
HF-2, Room 17-65
5600 Fishers Lane
Rockville, MD 20857
(800) 332-1088   FAX (800) 332-0178   (301) 443-0117
http://www.fda.gov/medwatch

The Medical Products Reporting Program reports safety warnings and recalls for products regulated by the FDA, such as drugs, medical devices, devices that emit radiation, special nutritional products, and biologics (blood, etc.). Users may access the information online. Health professionals are encouraged to report problems with the use of any of these products to Medwatch.

National Association for Continence (NAFC)
PO Box 8310
Spartanburg, SC 29305-8310
(800) 252-3337   (864) 579-7900   FAX (864) 579-7902
http://www.nafc.org

An information clearinghouse for consumers, family members, and medical professionals. Answers individual questions if self-addressed stamped envelope is enclosed with letter. Membership, $20.00, includes a quarterly newsletter, "Quality Care," a "Resource Guide: Products and Services for Continence" (nonmembers, $13.00), and a continence referral service. Free publications list.

National Association of Rehabilitation Professionals in the Private Sector (NARPPS)
1661 Worcester Road, #203
Framingham, MA 01701
(800) 240-4337   (508) 820-8889   FAX (508) 820-4337
e-mail: narpps@ix.netcom.com   http://www.narpps.org

A professional membership organization for rehabilitation professionals who work as private practitioners, for industry, or for private rehabilitation services. Holds annual meeting. Membership, $155.00; includes bimonthly newsletter, "NARPPS Journal and News," and bimonthly journal, "Rehabilitation Professional." "NARPPS National Directory," printed annually, is available online.

National Association of Sibling Programs (NASP)
Sibling Support Project
Children's Hospital and Medical Center
PO Box 5371
Seattle, WA 98105
(206) 368-4911   FAX (206) 368-4816
e-mail: dmeyer@chmc.org

Maintains a database of sibling programs across the U.S. Includes programs for young siblings of children with developmental disabilities, chronic illness, or for adult siblings.

National Center for Medical Rehabilitation Research (NCMRR)
Building 61E, Room 2A03
9000 Rockville Pike
Bethesda, MD 20892
(301) 402-2242   (301) 402-2554 (TT)
FAX (301) 402-0832   e-mail: tuels@box-t.nih.gov
http://silk.nih.gov/silk/NCMRR

A federal agency that conducts and supports research to develop ways of improving the lives of individuals with disabilities, including research to develop technology and assistive devices.

National Council on Disability (NCD)
1331 F Street, NW, Suite 1050
Washington, DC 20004-1107
(202) 272-2004   (202) 272-2074 (TT)   FAX (202) 272-2022
e-mail: mquigley@ncd.gov   http://www.ncd.gov

An independent federal agency mandated to study and make recommendations about public policy for people with disabilities. Holds regular meetings and hearings in various locations around the country. Publishes monthly newsletter, "NCD Bulletin," available in standard print, large print, braille, and computer disk. Free

National Health Information Center (NHIC)
Office of Disease Prevention and Health Promotion
PO Box 1133
Washington, DC 20013-1133
(800) 336-4797   In MD, (301) 565-4167   FAX (301) 984-4256
e-mail: nhicinfo@health.org   http://nhic-nt.health.org

Maintains a database of health organizations and a library. Provides referrals related to health issues for both professionals and consumers. Publications enable individuals to locate information and resources in the federal government. Free publications list; also available on the web site.

National Institute on Disability and Rehabilitation Research (NIDRR)
U.S. Department of Education
400 Maryland Avenue, SW
Washington, DC 20202
(202) 205-8134   (202) 205-8198 (TT)   FAX (202) 205-8515
http://www.ed.gov/OSERS/offices/NIDRR

A federal agency that supports research into various aspects of disability and rehabilitation, including demographic analyses, social science research, and the development of assistive devices.

National Kidney and Urologic Diseases Information Clearinghouse (NKUDIC)
3 Information Way
Bethesda, MD 20892-3580
(301) 654-4415   FAX (301) 907-8906
e-mail: nddic@info.niddk.nih.gov   http://www.niddk.nih.gov

Responds to requests from the public and professionals about diseases of the kidneys and urologic system. Publishes quarterly newsletter, "KU Notes," free. Free list of publications.

National Library of Medicine (NLM)
8600 Rockville Pike
Building 38, Room 2S-10
Bethesda, MD 20894
(888) 346-3656   (301) 594-5983   http://www.nlm.nih.gov

Operates "Medline," a computerized database of articles in major medical journals from around the world. Users may search for a specific health topic and receive citations and abstracts of articles online. Available directly at no charge over the Internet. ("Medline" is also available at most medical, public, and university libraries.) Additional databases such as DIRLINE, AIDSLINE, and AIDSDRUGS are also available. Also publishes clinical alerts online.

National Organization for Rare Disorders (NORD)
PO Box 8923
New Fairfield, CT 06812-8923
(203) 746-6518   FAX (203) 746-6481   (203) 746-6927 (TT)
e-mail: orphan@NORD-RDB.com   http://www.nord-rdb.com/~orphan

Federation of voluntary health organizations that serves individuals with rare or "orphan" diseases. Maintains a confidential patient networking program for individuals and family members who have been diagnosed with a rare disorder. Offers Medical Equipment Exchange on web site to link buyers and sellers of used medical equipment and a Medication Assistance Program. Membership, $30.00, includes newsletter, "Orphan Disease Update," published three times per year. Reprints of articles on rare diseases available for $7.50 per copy; abstracts available free on the web site.

National Organization on Disability (NOD)
910 16th Street, NW, Suite 600
Washington, DC 20006
(800) 248-2253 (Referral Line)   (202) 293-5960   (202) 293-5968 (TT)
FAX (202) 293-7999   e-mail: ability@nod.org   http://www.nod.org

An organization dedicated to achieving the full participation of people with disabilities in all aspects of community life. Works with a network of local agencies to achieve this goal. Provides technical assistance and maintains an informational database.

National Rehabilitation Association (NRA)
633 South Washington Street
Alexandria, VA 22314
(703) 836-0850   (703) 836-0849 (TT)
FAX (703) 836-0848   e-mail: info@nationalrehab.org
http://www.nationalrehab.org

A professional membership organization for rehabilitation professionals and independent living center affiliates. Includes special divisions for independent living, counseling, job placement, etc. Legislative alerts appear on NRA's web site. Regular membership, $91.00, includes "Journal of Rehabilitation" and newsletter, "Contemporary Rehab;" associate member, $61.00 (journal not included); student membership, $10.00.

National Rehabilitation Information Center (NARIC)
8455 Colesville Road, Suite 935
Silver Spring, MD 20910-3319
(800) 346-2742   (301) 588-9284   (301) 495-5626 (TT)
FAX (301) 587-1967   e-mail: naric@capaccess.org
http://www.naric.com/naric/home.html

A federally funded center that responds to telephone and mail inquiries about disabilities and support services. Maintains "REHABDATA," a database with publications and research references. Some NARIC publications are available on the web site.

National Self-Help Clearinghouse
Graduate School and University Center/CUNY
25 West 43rd Street, Room 620
New York, NY 10036
(212) 642-2944   FAX (212) 642-1956
http://www.selfhelpweb.com

Makes referrals to local self-help groups. Publishes quarterly newsletter "Self-Help Reporter," and a list of local self-help clearinghouses in the U.S. Free

Research and Training Center on Independent Living (RTC/IL)
University of Kansas
4089 Dole Human Development Center
Lawrence, KS 66045
(913) 864-4095 (V/TT)   FAX (913) 864-5063
http://www.lsi.ukans.edu/rtcil/rtcil.htm

A federally funded center that conducts research and training on the variables that affect independent living. Publications catalogue, free.

Research and Training Center on Rural Rehabilitation
52 Corbin Hall
University of Montana
Missoula, MT 59812
(888) 268-2743   (406) 243-2460
FAX (406) 243-2349   e-mail: gargoyle@selway.umt.edu
http://ruralinstitute.umt.edu/rtcrrural

A federally funded center that conducts research and training on issues that affect service delivery of rehabilitation in rural areas. Maintains a directory of rural disability services throughout the country.

Resources for Rehabilitation
33 Bedford Street, Suite 19A
Lexington, MA 02420
(781) 862-6455   FAX (781) 861-7517
e-mail: info@rfr.org   http://www.rfr.org

Provides training and information to professionals who serve people with disabilities and to the public. Publications, custom designed training programs, program evaluations, and needs assessments.

Sexual Health Network
Mitchell Tepper
3 Mayflower Lane
Shelton, CT 06484
(203) 924-4623   FAX (203) 924-4623
e-mail: mitch@sexualhealth.com   http://www.sexualhealth.com

Provides information, education, and training for individuals with disabilities. Sells books and videos. Maintains a referral network of multidisciplinary professions who will answer individuals' questions.

Sexuality Information and Education Council of the United States (SIECUS)
130 West 42nd Street, Suite 350
New York, NY 10036-7802
(212) 819-9770   FAX (212) 819-9776
e-mail: siecus@siecus.org   http://www.siecus.org

Provides information and education about sexuality through publications, database, library, symposia, and advocacy. Bimonthly journal, "SIECUS Report," $65.00. Publications catalogue, free.

Society for Disability Studies (SDS)
c/o Richard Scotch, School of Social Sciences
University of Texas at Dallas
Box 830688
Richardson, TX 75083-0688
(972) 883-4122 (V/TT)   e-mail: sdshq@utdallas.edu
http://www.wipd.com/sds

Membership organization of practitioners, clinicians, and social scientists interested in the study of issues related to disability. Holds an annual meeting. Membership fees vary by income level.

Society for the Scientific Study of Sexuality
PO Box 208
Mount Vernon, IA 52314-0208
(319) 895-8407   FAX (319) 895-6230
e-mail: TheSociety@worldnet.att.net
http://www.ssc.wisc.edu/ssss

A multidisciplinary society of professionals who conduct research on sex; includes a special interest group on disability. Membership, $125.00, includes "Journal of Sex Research;" nonmembers subscription, individuals, $88.00; institutions, $126.00; and quarterly newsletter, "Sexual Science."

Substance Abuse Resources & Disability Issues (SARDI)
Rehabilitation Research and Training Center on Drugs and Disability
Wright State University
Dayton, OH 45401-0927
(937) 259-1384
http://www.med.wright.edu/som/sardi

A federally funded research center that investigates the relationship between drug use and disabilities. Free newsletter.

TASH: The Association for Persons with Severe Handicaps
29 West Susquehanna Avenue, Suite 210
Baltimore, MD 21204
(410) 828-8274   (410) 828-1306 (TT)   FAX (410) 828-6706
e-mail: info@tash.org   http://www.tash.org

A national advocacy organization that disseminates information to improve the education and increase the independence of individuals with severe disabilities. Holds an annual conference. Publishes a quarterly journal, "Journal of the Association for Persons with Severe Handicaps" and the "TASH Newsletter" (both included with membership). Regular membership, $88.00; reduced fee membership for parents, self-advocates, and financial hardship, $45.00.

United Way of America (UWA)
701 North Fairfax Street
Alexandria, VA 22314-2045
(703) 836-7100   FAX (703) 683-7840
http://www.unitedway.org

An umbrella organization of local human service organizations. National office will direct callers to the local United Way, which in turn will provide referral to a specific local service agency.

Untangling the Web
International Center on Disability Information
Barron Drive, PO Box 1004
Institute, WV 25112-1004
(304) 766-2680   (304) 766-2697 (TT)   FAX (304) 766-2689
e-mail: rta@rtc2.icdi.wvu.edu   http://www.icdi.wvu.edu

This web site provides links to a wide variety of other web sites, organized by disability.

World Institute on Disability (WID)
510 16th Street, Suite 100
Oakland, CA 94612-1502
(510) 763-4100   (510) 208-9496 (TT)   FAX (510) 763-4109
e-http://www.wid.org

A public policy center founded and operated by individuals with disabilities, WID conducts research, public education, and training. It also develops model programs related to disability. It deals with issues such as personal assistance, public transportation, employment, and access to health care. WID's Research and Training Centers are federally funded centers that study personal assistance services, federal independent living initiatives, and community integration issues.

After the Diagnosis
by JoAnn LeMaistre
Alpine Guild
PO Box 4848
Dillon, CO 80435
(800) 869-9559   FAX (970) 262-9378

This book describes the emotional responses to health changes due to physical disabilities, chronic illness, and aging. $18.95 plus $2.00 shipping and handling

Alcohol, Disabilities, and Rehabilitation
by Susan A. Storti
Singular Publishing Group
401 West A Street, Suite 325
San Diego, CA 92101
(800) 521-8545   FAX (800) 774-8398
e-mail: singpub@mail.cerfnet.com http://www.singpub.com

This book discusses alcohol abuse in individuals with disabilities and chronic conditions. Includes treatment and rehabilitation strategies. $34.95 plus $6.00 shipping and handling

American Rehabilitation
Superintendent of Documents
PO Box 371954
Pittsburgh, PA 15250-7954
(202) 512-1800   FAX (202) 512-2250
http://www.access.gpo.gov/index.html

Published by the Rehabilitation Services Administration, this magazine provides information on rehabilitation programs, services, and publications. $8.00

Black Bird Fly Away: Disabled In An Able-Bodied World
by Hugh Gregory Gallagher
Vandamere Press
PO Box 5243
Arlington, VA 22205
(800) 551-7776   FAX (703) 536-9644

Written by a man, who is quadriplegic due to polio, this book describes his life with disability, including his accomplishments as well as coping with severe depression. He also describes the development of disability rights during the past 40 years. $21.95 plus $3.75 shipping and handling

Dictionary of Rehabilitation
by Myron G. Eisenberg
Springer Publishing Company
536 Broadway
New York, NY 10012
(212) 431-4370   FAX (212) 941-7842   http://springerpub.com

This book defines the core terms used in the rehabilitation field. $43.95 plus $3.50 shipping and handling

Disability Funding News
CD Publications
8204 Fenton Street
Silver Spring, MD 20910
(800) 666-6380   (301) 588-6380   FAX (301) 588-6385

This semimonthly publication contains information about funding opportunities from the federal government and private foundations. $239.00

Disability in America: Toward a National Agenda for Prevention
by Andrew M. Pope and Alvin R. Tarlow (eds.)
National Academy Press
2101 Constitution Avenue, NW
Lockbox 285
Washington, DC 20055
(800) 624-6242   (202) 334-3313   FAX (202) 334-2451
http://www.nap.edu

The report of a panel of experts, this book examines the magnitude of disability in the U.S., recommends a model to prevent disabilities, and makes a series of policy recommendations. $29.95 plus $4.00 shipping and handling. A 20% discount is offered to individuals who purchase books through the National Academy's Web Bookstore.

Disability in the United States: A Portrait from National Data
by Susan Thompson-Hoffman and Inez Fitzgerald-Storck (eds.)
Springer Publishing Company, New York, NY

This book is a collection of articles based on data collected from a variety of federal agencies. It presents an analysis of the relationship between a wide variety of demographic characteristics and disability with implications for future policy and research. Out of print

Disability Studies Quarterly
David Pfeiffer
Hawaii University Affiliated Program on Disabilities
University of Hawaii at Manoa
1776 University Avenue, UA 4-6
Honolulu, HI 96822
e-mail: sds@hexen.com   http://www.wipd.com/sds

A quarterly journal with reports on recent research findings, upcoming meetings, and grant solicitations. Reviews of books and audio-visual materials. Available in standard print, audiocassette, e-mail, and computer disk (PC). Individuals, $35.00; institutions, $45.00; students, $20.00; low income, "what you can afford."

Don't Worry, He Won't Get Far on Foot
by John Callahan
Random House, Order Department
400 Hahn Road, PO Box 100
Westminster, MD 21157
(800) 793-2665   http://www.randomhouse.com

Written by a nationally known cartoonist who experienced a spinal cord injury as a result of an accident caused by drinking and driving, this witty autobiographical account provides details of his rehabilitation and his life after his accident, including his return to sobriety. $12.00 plus $3.00 shipping and handling

Enabling Romance: A Guide to Love, Sex, and Relationships for the Disabled
by Ken Kroll and Erica Levy Klein
Woodbine House
6510 Bells Mill Road
Bethesda, MD 20817
(800) 843-7323   FAX (301) 897-5838
e-mail: info@woodbinehouse.com   http://www.woodbinehouse.com

Written by a man who has a disability and his wife who does not, this book provides examples of how people with a variety of disabilities have established fulfilling relationships. $15.95 plus $4.50 shipping and handling

Encyclopedia of Disability and Rehabilitation
by Arthur E. Dell Orto and Robert P. Marinelli (eds.)
Macmillan Library Reference
866 Third Avenue, 2nd Floor
New York, NY 10022
(800) 257-5157   http://www.mlr.com

Written by a variety of experts in the field of disability, this reference book includes articles ranging from AIDS to stroke, advocacy to wheelchairs, and aging to work. $105.00 plus $4.00 shipping and handling

Erection
by Goedele Liekens and Michael Perry
Focus International
1160 East Jericho Turnpike, Suite 15
Huntington, NY 11743
(800) 843-0305   (516) 549-5320   FAX (516) 549-2066
e-mail: Sex_Help@focusint.com   http://www.hip.com/focus

This videotape provides information about causes and treatment of erectile dysfunction. 53 minutes. $19.95 plus $6.00 shipping and handling

Federal Register
New Orders, Superintendent of Documents
PO Box 371954
Pittsburgh, PA 15250-7954
(202) 512-1800   FAX (202) 512-2250
e-mail: gpoaccess@gpo.gov   http://www.access.gpo.gov/su_docs/aces/aces140.html

A federal publication printed every weekday with notices of all regulations and legal notices issued by federal agencies. Domestic subscriptions, $607.00 annually for second class mailing of paper format; $220.00 annually for microfiche. Also available on the web site at no charge.

Flying Solo: Reimagining Manhood, Courage, and Loss
by Leonard Kriegel
Random House, Order Department
400 Hahn Road, PO Box 100
Westminster, MD 21157
(800) 793-2665   http://www.randomhouse.com

Written by a man who became paraplegic due to childhood polio, this book examines traditional views of manhood and how they sustained and stymied him. $22.00 plus $4.00 shipping and handling

Flying without Wings
by Arnold R. Beisser
Doubleday, New York, NY

This book is written by a physician who became a quadriplegic due to polio, shortly after graduating from medical school. He describes how he came to terms with disability and discusses acceptance and his efforts to make the most of his life. Out of print.

Foundations of the Vocational Rehabilitation Process
by Stanford E. Rubin and Richard T. Roessler
Pro-Ed
8700 Shoal Creek Boulevard
Austin, TX 78758
(800) 897-3202   (512) 451-3246   FAX (800) 397-7633
http://www.proedinc.com

A textbook with complete coverage of the development of vocational rehabilitation programs in the U.S., legislative history, and procedures used by professionals to conduct client assessments and deliver services. $37.00 plus 10% shipping and handling

Grants for Organizations Serving People with Disabilities
Research Grant Guides, Inc.
PO Box 1214
Loxahatchee, FL 33470
(561) 795-6129   FAX (561) 795-7794
http://www.researchgrant.com

This book provides profiles of foundations and federal sources of funding, including areas of interest and eligibility requirements. Includes chapters with advice on proposal writing. $59.50 plus $6.00 handling fee.

Health Promotion for Men 50+
American Association of Retired Persons (AARP)
601 E Street, NW
Washington DC 20049
(800) 441-2277   (202) 434-2277   http://www.aarp.org

This booklet provides information about how to do outreach to men; how to implement a community program; and resources that provide information about the health needs of men over 50. Free

If I Can't Do It
by Walter Brock
Fanlight Productions
47 Halifax St.
Boston, MA 02130
(800) 937-4113   (617) 524-0980   FAX (617) 524-8838
e-mail: fanlight@fanlight.com   http://www.fanlight.com

This videotape tells the story of a man, born with cerebral palsy, who struggles to live independently and becomes a disability activist. 57 minutes. Purchase, $245.00; rental for one day, $50.00; rental for one week, $100.00; plus $9.00 shipping charge.

Impotence: A Matter Most Delicate
Focus International
1160 East Jericho Turnpike, Suite 15
Huntington, NY 11743
(800) 843-0305   (516) 549-5320   FAX (516) 549-2066
http://www.hip.com/focus   e-mail: Sex_Help@focusint.com

This videotape describes treatments for impotence, including drugs, implants, and prostheses. 26 minutes. $29.95 plus $6.00 shipping and handling

Journal of Disability Policy Studies
Department of Rehabilitation Education and Research
346 North West Avenue
Fayetteville, AR 72701
(501) 575-6420 (V/TT)   FAX (501) 575-3253
http://comp.uark.edu/~rehab

A journal, published twice a year, with articles related to legislative policy and regulatory matters as well as articles from a range of academic disciplines. $24.00

Journal of Rehabilitation Research and Development (JRRD)
Scientific and Technical Publications Section
Rehabilitation Research and Development Service
103 South Gay Street, 5th floor
Baltimore, MD 21202
(410) 962-1800   FAX (410) 962-9670   e-mail: pubs@vard.org
http://www.vard.org

A quarterly journal that includes articles on disability, rehabilitation, sensory aids, gerontology, and disabling conditions. Includes abstracts of literature, book reviews, and calendar of events. Annual supplements provide research progress reports. Clinical supplements report on specific topics. Free

Kaleidoscope
United Disability Services
701 South Main Street
Akron, OH 44311-1019
(330) 762-9755   (330) 379-3349 (TT)   FAX (330) 762-0912

A magazine that explores disability through articles of fiction, poetry, and fine art. Contributions by individuals with disabilities and individuals without disabilities. Two issues per year. Individuals, $9.00; institutions, $14.00.

Life Services Planning for the Elderly and Persons with Disabilities
Commission on Mental and Physical Disability Law
American Bar Association
740 15th Street, NW, 9th Floor
Washington, DC 20005
(202) 662-1570   (202) 662-1012   FAX (202) 662-1032
e-mail: cmpdl@attmail.com   http://www.abanet.org

This three book series provides guidance for individuals, families, and service providers about estates, financial issues, health care, and government benefits. $20.00 plus $5.00 shipping and handling

Mainstream
2973 Beach Street
San Diego, CA 92102
(619) 234-3138   FAX (619) 234-3155
http://www.mainstream-mag.com

A magazine with articles, information about products, and a calendar of events. Ten issues per year. One year, $24.00; two years, $44.00.

Making Disability
by Paul Higgins
Charles C. Thomas, Publisher
2600 South First Street
Springfield, IL 62794-9265
(800) 258-8980   (217) 789-8980   FAX (217) 789-9130
e-mail: books@ccthomas.com   http://www.ccthomas.com

Written by a sociologist, this book examines disability as a social phenomenon rather than a defect. It discusses the depiction of disability, experiencing disability, serving individuals with disabilities, and developing disability policy. Hardcover, $54.95; softcover, $35.95; plus $5.50 shipping and handling.

Making Wise Medical Decisions: How to Get the Information You Need
Resources for Rehabilitation
33 Bedford Street, Suite 19A
Lexington, MA 02420
(781) 862-6455   FAX (781) 861-7517
e-mail: info@rfr.org   http://www.rfr.org

This book includes information about where to go and what to read in order to make informed, rational, medical decisions. It describes how to obtain relevant health information and evaluate medical tests and procedures, health care providers, and health facilities. Includes chapters on protecting the health of children who are ill; special issues facing elders; and people with chronic illnesses and disabilities and the health care system. $39.95 plus $5.00 shipping and handling (See order form on last page of this book.)

Missing Pieces: A Chronicle of Living with a Disability
by Irving Zola
Temple University Press
1601 North Broad Street
Philadelphia, PA 19122
(800) 447-1656   FAX (215) 204-4719
e-mail: tempress@astro.ocis.temple.edu
http://www.temple.edu/tempress

Written by a sociologist with mobility impairment due to polio and an automobile accident, this book was inspired by his stay at a special residential village for people with disabilities in the Netherlands. It includes analysis of what it is like to be a person with a disability in a society designed for those who are healthy. $22.95 plus $4.00 shipping and handling

Moving Violations: War Zones, Wheelchairs, and Declarations of Independence
by John Hockenberry
Time-Warner Trade Publishing
Attn: Order Department
3 Center Plaza
Boston, MA 02108
(800) 759-0190   FAX (800) 286-9471   (617) 227-0730

Written by a television reporter who became a paraplegic at the age of 19 as a result of an automobile accident, this book describes his adjustment to disability, rehabilitation, jobs in radio and television, and the stories of other family members with disabilities. Hardcover, $24.45; softcover, $14.45.

My Body Is Not Who I Am
Aquarius Health Care Videos
5 Powderhouse Lane
PO Box 1159
Sherborn, MA 01770
(508) 651-2963   FAX (508) 650-4216
e-mail: aqvideos@tiac.net   http://www.aquariusproductions.com

In this videotape, individuals discuss the effects that disability has had on their lives. Includes family relationships, sexuality, and health care. 35 minutes. $195.00 plus $9.00 shipping and handling

No Pity: People with Disabilities Forging a New Civil Rights Movement
by Joseph P. Shapiro
Random House, Order Department
400 Hahn Road, PO Box 100
Westminster, MD 21157
(800) 793-2665   http://www.randomhouse.com

This book describes the evolution of the disability rights movement and profiles its leaders. $15.00 plus $4.00 shipping and handling

NORD Resource Guide
National Organization for Rare Disorders (NORD)
PO Box 8923
New Fairfield, CT 06812-8923
(203) 746-6518   FAX (203) 746-6481   (203) 746-6927 (TT)
e-mail: orphan@NORD-RDB.com   http://www.nord-rdb.com/~orphan

This directory lists organizations that support individuals with rare diseases and disabilities. $39.95 plus $5.00 shipping and handling

Nothing About Us Without Us: Disability Oppression and Empowerment
by James I. Charlton
University of California Press
California Princeton Fulfillment Service
1445 Lower Ferry Road
Ewing, NJ 08618
(800) 777-4726   FAX (800) 999-1958   (609) 883-1759
FAX (609) 883-7413   e-mail: orders@cpfs.pupress.princeton.edu
http://www.ucpress.berkeley.edu

Written by a man who has worked in the disability rights and independent living movement, this book discusses how individuals with disabilities need to have the right to make their own decisions and be treated as equal members of society. $27.50 plus $3.75 shipping and handling

Ragged Edge
Advocado Press Inc.
Box 145
Louisville, KY 40201
e-mail: editor@ragged-edge-mag.com
http://www.ragged-edge-mag.com

This bimonthly magazine reports on disability issues from the perspective of disability rights activists. Individuals, $17.50; institutions, $35.00. The "Electronic EDGE" is available at no charge on the web site.

Report on Disability Programs
Business Publishers
951 Pershing Drive
Silver Spring, MD 20910
(800) 274-0122   (301) 587-6300   FAX (301) 589-8493
e-mail: bpinews@bpinews.com   http://www.bpinews.com

A biweekly newsletter with information on policies promulgated by federal agencies, laws, and funding sources. $297.00

Reproductive Issues for Persons with Physical Disabilities
by Florence P. Haseltine, Sandra S. Cole, and David B. Gray (eds.)
Brookes Publishing Company
PO Box 10624
Baltimore, MD 21285-0624
(800) 638-3775   FAX (410) 337-8539
e-mail: custserv@pbrookes.com   http://www.pbrookes.com

This book provides an overview of sexuality, disability, and reproductive issues across the lifespan for individuals with disabilities including multiple sclerosis and spinal cord injury. Includes academic articles as well as personal narratives written by individuals with disabilities. $34.95

The Self-Help Sourcebook: Your Guide to Community and Online Support Groups
American Self-Help Clearinghouse
Northwest Covenant Medical Center
Pocono Road
Denville, NJ 07834
(973) 625-9565   (973) 625-9053 (TT)   FAX (973) 625-8848
http://www.cmhc.com/selfhelp

A directory of national and model self-help groups. $10.00 plus $2.00 shipping and handling; also available on the web site.

Sexual Concerns When Illness or Disability Strikes
by Carol L. Sandowski
Charles C. Thomas Publisher
2600 South First Street
Springfield, IL 62794
(800) 258-8980   (217) 789-8980   FAX (217) 789-9130
e-mail: books@ccthomas.com   http://www.ccthomas.com

Written by a social worker who is a certified sex counselor, this book discusses sexuality and issues of self-esteem that arise with illness or disability. $41.95 plus $5.50 shipping and handling

Sexuality and Disability
Plenum Publishing Company, Attention: Journal Department
Human Sciences Press
233 Spring Street
New York, NY 10013-1578
(800) 221-9369   (212) 620-8000   FAX (212) 807-1047
http://www.plenum.com

A quarterly journal with articles on the medical and rehabilitation aspects of sexuality for individuals who have experienced a disability. Individuals, $55.00; institutions, $295.00.

Sexuality and Disability
Sexuality Information and Education Council of the United States (SIECUS)
130 West 42nd Street, Suite 350
New York, NY 10036-7802
(212) 819-9770   FAX (212) 819-9776
e-mail: siecus@siecus.org   http://www.siecus.org

This annotated bibliography lists general books, books for professionals, curricula, journals and newsletters, teaching aids, databases, and organizations that provide information about sexuality for individuals with disabilities. $2.00 Also available on the web site, free.

Staring Back: The Disability Experience from the Inside Out
by Kenny Fries (ed.)
Penguin Putnam
PO Box 12289
Newark, NJ 07101
(800) 253-6476   FAX (201) 896-8569
http://www.penguin.com

This anthology includes essays, poems, and works of fiction written by individuals who have a broad range of disabilities. $15.95 plus $2.00 shipping and handling

That All May Worship
National Organization on Disability (NOD)
910 16th Street, NW, Suite 600
Washington, DC 20006
(800) 248-2253 (Referral Line)   (202) 293-5960   (202) 293-5968 (TT)
FAX (202) 293-7999   e-mail: ability@nod.org http://www.nod.org

This interfaith guide helps congregations make their facilities accessible to people with disabilities. $10.00.

Treating Erectile Problems
by Joseph Lo Piccolo and Jerry Friedman
Focus International
1160 East Jericho Turnpike, Suite 15
Huntington, NY 11743
(800) 843-0305   (516) 549-5320   FAX (516) 549-2066
e-mail: Sex_Help@focusint.com   http://www.hip.com/focus

This videotape explores the communication problems that can lead to erectile dysfunction and demonstrates various techniques for sexual pleasure without an erection. 20 minutes. $14.95 plus $6.00 shipping and handling

Us and Them
by Fred Simon and Janet Kamien
Fanlight Productions
47 Halifax St.
Boston, MA 02130
(800) 937-4113   (617) 524-0980   FAX (617) 524-8838
e-mail: fanlight@fanlight.com   http://www.fanlight.com

This videotape is about relationships between people who have disabilities and those who do not. 32 minutes, black and white. Purchase, $69.00; rental for one day, $50.00; plus $9.00 shipping charge.

Wheelchairs: Your Options and Rights Guide to Obtaining Wheelchairs from the Department of Veterans Affairs
PVA Distribution Center
PO Box 753
Waldorf, MD 20604-0753
(888) 860-7244   (301) 932-7834   FAX (301) 843-0159
http://www.pva.org

This booklet provides information on eligibility criteria, lists the types of wheelchairs available, and describes DVA procedures. Available in English and Spanish. Free

Chapter 2

COPING WITH DAILY ACTIVITIES

Men in our society carry out a variety of roles and responsibilities. In addition to performing the required tasks of their chosen occupational field, they are husbands, fathers, and caregivers for sick or disabled partners, parents, and children. For men with disabilities, these activities may become a challenge. Although the number of products to help people with disabilities live independently has increased dramatically in recent years, especially with the advent of the personal computer, the everyday tasks performed by men with disabilities are often more time consuming than they are for healthy men. The sections that follow provide information about everyday activities in the family, providing care for others with disabilities, working with a disability, using environmental adaptations, locating accessible housing, and recreation and travel.

HOW DISABILITIES AND CHRONIC CONDITIONS AFFECT THE FAMILY

Diagnosis of a disability or chronic condition in a family member can cause disruption in the healthiest of families. Coping with a crisis situation puts strain on any relationship; coping with the inevitability of a permanent change causes strain between marital partners and places great stress upon children. Stress may be related to providing adequate health care, financial concerns, disruption of familiar patterns of everyday living and work, and sexual relations.

Children in the family are often not told the details of the situation, as parents do not want to frighten them. Without information, however, their imaginations may picture a situation far worse than reality. During the initial crisis, when a father is in the hospital, the children are often deprived not only of his company but also of their mother, who is tending to the father's emotional and physical needs (Rustad: 1984).

It is crucial that family members understand the nature of the condition and its effects on daily functioning. Holding realistic expectations for what the affected family member can and cannot do contributes to the individual's ability to cope with the situation. Being overly protective and trying to do everything for the affected family member may result in diminished self-esteem and independence. On the other hand, expecting the individual to carry out activities that are unrealistic or implying that the limitations are "only in the head" creates a great deal of additional stress. People with disabilities and chronic conditions often express the fear of being a burden on family members; when their relatives suggest that they can accomplish tasks that are physically impossible for them, the affected individuals will be reluctant to ask for assistance at any time.

Following the onset of a disability or chronic condition, all family members must be prepared for role changes and accommodations. The man who has been affected may find that he can no longer carry out the roles in the family that he was accustomed to. For example, if he is no longer able to drive, he will not be able to transport children to activities or go grocery shopping on his own. His partner or spouse will need to take on additional roles. Children who are old enough should be encouraged to take on some additional household responsibilities. When it is financially feasible, hiring household help can alleviate some of the burdens placed on family members. Some families may qualify for homemaker services provided by government agencies or voluntary organizations.

Often the assistance of a social worker or a psychologist is necessary to help the family restructuring that takes place following the development of a disability or chronic condition. The emotional needs of the spouse or partner must also be considered. Since the spouse or partner has the additional role of providing emotional and physical support for the individual who has developed a disability or chronic condition, he or she will likely need support also. Self-help groups of other caregivers in similar situations may prove helpful. Hulnick and Hulnick (1989) suggest that counselors can help family members "reframe" the context of the situation so that they respond positively, learn and grow from the new situation, and empower themselves to make choices. Local and state governments, private agencies that provide case management services, and voluntary organizations that are dedicated to one disease or disability often have programs to help family members as well as the individuals with disabilities and chronic conditions.

CARING FOR OTHERS WITH DISABILITIES

Both single fathers and husbands of women who have become disabled have special needs that must be addressed. Those men who are part of two parent intact families must learn to equitably share the caregiving chores with their wives. Stoller (1990) points out that 28% of caregivers are men. These men care for spouses, parents, children, other relatives, and friends. Kaye and Applegate's (1995) study of older male caregivers found that over 40% had their own health problems and about the same proportion was depressed. Yet the role of men as caregivers is neglected in both the literature and in programs designed to help caregivers.

Support groups for men who are caregivers may provide both emotional support and practical suggestions to solve problems. Yet many men may be reluctant to attend because they have been socialized to be independent and to keep their feelings to themselves. In addition, caregivers may find that their time is limited and may be reluctant to leave the care recipient alone. Nonetheless, those men who have attended groups for caregivers have found them beneficial; they received information on community services, learned how to deal with their emotions, and provided help to others (Jacobs: 1989).

Short term respite programs that enable caregivers to have time to themselves, adult day care programs, utilization of personal attendants or home health aides, and special programs for children and elders have been developed as a way for caregivers to give adequate care and also tend to their own personal needs. Meeting the financial needs of dependent family members often requires the help of an attorney who specializes in family law. In addition, the federal Family and Medical Leave Act requires employers to permit employees to take leave from their jobs in order to care for sick relatives (see Chapter 3, "Laws that Affect Men with Disabilities").

References

Hulnick, Mary R. and H. Ronald Hulnick
1989 "Life's Challenges: Curse or Opportunity? Counseling Families of Persons with Disabilities" Journal of Counseling and Development 68(November/December):166-170

Jacobs, Geraldine
1989 Involving Men in Caregiver Support Groups: A Practical Guidebook Bryn Mawr, PA: Graduate School of Social Work and Social Research, Bryn Mawr College

Kaye, Lenard W. and Jeffrey S. Applegate
1995 "Men's Style of Nurturing Elders" pp. 205-221 in Donald Sabo and David Frederick Gordon (eds.) Men's Health and Illness: Gender, Power, and the Body Newbury Park, CA: Sage Publications

Rustad, Lynne C.
1984 "Family Adjustment to Chronic Illness and Disability in Mid-Life" pp. 222-242 in Myron G. Eisenberg, LaFaye C. Sutkin, and Mary A. Jansen (eds.) Chronic Illness and Disability through the Life Span New York, NY: Springer Publishing Company

Stoller, Eleanor Palo
1990 "Males as Helpers: The Role of Sons, Relatives, and Friends" The Gerontologist 30:2:228-235

<u>Children of Aging Parents</u> (CAPS)
Woodbourne Office Campus, Suite 302A
1609 Woodbourne
Levittown, PA 19057
(800) 227-7294   (215) 945-6900   http://www.experts.com

Helps caregivers find the appropriate care and support for elders as well as for themselves. Sponsors a network of support groups for caregivers. Publishes a variety of training and resource materials for support groups, a national directory of geriatric case managers, and a newsletter, "CAPSule." Membership, individuals, $20.00; professionals and organizations, $100.00.

<u>National Family Caregivers Association</u>
10605 Concord Street, Suite 501
Kensington, MD 20895-2504
(800) 896-3650   (301) 942-6430   FAX (301) 942-2302
http://www.nfcacares.org

A membership organization for individuals who provide care for others at any stage of their lives or with any disease or disability. Maintains an information clearinghouse and a network of individuals who would like to provide and receive support from others in similar situations. Membership, individuals, $20.00; professionals, $30.00; nonprofit organizations, $50.00; group medical practices, home health agencies, etc., $100.00; hospitals and corporate providers, $200.00.

<u>National Fathers' Network</u>
Kindering Center
16120 NE 8th Street
Bellevue, WA 98008-3937
(425) 747-4004   FAX (425) 747-1069
e-mail: jmay@fathersnetwork.org   http://www.fathersnetwork.org

A network of fathers, professionals, and others interested in sharing ideas about caring for children with disabilities. Provides training for individuals who want to establish support groups for fathers. Membership is free, but donations are requested; individuals, $10.00, organizations, $30.00. Newsletters, "National Fathers' Network Newsletter" and "DADS - - Dads Advocating for Dads," published twice a year, free.

National Resource Center for Parents with Disabilities
Through the Looking Glass
2198 Sixth Street, Suite 100
Berkeley, CA 94710-2204
(800) 644-2666   (800) 804-1616 (TT)   (510) 848-1112
FAX (510) 848-4445   e-mail: TLG@lookingglass.org
http://www.lookingglass.org

A federally funded center that conducts research on the needs of parents with disabilities. Conducts research on special equipment and techniques of caring for babies. Maintains a national network of parents with disabilities, their families, researchers, and service providers. Convenes a National Task Force on Parents with Disabilities and Their Families, which meets annually. "Keeping Our Families Together," a report of the first Task Force meeting is available in print, large print, braille, and audiocassette; $2.00. Publishes quarterly newsletter, "Parenting with a Disability," which provides information about the center's activities, publications in the field, and practical suggestions for parents. Available in print, large print, braille, and audiocassette. Free

Well Spouse Foundation
610 Lexington Avenue, Suite 814
New York, NY 10022
(800) 838-0879   (212) 644-1241   FAX (212) 644-1338
e-mail: wellspouse@aol.com

A network of support groups that provide emotional support to spouses and children of people who are chronically ill. Membership, individuals, $20.00; professionals, $50.00; includes bimonthly "Well Spouse Foundation Newsletter."

Family Challenges: Parenting with a Disability
Aquarius Health Care Videos
5 Powderhouse Lane
PO Box 1159
Sherborn, MA 01770
(508) 651-2963   FAX (508) 650-4216
e-mail: aqvideos@tiac.net   http://www.aquariusproductions.com

In this videotape, the children and spouses of parents with disabilities describe their relationships and coping strategies. Includes two fathers, one with a spinal cord injury and one with a neuromuscular disease. 25 minutes. $195.00 plus $9.00 shipping and handling

Helping Yourself Help Others: A Book for Caregivers
by Rosalynn Carter with Susan K. Golant
Random House, Order Department
400 Hahn Road, PO Box 100
Westminster, MD 21157
(800) 793-2665   http://www.randomhouse.com

This book focuses on family caregivers, offering suggestions for everyday problems such as physical and emotional needs, isolation, burnout, and dealing with professional caregivers. Lists of organizations, books, and resources included. $14.00

How to Help Children Through a Parent's Serious Illness
by Kathleen McCue with Ron Bonn
St. Martin's Griffin
c/o VHPS
175 Fifth Avenue
New York, NY 10010
(800) 321-9299   http://www.stmartins.com

This book presents practical guidelines to help parents explain their illness to children of different ages, how to understand the children's reactions, and how to seek professional help. Includes a chapter on chronic illness. $11.95 plus $3.75 shipping and handling

Mainstay: For the Well Spouse of the Chronically Ill
by Maggie Strong
Bradford Books
160 Main Street
Northampton, MA 01060-3134
(413) 584-4597   http://gcim.com/mainstay

Written by a woman whose husband was diagnosed with multiple sclerosis at age 46, this book provides her personal account and others' stories, practical suggestions, and advice from health care professionals. $15.00 plus $3.00 shipping and handling

Special Kids, Special Dads: Fathers of Children with Disabilities
National Fathers' Network
Kindering Center
16120 NE 8th Street
Bellevue, WA 98008-3937
(425) 747-4004   FAX (425) 747-1069
e-mail: jmay@fathersnetwork.org   http://www.fathersnetwork.org

This videotape explores the emotional needs of fathers of children with special needs and how to support them in parenting. Discussion guide included. 23 minutes. $80.00 plus $5.00 shipping and handling

To Everything There is a Season: A Guide for Caregivers of Farmers and Ranchers with Disabilities
Breaking New Ground Resource Center
Purdue University
1146 ABE Building
West Lafayette, IN 47907-1146
(800) 825-4264   (765) 494-5088 (V/TT)   FAX (765) 496-1356
http://abe.www.ecn.purdue.edu/ABE/Extension/BNG/Index.html

This resource kit is targeted to rural caregivers. Includes a videotape, brochure, and written resources. Entire resource kit, $75.00; videotape only, $65.00; written resources only, $12.00; brochure only, $.75.

Uncommon Fathers: Reflections on Raising a Child with a Disability
by Donald J. Meyer (ed.)
Woodbine House
6510 Bells Mill Road
Bethesda, MD 20817
(800) 843-7323   FAX (301) 897-5838
e-mail: info@woodbinehouse.com   http://www.woodbinehouse.com

Written by fathers of children with developmental disabilities, the essays in this book describe the fathers' perspectives of the impact children with disabilities have on their families. $14.95 plus $4.50 shipping and handling

Unending Work and Care: Managing Chronic Illness at Home
by Juliet M. Corbin and Anselm Strauss
Jossey-Bass Inc., San Francisco, CA

An analysis of the issues that affect the lives of individuals with chronic illness and their family members. Describes physical and emotional needs; the role of health care personnel; and the means to manage chronic illness effectively. Out of print.

Three-fifths (59.1%) of men with disabilities are employed (McNeil: 1993). Individuals in higher paying, white collar positions are more likely to retain their jobs after disability. Men of working age (16 to 64) have higher levels of work disability than women in all age groups, although the difference is small in some age groups; overall 8.7% of men have work disabilities (Kraus and Stoddard: 1991).

Since men are socialized at an early age to be successful in their careers, the inability to work or a decrease in job status and salary may prove devastating to a man's ego. Rehabilitation programs to adapt the workplace or retraining for a new position may enable a man to continue working and maintain his self-esteem. (See Chapter 1, p. 18 for a description of rehabilitation programs.)

Men with recently acquired disabilities should think carefully about the type of work they would like to do, being realistic about their physical abilities and their stamina. Vocational assessment and counseling may prove useful to men whose conditions require a position change. Physical location of the place of employment, transportation, and work schedule are all important considerations regarding a particular position. For some men, disability may mean changing to a different specialty within the same general field; for example, a surgeon who is no longer able to carry out surgery may train for a specialty that does not require the use of his hands, such as psychiatry.

Learning to delegate responsibility may be difficult at first for those men who are used to doing everything themselves. Allowing others to take on additional responsibilities and avoiding the most stressful daily business operations enable many men to continue working. A small business owner who was diagnosed with multiple sclerosis was not only able to continue to work from his home, but he also believed that the change in his business operation opened up new opportunities:

> This experience forced me to let go of a lot of things, and now that
> I let go, it gives the business an opportunity to grow (Norman:
> 1996, D4).

The Americans with Disabilities Act requires that employers make "reasonable accommodations" for people with disabilities (see Chapter 3, "Laws that Affect Men with Disabilities"). Advances in technology, especially in computer technology that is the core of most office work, have produced a variety of adapted equipment that enables even those with the most limited mobility to continue working. Men with minimal mobility can control their environment through the use of switches, headpointers, joysticks, and sip-and-puff switches; these devices are used in conjunction with special software or adapted hardware. For example, men with high quadriplegia are able to turn electrical devices on and off through the use of a sip-and-puff device. Switches that may be operated by a toe, a foot, or a hand permit entry of data into computers. Headpointers are attached to a headset and consist of pointers with rubber tips that are used to control keys on the keyboard. Joysticks enable men with limited motion to simulate the movement of a mouse.

Speech recognition systems enable men who are severely limited in their mobility to use personal computers in a variety of situations. These systems recognize the user's voice as an alternative way of entering data into computers and may be used to write and to carry out conversations, both on the job and in other settings.

Barrier-free design ensures that men with disabilities can enter and exit the building easily and safely; that bathroom facilities, water fountains, and employee dining rooms are accessible; that aisles and entryways are wide enough to accommodate wheelchairs; that ramps are placed where needed; and that floor coverings are amenable to the use of wheelchairs. Special paint or grit strip paint applied to slippery surfaces or inclines reduces the risk of accidents. Mirrors mounted at hallway intersections and see-through panels in doors may help prevent accidents for employees traveling in wheelchairs. Elevator buttons, public telephones, and light switches should also be accessible to people who use wheelchairs. Staff members who are not disabled should be assigned the responsibility for helping men with disabilities to exit the building in case of an emergency, such as a fire, bomb threat, or toxic leak.

The space underneath the desk should be large enough to accommodate a wheelchair; file cabinets should be lateral so that they are within reach. Special desks and workstations are available to accommodate wheelchairs and adjust to the required height of the user. Where carpets are used, they should be low level pile to allow for easier mobility, and elevators should be large enough to accommodate wheelchairs. Some individuals use standing wheelchairs that offer flexibility in adapting to the workplace as well as improved circulation, reduced pressure sores, and direct eye contact with colleagues without looking up from a seated position.

Transportation has often been a barrier to employment for men with disabilities. Some men with disabilities may be able to operate their own automobiles or vans. Many car manufacturers offer specially adapted vans to carry wheelchairs. Some of these companies also have special purchase or loan programs for people with disabilities. General Motors, Ford, Chrysler, and Saturn offer financial assistance for the purchase of adaptive equipment such as hand controls, a ramp, or a lift to be installed in vehicles (see "ORGANIZATIONS" section under Recreation and Travel in this chapter). Public transportation systems may have regular buses with special equipment to lift wheelchairs, or they may offer transportation in vehicles specially designed for people with disabilities. The entry from the parking lot should provide enough space for wheelchairs to be removed from the vehicle. Level ground or ramps should lead into the building.

Men who require continued medical supervision to manage their conditions should be allowed time to schedule doctors' appointments. Flexibility is often the key, enabling men to work through lunch or later hours one day in order to take time off for medical care another day. Employers who cooperate to accommodate the special needs of men with disabilities and chronic conditions will contribute to a more productive workforce.

References

Kraus, Lewis E. and Susan Stoddard
1991 Chartbook on Work Disability in the United States Washington, DC: National Institute on Disability and Rehabilitation Research

McNeil, John M.
1993 <u>Americans With Disabilities 1991-1992</u>, Washington, DC: U.S. Bureau of the Census
    Current Population Reports P70-33

Norman, Jan
1996 "Down But Clearly Not Out" <u>The Boston Globe</u> July 31

ORGANIZATIONS

Breaking New Ground Resource Center
Department of Agricultural Engineering
Purdue University
1146 ABE Building
West Lafayette, IN 47907-1146
(800) 825-4264   (765) 494-5088 (V/TT)   FAX (765) 496-1356
http://abe.www.ecn.purdue.edu/ABE/Extension/BNG/Index.html

A federally funded research center that investigates ways to improve opportunities for employment of farmers with disabilities. Provides assistive technology and outreach. Newsletter, "Breaking New Ground," available in standard print and on audiocassette. Free

Equal Employment Opportunity Commission (EEOC)
1801 L Street, NW, 10th floor
Washington, DC 20507
(800) 669-3362 to order publications
(800) 669-4000 to speak to an investigator
(800) 800-3302 (TT)
In the Washington, DC metropolitan area, (202) 275-7377
(202) 275-7518 (TT)   http://www.eeoc.gov

Responsible for promulgating and enforcing regulations for the employment section of the ADA. Copies of its regulations are available in standard print, large print, braille, computer disk, and audiocassette.

Job Accommodation Network (JAN)
West Virginia University
918 Chestnut Ridge Road, Suite 1
PO Box 6080
Morgantown, WV 26506-6080
(800) 526-7234   (800) 232-9675 (V/TT)
FAX (304) 293-5407   http://janweb.icdi.wvu.edu

Maintains database of products that facilitate accommodation in the workplace. Provides information to employers about practical accommodations which enable them to employ individuals with disabilities.

President's Committee on Employment of People with Disabilities (PCEPD)
1331 F Street, NW
Washington, DC 20004
(202) 376-6200   (202) 376-6205 (TT)   FAX (202) 376-6219
e-mail: info@pcepd.gov   http://www.pcepd.gov

A federal agency that fosters communication among state and local agencies, labor unions, and private enterprises that work toward improved employment opportunities for people with disabilities. Operates Workforce Recruitment Program to connect public and private sector employers with postsecondary students and graduates with disabilities who are seeking employment. Holds an annual conference and sponsors studies.

Rehabilitation Engineering and Assistive Technology Society of North America/RESNA
1700 North Moore Street, Suite 1540
Arlington, VA 22209-1903
(703) 524-6686   (703) 524-6639 (TT)   FAX (703) 524-6630
e-mail: nationaloffice@resna.org   http://www.resna.org

Multidisciplinary professional membership organization for people involved with improving technology for people with disabilities. Conducts a variety of projects, including research in the area of assistive technology and rehabilitation technology service delivery and technical assistance to statewide programs to develop technology. Membership, regular, $120.00; institutional, $275.00; corporate, $525.00; includes semi-annual journal, "Assistive Technology" and "RESNA News." Special membership rates for consumers and for students, $50.00 without journal; $80.00 with journal.

Rehabilitation Technology Associates
West Virginia Rehabilitation Research and Training Center
5088 Washington Street, West, Suite 200
Cross Lanes, WV 25313
(304) 759-0716 (V/TT)   FAX (304) 759-0726
e-mail: rta@rtc2.icdi.wvu.edu   http://www.icdi.wvu.edu/rta.htm

A membership organization for professionals in the rehabilitation field who use technology in the performance of their jobs. Holds an annual meeting. Membership is free.

Vocational Rehabilitation Services
Veterans Benefits Administration
Department of Veterans Affairs (VA)
810 Vermont Avenue, NW
Washington, DC 20420
(202) 273-5400   (800) 827-1000 (connects with regional office)
FAX (202) 273-7485   http://www.va.gov

Provides education and rehabilitation assistance and independent living services to veterans with service related disabilities through offices located in every state as well as regional centers, medical centers, and insurance centers. Medical services are provided at VA Medical Centers, Outpatient Clinics, Domiciliaries, and Nursing Homes.

Adaptive Technologies for Learning & Work Environments
by Joseph J. Lazzaro
Customer Service
American Library Association
155 North Wacker Drive
Chicago, IL 60606
(800) 545-2433   http://www.ala.org/market/books/bookstore.htm

This book explores adaptive technology for those with motor and/or speech impairments, visual impairment, and hearing impairment. It focuses on personal computer hardware, software, computer networks, and online services. It also lists funding sources, training and technical support resources, and vendors. $45.00 plus $7.00 shipping and handling

Americans with Disabilities Act: Questions and Answers
Department of Justice, Civil Rights Division, Disability Rights Section
PO Box 66738
Washington, DC 20035-6738
(800) 514-0301 Information Line
(800) 514-0383 (TT) Information Line
FAX (202) 307-1198   http://www.usdoj.gov/crt/ada/adahom1.htm

This booklet's question and answer format provides explanations of the ADA's effects on employment, state and local governments, and public accommodations. Available in standard print, large print, audiocassette, braille, disk, automated fax system, and on the web site. Free

Careers and the Disabled
Equal Opportunity Publications
1160 East Jericho Turnpike, Suite 200
Huntington, NY 11743
(516) 421-9421   e-mail: info@EOP.com

This quarterly magazine features career guidance articles, role model profiles, and lists of companies looking for qualified job candidates. Pre-paid subscription, $10.00; invoiced, $12.00.

Computer Resources for People with Disabilities
by the Alliance for Technology Access
Hunter House Inc., Publishers
PO Box 2914
Alameda, CA 94501-0914
(510) 865-5282   FAX (510) 865-4295
e-mail: hhi@hunterhouse.com

This book describes assistive technology and discusses what to consider when making a purchase, the support team members that can provide assistance, and information on sources of funding for purchases. $17.95 plus $4.50 shipping and handling

Meeting the Needs of Employees with Disabilities
Resources for Rehabilitation
33 Bedford Street, Suite 19A
Lexington, MA 02420
(781) 862-6455   FAX (781) 861-7517
e-mail: info@rfr.org   http://www.rfr.org

This book provides information to help people with disabilities retain or obtain employment. Information on government programs and laws, supported employment, training programs, environmental adaptations, and the transition from school to work are included. Chapters on mobility, vision, and hearing and speech impairments include information on organizations, products, and services that enable employers to accommodate the needs of employees with disabilities. $42.95 plus $5.00 shipping and handling (See order form on last page of this book.)

Part of the Team - People with Disabilities in the Workforce
National Easter Seal Society
Communications Department
230 West Monroe Street, Suite 1800
Chicago, IL 60606
(800) 221-6827   (312) 726-6200   (312) 726-4258 (TT)
FAX (312) 726-1494   http://www.easter-seals.org

This videotape profiles ten individuals who have overcome physical barriers to employment with cooperation and communication with their employers. $15.00 plus $4.95 shipping and handling

Housing plays an important role in a man's ability to remain independent. Most men with disabilities will opt to live in their own home whenever possible. Often this requires financial assistance, household help, environmental modifications, or moving to a more accessible building. The government has provided a number of programs to assist people with disabilities with affordable housing and to protect them from discrimination.

The *Fair Housing Amendments Act of 1988* (P.L. 100-430) requires that multifamily dwellings of four or more units first occupied after March 13, 1991 be accessible to individuals with disabilities. Tenants with disabilities have the legal right to make modifications to rental housing at their own expense in order to meet their needs. However, the residence must be restored to its original condition "within reason" when the tenant moves. In addition, HUD has established programs to house individuals with disabilities who are homeless.

Public housing is a major resource for men with disabilities and older men with low income. *Section 8* Certificates and Vouchers provide federal subsidies to income-eligible households to help defray housing costs in the private rental market. Section 8 subsidies may also be used in group residences. Local public housing authorities administer the program. *Section 803* of the National Affordable Housing Act of 1990, HOPE for Elderly Independence, combines tenant-based rental housing certificates and rental vouchers with supportive services to enable frail elders who have not been receiving any form of housing assistance to continue living in the community.

Section 202 of the *Housing and Community Development Act of 1987,* Direct Loan Program for Housing for the Elderly or Handicapped, provides loans to nonprofit organizations to sponsor development of housing for elders and persons with disabilities, including units eligible for Section 8 rent subsidies. Under amendments to the *Housing and Community Development Act of 1987* (P.L. 100-242), the Department of Housing and Urban Development provides direct loans for the development of projects for elders and individuals with disabilities. These developments may consist of apartments or group homes for up to 15 residents.

Home Equity Conversion Mortgages, sometimes called reverse mortgages, allow elders to convert the equity in their homes into cash that will enable them to meet housing expenses. These mortgages are insured by HUD in the event that the lender defaults. The reverse mortgage does not have to be repaid until the mortgagee moves or dies. Homeowners must be age 62 or older, occupy their own home as a principal residence, and own the home free and clear or nearly so. Reverse mortgage payment options include "tenure," monthly payments to homeowners as long as they use their homes as principal residences; "term," which provides monthly payments for a specified period; and "line-of-credit," which allows homeowners to draw on their equity up to a maximum amount. HUD USER [(800) 245-2691] can provide more information on this program.

Individuals who feel that they have experienced discrimination in housing may file complaints with HUD or a state or local fair housing agency, or they may file a civil suit.

Other housing options for men with disabilities include assisted living facilities, such as board and care homes, adult care homes, and residential care facilities. Many cities have residential hotels for older men with services, such as housekeeping, security, and social activities. Continuing care retirement communities provide housing choices ranging from independent apartment living with services, such as congregate meals and activities, to 24-hour nursing care. Shared housing programs include shared group residences and programs which match elders who need some assistance to remain at home with younger people who need inexpensive housing. Accessory housing, independent housing units built on to single family homes or erected on the property of a single family home, is another option for elders who wish to live independently but need supportive services.

Environmental adaptations for the home range from a ramp or simple tactile markings on appliances to major renovations, which include the installation of elevators and redesign of kitchens. Lowered kitchen counters and appliances facilitate cooking for men who use wheelchairs. Other adaptive design features include accessible routes, light switches, electrical outlets, and thermostats; bathrooms with walls sturdy enough to install grab bars; and kitchens, bathrooms, and entryways with sufficient space to maneuver wheelchairs.

Many architects now specialize in designing buildings and dwelling units that meet the needs of people with disabilities. The state office on disability, the architectural access board, or the local or state professional society of architects should be able to provide a list of qualified architects.

Assistive devices for dressing, such as elastic shoelaces, velcro closures, and buttoning aids, are especially useful for men with mobility impairments. Foam hair rollers, water pipe foam insulation, or layers of tape are used to build up the handles of items as varied as toothbrushes, pens, pencils, eating utensils, paint brushes, and crochet hooks.

Remote controls turn on and off lights and televisions and open and close garage doors. Telephones with voice dialers permit the storage of frequently called telephone numbers and automatic dialing. Speaker phones allow individuals with poor motor control or tremors to carry on a telephone conversation comfortably.

Although some of the publications described below mention a specific disability or age, they include suggestions that are applicable for individuals of all ages and with a variety of conditions. Suppliers of personal and home health care aids, recreational products, and mobility aids for more than one type of condition or disability are listed. Many hospital pharmacies as well as large department and discount stores now sell home health products such as wheelchairs, bathroom safety devices, canes, and walkers. Some of this equipment may also be available on a rental or loan basis from community health agencies.

ORGANIZATIONS

<u>ABLEDATA</u>
National Rehabilitation Information Center (NARIC)
8455 Colesville Road, Suite 935
Silver Spring, MD 20910-3319
(800) 346-2742   (301) 588-9284   (301) 495-5626 (TT)
FAX (301) 587-1967   e-mail: naric@capaccess.org
http://www.naric.com/naric/home.html

A database of disability-related products for personal care, recreation, and transportation is available on the web site. Searches will be done for individuals who do not have access to the web; first 50 items from database searches, free; a fee is charged for longer searches.

<u>Architectural and Transportation Barriers Compliance Board</u> (ATBCB)
1331 F Street, NW, Suite 1000
Washington, DC 20004-1111
(800) 872-2253   (800) 993-2822 (TT)   (202) 272-5434
(202) 272-5449 (TT)   FAX (202) 272-5447
e-mail: info@access-board.gov   http://www.access-board.gov

A federal agency charged with developing standards for accessibility in federal facilities, public accommodations, and transportation facilities as required by the Americans with Disabilities Act and other federal laws. Publishes the "Uniform Federal Accessibility Standards," which describes accessibility standards for buildings and dwelling units developed for four federal agencies. Provides technical assistance, sponsors research, and distributes publications. Publishes a free quarterly newsletter, "Access America." Publications available in standard print, large print, braille, audiocassette, computer disk, and on the web site.

<u>Association of Home Appliance Manufacturers</u>
20 North Wacker Drive
Chicago, IL 60606
(312) 984-5800   FAX (312) 984-5823   http://www.aham.org

Provides referral to the major home appliance manufacturers for information on modifications for their products. Distributes "Do Your PART (Protect Against Range Tipping), a booklet describing safety measures to avoid kitchen accidents. Free

Center for Universal Design
North Carolina State University
Box 8613
Raleigh, NC 27695-8613
(800) 647-6777   (919) 515-3082 (V/TT)   FAX (919) 515-3023
e-mail: cud@ncsu.edu   http://www.ncsu.edu/ncsu/design/cud

A federally funded research and training center that works toward improving housing and product design for people with disabilities. Provides technical assistance, training, and publications. Some publications are available on the web site.

Compliance/Disability Rights Support Division
Department of Housing and Urban Development (HUD)
451 7th Street, SW, Room 5240
Washington, DC 20410
(202) 708-0404   FAX (202) 708-1251   http://www.hud.gov
HUD Discrimination Hotline: (800) 669-9777; (800) 927-9275 (TT)

Operates programs to make housing accessible, including loans for developers of independent living and group homes and loan and mortgage insurance for rehabilitation of single or multifamily units. Individuals who feel their rights have been violated may file a complaint with one of the ten regional offices located throughout the country.

Fair Housing Information Clearinghouse
Department of Housing and Urban Development (HUD)
PO Box 9146
McLean, VA 22102
(800) 343-3443   (800) 290-1617 (TT)   FAX (703) 821-2098
e-mail: fairhousing@circsol.com   http://www.circsol.com/fairhousing

Provides technical assistance on accessibility requirements mandated by federal law. Distributes information about federal laws and regulations and educational materials that discuss prohibition of discrimination in housing. Many brochures are free. Information kit and publications list, free. Individuals who feel that they have been discriminated against should call the National HUD Discrimination Hotline, (800) 669-9777; (800) 927-9275 (TT).

GE Answer Center
9500 Williamsburg Plaza
Louisville, KY 40222
(800) 626-2000   (800) 833-4322 (TT)

This consumer information center provides assistance to individuals with disabilities as well as to the general public. Appliance controls marked with braille or raised dots are available for individuals who are blind or visually impaired, free. Two brochures, "Appliance Help for

Those with Special Needs," and "Basic Kitchen Planning for the Physically Handicapped," are free. The center is open 24 hours a day, seven days a week.

National Association of Home Builders (NAHB)
National Research Center, Economics and Policy Analysis Division
400 Prince George's Boulevard
Upper Marlboro, MD 20772-8731
(301) 249-4000   FAX (301) 249-0305   http://www.nahbrc.org

The research section of the home building industry trade organization produces publications and provides training on housing and special needs.

Adaptable Dwellings
HUD USER
PO Box 6091
Rockville, MD 20850
(800) 245-2691   In MD, (301) 519-5154   FAX (301) 519-5767
e-mail: huduser@aspensys.com   http://www.huduser.org

Presents the findings of a research study of the perceptions individuals with disabilities and those without disabilities have toward a variety of adaptations and recommendations that emanated from the study. $10.00

Adapting the Home for the Physically Challenged
A/V Health Services
PO Box 20271
Roanoke, VA 24018-0028
(540) 725-9288 (Voice and FAX)   e-mail: avhealth4u@aol.com

This videotape helps individuals who use wheelchairs or walkers to modify their homes. Ramp construction and modifications for every room are explained. 30 minutes. $90.00

A Consumer's Guide to Home Adaptation
Adaptive Environments Center
374 Congress Street, Suite 301
Boston, MA 02210
(800) 949-4232 (V/TT)   (617) 695-1225 (V/TT)   FAX (617) 482-8099
e-mail: adaptive@adaptenv.org http://www.adaptenv.org

This workbook enables people with disabilities to plan the modifications necessary to adapt their homes. Describes how to widen doorways, lower countertops, etc. $12.00

Designs for Independent Living
Appliance Information Service (AIS)
Whirlpool Corporation
Administrative Center
Benton Harbor, MI 49022
(800) 253-1301   (800) 334-6889 (TT)
http://www.whirlpool.com

This brochure provides information on adaptations for the home environment and major appliances. Free

The Do-Able Renewable Home
by John P. S. Salmen
American Association of Retired Persons (AARP)
601 E Street, NW
Washington, DC 20049
(800) 441-2277   (202) 434-2277   http://www.aarp.org

This booklet describes how individuals with disabilities can modify their homes for independent living. Room-by-room modifications are accompanied by illustrations. Free

Easy Things to Make--To Make Things Easy: Simple Do-It-Yourself Home Modifications for Older People and Others with Physical Disabilities
by Doreen Greenstein
Brookline Books
PO Box 1047
Cambridge, MA 02238-1047
(800) 666-2665   (617) 868-0360   FAX (617) 868-1772
e-mail: brooklinebk@delphi.com

This book describes low-cost home modifications and suggests adaptations for everyday activities. Large print. $15.95

Eighty-Eight Easy-To-Make Aids for Older People & for Special Needs
by Don Caston
Hartley & Marks, Publishers
Box 147
Point Roberts, WA 98281
(604) 739-1771   Orders (800) 277-5887   FAX (800) 707-5887
e-mail: hartmark@direct.ca

This book provides practical adaptations for the home with step-by-step instructions. These suggestions would be useful to many individuals with disabilities, regardless of age. $12.95 plus $3.50 shipping and handling

Fair Housing Accessibility Guidelines
Fair Housing Information Clearinghouse
Department of Housing and Urban Development (HUD)
PO Box 9146
McLean, VA 22102
(800) 343-3443   (800) 290-1617 (TT)   FAX (703) 821-2098
e-mail: fairhousing@circsol.com   http://www.circsol.com/fairhousing

This videotape describes the Fair Housing Act's design and construction requirements for new multifamily housing, design techniques, and construction methods. 27 minutes. Free

<u>The Less Challenging Home</u>
Appliance Information Service
Whirlpool Corporation
Benton Harbor, MI 49022
(800) 253-1301   (800) 334-6889 (TT)
http://www.whirlpool.com

This booklet provides suggestions for incorporating accessible design when building or remodeling kitchens and bathrooms. Describes building materials and appliances and includes charts indicating appliance features that are helpful to users with disabilities. Free

<u>Retrofitting Homes for a Lifetime</u>
National Association of Home Builders (NAHB)
National Research Center, Economics and Policy Analysis Division
400 Prince George's Boulevard
Upper Marlboro, MD 20772-8731
(301) 249-4000   FAX (301) 249-0305   http://www.nahbrc.org

This publication enables remodelers and homeowners to assess needed modifications; provides an accessibility checklist; suggests financing alternatives; and makes recommendations for working with builders. $10.00

<u>What Does Fair Housing Mean to People with Disabilities?</u>
Fair Housing Information Clearinghouse (FHIC)
Department of Housing and Urban Development (HUD)
PO Box 9146
McLean, VA 22102
(800) 343-3443   (800) 483-2209 (TT)   FAX (703) 821-2098
http://www.hud.gov

This booklet describes the Fair Housing Act and the rights of individuals with disabilities, including definitions and examples of "reasonable accommodation" and building modifications, where to get help, and how to file a complaint. Free

RESOURCES FOR ASSISTIVE DEVICES

The following vendors sell assistive devices that help people remain independent. Those that specialize in a specific type of product have a notation under the listing. Otherwise, their product line is broad, usually including personal, health care, and aids and devices for the home. Unless otherwise noted, the catalogues are free.

Access with Ease
PO Box 1150
Chino Valley, AZ 86323
(800) 531-9479   (520) 636-9469
e-mail: kmjc@morthlink.com

adaptAbility
Norwich Avenue
Colchester, CT 06415-0515
(800) 243-9232   FAX (800) 566-6678
e-mail: service@snswwide.com   http://www.snswwide.com

Enrichments
Sammons Preston
PO Box 5071
Bolllingbrook, IL 60440
(800) 323-5547   FAX (800) 547-4333
e-mail: sp@sammonspreston.com

Independent Living Aids, Inc. (ILA)
27 East Mall
Plainview, NY 11803
(800) 537-2118   (516) 752-8080
e-mail: indlivaids@aol.com   http://www.independentliving.com

LS & S Group
PO Box 673
Northbrook, IL 60065
(800) 468-4789   (847) 498-9777
e-mail: lssgrp@aol.com   http://www.lssgroup.com

Making Life Better: A Catalog of Catalogs
National Easter Seal Society
230 West Monroe Street, Suite 1800
Chicago, IL 60606-4802
(800) 221-6827   (312) 726-6200   (312) 726-4258 (TT)
FAX (312) 726-1494   http://www.easter-seals.org

Features 48 retailers of assistive and adaptive equipment. $10.00, includes $5.00 certificate for National Easter Seal Society resources.

Medic Alert
PO Box 819008
Turlock, CA 95381-9008
(800) 344-3226   In CA, (209) 668-3333   FAX (209) 669-2450
http://www.medicalert.org

Medical identification bracelet for people with chronic conditions.

Radio Shack/Tandy Corporation
500 One Tandy Center, 100 Throckmorton Street
Fort Worth, TX 76102
(817) 390-3700   http://www.tandy.com

Radio Shack products for individuals with disabilities, such as talking watches and clocks and assistive listening aids, are included in the company's regular catalogues.

Sears Home HealthCare Catalog
3737 Grader Street, Suite 110
Garland, TX 75041
(800) 326-1750   (800) 733-7249 (TT)

Sells health care and rehabilitation products.

Both travel and recreation provide relief from tension, relaxation, and social interactions. Individuals who participate in recreational activities have an increased sense of self-worth and well-being. For individuals who are seriously ill, recreation diverts attention from the illness and provides opportunities for socialization. Some individuals with disabilities need assistance in order to continue with their favorite recreational pastimes. Others may develop an interest in new activities more appropriate to their current condition.

In the aftermath of World War II, rehabilitation programs were developed to treat the men returning home with physical and mental disabilities. Competitive sports were included in the program of the first spinal cord injury center opened in England in 1944 (DePauw and Gavron: 1995). During the 1950's, wheelchair sports expanded throughout Europe to the United States, and individuals with other disabilities became involved in national and international sports organizations. For men who have engaged in sports throughout their lives, the advent of disability seems to signal an end to valued activities. Those who receive care in rehabilitation facilities are more apt to discover the adaptations available in equipment and techniques that make sports opportunities accessible. Sports enthusiasts may choose activities such as skiing, basketball, running, golf, scuba diving, baseball, horseback riding, archery, and sailing, to name just a few examples.

The Americans with Disabilities Act (ADA) of 1990 mandates accessibility to recreation facilities and athletic programs, from aerobic training classes and local parks to football stadiums and other venues. Advances in technology have led to the development of racing wheelchairs, special hand and foot prostheses, and adapted ski equipment such as sit-skis. All-terrain vehicles (ATVs), adapted with lifts, hand controls, or safety harnesses, enable individuals with mobility impairments to participate in many outdoor recreation activities. Organizations that specialize in adaptive recreation programs are listed below (see "ADAPTIVE SPORTS AND RECREATION ORGANIZATIONS"). The ADA also requires that fixed route buses and rail transportation be accessible and usable by individuals with disabilities. However, deadlines for implementation of the ADA's regulations vary from six to seven years for private intercity transit to as long as 20 years for Amtrak and commuter rail stations.

The Federal Aviation Administration requires each airline to submit a company-wide policy for travelers with disabilities. Passengers may call ahead to request early boarding, special seating, or meals which meet dietary restrictions. Airport facilities are designed to offer accessible restrooms, elevators, electric carts or wheelchairs, and first aid stations. The Air Carrier Access Act of 1986 (ACAA) includes regulations that cover the needs of travelers with disabilities, such as access to commuter planes, accessible lavatories, wheelchair storage, and sensitivity training for all airline personnel. Contact the airlines to obtain a written statement of the special services they provide. Individuals who believe that their rights have been denied may file a complaint within 45 days of the incident with the Aviation Protection Division, U.S. Department of Transportation, C-75 Room 4107, Washington, DC 20590, (202) 366-2220; (202) 765-7687 (TT); e-mail: airconsumer@ost.dot.gov.

Amtrak offers a 15% discount on most one-way, round trip, and All Aboard America rail fares for individuals with disabilities. Passengers must present proof of disability, such as a certificate of legal blindness or a letter from a physician specifying the nature of the disability. Greyhound allows passengers with disabilities requiring assistance with personal hygiene, eating, medications, or while the bus is in motion to request a free ticket for a companion (certain restrictions apply). There is no charge for guide dogs for individuals who are visually impaired, blind, or deaf.

Travel agencies that plan special trips for people with disabilities are available throughout North America. Many major hotel chains, airlines, and car rental companies provide special assistance to people with disabilities and often have special toll-free numbers for users of text telephones (TTs). Some companies offer specially trained travel companions to people with disabilities who need an escort. In the United States, many state tourism offices provide information about accessible attractions for prospective visitors with disabilities. Auto clubs both here and abroad are also good sources for such information.

Individuals with disabilities and elders are eligible for special entrance passes to federal recreation facilities. The *Golden Access Passport* is a free lifetime pass available to any U.S. citizen or permanent resident, regardless of age, who is blind or permanently disabled. It admits the permit holder and passengers in a single, private, noncommercial vehicle to any parks, monuments, historic sites, recreation areas, and wildlife refuges which usually charge entrance fees. If the permit holder does not enter by car, the Passport admits the permit holder, spouse, and children. The permit holder is also entitled to a 50% discount on charges such as camping, boat launching, and parking fees. Fees charged by private concessionaires are not discounted. Golden Access Passports are available only in person, with proof of disability, such as a certificate of legal blindness. Since the Passport is available at most federal recreation areas, it is not necessary to obtain one ahead of time. A *Golden Age Passport* offers the same benefits to persons age 62 or older, with proof of age.

Rehabilitation hospitals and centers offer driver evaluation services such as clinical testing and observation to determine an individual's need for adaptive equipment or training. Many Department of Veterans Affairs Medical Centers (VAMC) offer driver evaluation services, driver training, and information services to veterans with disabilities through the Rehabilitation Medicine Service at their facilities. The Internal Revenue Service allows individuals to include in medical expenses the cost of special hand controls and other special equipment installed in a car to be used by a person with a disability. Individuals may also consider as a medical expense the difference between the cost of a car designed to hold a wheelchair and the cost of the car without modification. Contact the Internal Revenue Service (see "ORGANIZATIONS" section below) to obtain Publication 502 "Medical and Dental Expenses." Major automobile manufacturers offer reimbursement for adaptive equipment installed on new vehicles. Programs for special adaptive equipment offered by automobile manufacturers are listed in the "ORGANIZATIONS" section below.

References

DePauw, Karen P. and Susan J. Gavron
1995 Disability and Sport Champaign, IL: Human Kinetics

ORGANIZATIONS

Access-Able
PO Box 1796
Wheat Ridge, CO 80034
(303) 232-2979   FAX (303) 239-8486
e-mail: bill@access-able.com   http://www.access-able.com

Provides information on accommodations, access guides, entertainment, tours, and transportation.

Amtrak
(800) 872-7245   (800) 523-6590 (TT)

Provides 15% discount on most fares for individuals with disabilities. On-board services and special meals available upon request with advance notice.

Architectural and Transportation Barriers Compliance Board (ATBCB)
1331 F Street, NW, Suite 1000
Washington, DC 20004-1111
(800) 872-2253   (800) 993-2822 (TT)   (202) 272-5434
(202) 272-5449 (TT)   FAX (202) 272-5447
e-mail: info@access-board.gov   http://www.access-board.gov

Maintains a database on accessible transportation, including a computerized, annotated bibliography. Publishes brochures on subjects such as "Air Carrier Policies on Transport of Battery Powered Wheelchairs."

Association of Driver Educators for the Disabled
PO Box 49
Edgerton, WI 53534
(608) 884-8833   FAX (608) 884-4851
http://www.driver-ed.org

Certifies members to conduct driver evaluation and training for individuals with disabilities.

Automobility
Chrysler Corporation
1220 Rankin Street
Troy, MI 48083-6004
(800) 255-9877   (800) 922-3826 (TT)
FAX (810) 597-3501   http://automobility.chrysler.com

Provides $750 to $1000 reimbursement (on eligible models) on the purchase of alerting devices for people who are deaf or hard of hearing and adaptive equipment for vehicles purchased to transport individuals who use wheelchairs.

Ford Mobility Motoring Program
(800) 952-2248   (800) 833-0312 (TT)   FAX (810) 540-7039
http://www.ford.com/showrooms/pavilion

This program funds adaptive equipment conversion up to $1000. Provides toll-free information line, list of assessment centers that determine equipment needs, and referrals to sources for additional assistance.

General Motors Mobility Assistance Center
PO Box 9011
Detroit, MI 48202
(800) 323-9935   (800) 833-9935 (TT)   (800) 263-3830 (TT)
http://www.gm.com

This program reimburses customers up to $1000 for vehicle modifications or adaptive driving devices for new or demo vehicles. Includes alerting devices for drivers who are deaf or hearing impaired such as emergency vehicle siren detectors and enhanced turn signal reminders.

Greyhound Lines, Inc.
PO Box 660362
Dallas, TX 75266-0362
(800) 231-2222 (General Information)
(800) 752-4841 (ADA Assist Line)
(800) 345-3109 (TT)   http://www.Greyhound.com

Provides assistance to travelers with disabilities upon request. Call ADA Assist line at least 48 hours in advance of travel.

Internal Revenue Service (IRS)
(800) 829-1040   (800) 829-4059 (TT)
http://www.irs.ustreas.gov

The IRS provides technical assistance about tax credits and deductions related to accommodations for disabilities. To request Publication 502, "Medical and Dental Expenses," call (800) 829-3676; (800) 829-4059 (TT).

Mobility International USA (MIUSA)
PO Box 10767
Eugene, OR 97440
(541) 343-1284 (V/TT)   FAX (541) 343-6812
e-mail: info@miusa.miusa.org   http://www.miusa.org

Promotes the participation of individuals with disabilities in international and educational exchange programs, such as workcamps, conferences, and internships. Membership, $35.00, includes quarterly newsletter, "Over the Rainbow."

National Mobility Equipment Dealers Association
909 East Skagway Avenue
Tampa, FL 33604
(800) 833-0427   (813) 932-8566   FAX (813) 931-4683
e-mail: nmeda@aol.com   http://www.nmeda.org

The members of this organization are car dealers, manufacturers, driver evaluators, and insurance companies. Provides local referrals to members who are adaptive equipment dealers and rates members' competencies in equipment installation and conversion.

National Park Service
Department of the Interior, Office of Public Affairs
PO Box 37127
Washington, DC 20013-7127
(202) 208-4747   http://www.nps.gov

Operates the Golden Access Passport program for people who have disabilities. Free brochure.

Saturn Mobility Program
100 Saturn Parkway, Mail Drop S-24
Spring Hill, TN 37174
(800) 522-5000   (800) 833-6000 (TT)   http://www.saturn.com

This program reimburses customers up to $1000 for adaptive equipment costs when an eligible new Saturn is purchased or leased.

Society for the Advancement of Travel for the Handicapped (SATH)
347 Fifth Avenue, Suite 610
New York, NY 10016
(212) 447-1928

Advocates for accessibility for individuals with disabilities and serves as a clearinghouse for information on barrier-free travel. Membership, individuals, $45.00; seniors and students, $30.00.

Travelin' Talk
PO Box 3534
Clarksville, TN 37043-3534
(931) 552-6670   FAX (931) 552-1182

A network of individuals and organizations that provides assistance to travelers with disabilities. One time registration fee varies according to income. Publishes resource directory for travelers with disabilities; members, $27.50; nonmembers, $32.50; plus $2.50 shipping and handling.

Very Special Arts
1300 Connecticut Avenue, NW, Suite 700
Washington, DC 20036
(800) 933-8721   (202) 628-2800   (202) 737-0645 (TT)
FAX (202) 737-0725   http://www.vsarts.org

Provides opportunities for individuals with disabilities to participate in fine and performing arts.

Wheelers Accessible Van Rental
(800) 456-1371   http://www.wheelerz.com

Rents mini-vans accessible to wheelchair users throughout the country.

Wilderness Inquiry
1313 5th Street, SE, Box 84
Minneapolis, MN 55414-1546
(800) 728-0719 (V/TT)   In Minneapolis and St. Paul, (612) 379-3858 (V/TT)
FAX (612) 379-5972   http://www.wildernessinquiry.org

Sponsors trips into wilderness areas for individuals with disabilities or chronic conditions. Request schedule of current trips.

ADAPTIVE SPORTS AND RECREATION ORGANIZATIONS

Achilles Track Club
42 West 38th Street, 4th Floor
New York, NY 10018
(212) 354-0300   FAX (212) 354-3978
e-mail: achillestc@aol.com

Promotes running as a recreational activity and competitive sport for individuals with disabilities. Chapters in many states and foreign countries. Membership is free. Publishes newsletter, "The Achilles Heel."

American Canoe Association
7432 Alban Station Boulevard, Suite B-232
Springfield, VA 22150
(703) 451-0141   FAX (703) 451-2245
e-mail: acadirect@aol.com   http://www.aca-paddler.org

Certifies instructors in adaptive paddling course for canoeing, kayaking, and coastal kayaking. Will refer individuals with disabilities to certified instructors in local area. Provides information on equipment adaptations.

Breckenridge Outdoor Education Center
PO Box 697
Breckenridge, CO 80424
(800) 383-2632   (970) 453-6422   FAX (970) 453-4676
e-mail: boec@boec.org   http://www.boec.org

Offers year-round adaptive outdoor learning experiences for children and adults with disabilities and provides training for therapists and educators.

Disabled Sports, U.S.A.
451 Hungerford Drive, Suite 100
Rockville, MD 20850
(301) 217-0960   (301) 217-0963 (TT)   FAX (301) 217-0968

Nationwide network of chapters sponsors recreational activities such as skiing, camping, hiking, biking, horseback riding, and mountain climbing. Offers adaptive fitness instructor training to therapists, exercise instructors, and program directors. Membership, $25.00, includes subscription to "Challenge Magazine."

Fishing Has No Boundaries
PO Box 175
Hayward, WI 54843
(800) 243-3462   (715) 634-3185
e-mail: fhnbinc@win.bright.net

Provides opportunities for individuals with disabilities to fish and teaches them about adaptive devices for fishing. Events sponsored by community organizations.

Handicapped Scuba Association
1104 El Prado
San Clemente, CA 92672-4637
(949) 498-6128   e-mail: hsahdq@compuserve.com
http://ourworld.compuserve.com/homepages/hsahdq

This organization trains and certifies scuba diving instructors to work with individuals with disabilities; teaches able-bodied divers to accompany divers with disabilities; and certifies divers with disabilities in "open water" diving. All contributors become members.

National Ability Center
PO Box 682799
Park City, UT 84068-2779
(435) 649-3991 (V/TT)   FAX (435) 658-3992
e-mail: nac@xmission.com   http://www.nationalabilitycenter.org

Offers year-round sports and recreation experiences for children and adults with disabilities.

National Foundation of Wheelchair Tennis
940 Calle Amanecer, Suite B
San Clemente, CA 92673
(714) 361-3663   FAX (714) 361-6603
http://www.nfwt.org

Provides tournaments for disabled athletes. Publishes monthly newsletter.

National Sports Center for the Disabled
PO Box 1290
Winter Park, CO 80482
(970) 726-1540   FAX (970) 726-4112
http://www.nscd.org/nscd

Offers year round recreation programs for children and adults with disabilities and offers training programs for recreation professionals.

National Wheelchair Basketball Association
c/o Charlotte Institute of Rehabilitation
1100 Blythe Boulevard
Charlotte, NC 28203
(704) 355-1064   FAX (704) 446-4999
e-mail: nwba@carolinas.org   http://www.nwba.org

This organization of more than 175 teams across the U.S. and Canada provides opportunities for organized competition in men's, women's, and youth divisions.

North American Riding for the Handicapped Association (NARHA)
PO Box 33150
Denver, CO 80233
(800) 369-7433   (303) 452-1212   FAX (303) 252-4610
http://www.narha.org

This professional association promotes therapeutic horseback riding for individuals with disabilities and accredits riding programs. Membership, $35.00, includes membership directory and subscription to two newsletters, "NARHA Strides," published quarterly, and "NARHA News," published eight times a year.

Universal Wheelchair Football Association
c/o John B. Kraimer
6641 Woodland Trace Court
Middletown, OH 45044
(513) 755-2427

Promotes the playing of football by individuals with disabilities. Provides rules upon request.

Wheelchair Sports, USA
3595 East Fountain Boulevard, Suite L-1
Colorado Springs, CO 80910
(719) 574-1150   FAX (719) 574-9840   e-mail: wsusa@aol.com
http://www.wsusa.org

This organization provides opportunities for individuals who use wheelchairs to compete in team and individual sports at local, regional, and international levels. The sports are archery, track and field, basketball, fencing, quad rugby, racquetball, shooting, sled hockey, swimming, table tennis, waterskiing, and weightlifting. Membership, $25.00; includes a quarterly newsletter.

Accessible Gardening for People with Physical Disabilities: A Guide to Methods, Tools, and Plants
by Janeen R. Adil
Woodbine House
6510 Bells Mill Road
Bethesda, MD 20817
(800) 843-7323   FAX (301) 897-5838
e-mail: info@woodbinehouse.com   http://www.woodbinehouse.com

Written for people with a variety of mobility impairments, this book provides information on making existing gardens more accessible and creating new gardens. Sources for obtaining supplies are included. $16.95 plus $4.50 shipping and handling

Access Travel: Airports
Consumer Information Center
PO Box 100
Pueblo, CO 81002
Order Line (888) 878-3256   FAX (719) 948-9724
e-mail: cic.info@pueblo.gsa.gov   http://www.pueblo.gsa.gov

This brochure lists facilities and services for people with disabilities in airport terminals worldwide. Free. Also available on the web site.

Directory of Travel Agencies for the Disabled $19.95
Travel for the Disabled: A Handbook of Travel Resources and 500 Worldwide Access Guides $19.95
by Helen Hecker
Twin Peaks Press
PO Box 129
Vancouver, WA 98666-0129
(800) 637-2256 (Order Line only)   (360) 694-2462   FAX (360) 696-3210
e-mail: 73743.2634@compuserve.com

The "Directory" lists travel agents who specialize in arrangements for people with disabilities in the U.S., Canada, and abroad. The "Handbook" lists access guides and accessible places plus travel tips. Both titles available in standard print or on audiocassette. Shipping, $4.00 first book, $1.50 additional book.

Disability and Sport
by Karen P. DePauw and Susan J. Gavron
Human Kinetics
1607 North Market Street
PO Box 5076
Champaign, IL 61825-5076
(800) 747-4457   (217) 351-5076   FAX (217) 351-2674
http://www.humankinetics.com

This book reviews the development of the sports movement for individuals with disabilities.
Describes sports modifications, lists disability sports organizations, discusses coaching athletes
with disabilities, and provides information about publications. Includes biographies of athletes
with disabilities. $35.00 plus $3.75 shipping and handling

The Disabled Driver's Mobility Guide
c/o Kay Hamada, Traffic Safety and Engineering
American Automobile Association (AAA)
1000 AAA Drive
Heathrow, FL 32746-5063
(407) 444-7961   FAX (407) 444-7956

This book provides information about adaptive equipment, driver training, and travel
information services. $5.95 plus $3.00 shipping and handling

Easy Access to National Parks: The Sierra Club Guide for People with Disabilities
by Wendy Roth and Michael Tompane
Random House, Order Department
400 Hahn Road, PO Box 100
Westminster, MD 21157
(800) 793-2665   http://www.randomhouse.com

This book reviews accessibility of 50 national parks for individuals with vision, hearing, or
mobility impairments. $16.00 plus $4.00 shipping and handling

Fodor's Great American Vacations For Travelers with Disabilities
Random House, Order Department
400 Hahn Road, PO Box 100
Westminster, MD 21157
(800) 793-2665   http://www.randomhouse.com

This book includes accessibility information for hotels, restaurants and attractions. $19.50
plus $4.00 shipping and handling

Games for People with Sensory Impairments: Strategies for Including Individuals of All Ages
by Lauren J. Lieberman and Jim F. Cowart
Human Kinetics
1607 North Market Street
PO Box 5076
Champaign, IL 61825-5076
(800) 747-4457   (217) 351-5076   FAX (217) 351-2674
http://www.humankinetics.com

This book describes program adaptations and instructional strategies for 70 games for individuals with vision or hearing impairment. $17.00 plus $3.75 shipping and handling

New Horizons for the Air Traveler with a Disability
Consumer Information Center
PO Box 100
Pueblo, CO 81002
Order Line (888) 878-3256   FAX (719) 948-9724
e-mail: cic.info@pueblo.gsa.gov   http://www.pueblo.gsa.gov

This booklet provides information about the Air Carrier Access rules and other regulations that affect air travelers. Free. Also available on the web site.

Sports 'N Spokes
2111 East Highland Avenue, Suite 180
Phoenix, AZ 85016-9611
(888) 888-2201   (602) 224-0500   FAX (602) 224-0507
e-mail: pvapub@aol.com

A bimonthly magazine that features articles about sports activities for people who use wheelchairs. $12.00

A World of Options: A Guide to International Exchange, Community Service, and Travel for Persons with Disabilities
by C. Bucks (ed.)
Mobility International USA (MIUSA)
PO Box 10767
Eugene, OR 97440
(541) 343-1284 (V/TT)   FAX (541) 343-6812
e-mail: info@miusa.miusa.org   http://www.miusa.org

This book lists educational exchange programs, international workcamps, and accessible travel opportunities. Personal experiences are used to describe these programs. Individuals, $35.00; organizations, $45.00.

RESOURCES FOR ASSISTIVE DEVICES

The following vendors sell assistive devices that help people with disabilities enjoy sports and recreational activities, such as swimming aids, fishing equipment, fitness equipment and home gyms, golf clubs, wheelchair ramps, bowling aids, and adapted games. Unless otherwise noted, the catalogues are free.

Abilitations
One Sportime Way
Atlanta, GA 30340
(800) 850-8602   FAX (800) 845-1535
http://www.abilitations.com

Access to Recreation
8 Sandra Court
Newbury Park, CA 91320
(800) 634-4351   (805) 498-7535   FAX (805) 498-8186
e-mail: krebs@westworld.com

Sells assistive devices that help people with disabilities enjoy sports and recreational activities, such as swimming aids, fishing equipment, fitness equipment and home gyms, golf clubs, wheelchair ramps, bowling aids, and adapted games.

adaptAbility
Norwich Avenue
Colchester, CT 06415-0515
(800) 243-9232   FAX (800) 566-6678
e-mail: service@snswwide.com   http://www.snswwide.com

Worldwide Games
PO Box 517
Colchester, CT 06415-0517
(800) 243-9232   FAX (800) 566-6678
e-mail: service@snswwide.com   http://www.worldwidegames.com

Catalogue of games and crafts. Free catalogue.

Chapter 3

LAWS THAT AFFECT MEN WITH DISABILITIES

(For laws related to housing, see Chapter 2, "Coping with Daily Activities")

Laws affecting men with disabilities cover a wide range of issues, including health care, financial benefits, rehabilitation, civil rights, transportation, access to public buildings, and employment. For those who are not specialists in the law, it is sometimes difficult to keep abreast of the laws and their amendments. At the same time, men with disabilities may be able to continue living independently if they are aware of their rights and know how to locate the proper equipment and professional services. In many instances, government programs provide financial assistance for their needs.

In 1990, the *Americans with Disabilities Act* (ADA) was passed. Considered the most important piece of civil rights legislation in recent years, the ADA (P.L. 101-336) increased the steps employers must take to accommodate employees with disabilities and required that new buses and rail vehicles, facilities, and public accommodations be accessible. The ADA defines disability as "a physical or mental impairment that substantially limits one or more of the major life activities..." [such as speaking, hearing, seeing, or walking]; "a record of such impairment;" or "being regarded as having such an impairment." Thus individuals who have been cured of cancer or mental illness may still be regarded by others as having a disability and may experience discrimination. Others may have a physical condition that does not limit activity, such as disfiguring scars from injuries incurred in an automobile accident, but are regarded as disabled. Individuals in these situations are covered by the law.

The major provisions of the ADA are as follows:

• Title I prohibits discrimination against individuals with disabilities who are otherwise qualified for employment and requires that employers make "reasonable accommodations." "Reasonable accommodations" include making existing facilities accessible and job restructuring (e.g., reassignment to a vacant position, modification of equipment, training, provision of interpreters and readers). Employers are protected from "undue hardship" in complying with this provision; the financial situation of the employer and the size and type of business are considered when determining whether an accommodation would constitute "undue hardship." The provisions of this section apply to employers with 15 or more employees. (For a more detailed discussion of the employment aspects of the ADA, see "Meeting the Needs of Employees with Disabilities," described in "PUBLICATIONS" section below).

• Title II prohibits discrimination by public entities (i.e., local and state governments) and requires that individuals with disabilities be entitled to the same rights and benefits of public programs as other individuals. For example, local programs for elders may not discriminate against those elders who have visual impairments or other disabilities; they are entitled to receive the same benefits of the programs as elders who do not have disabilities.

• Title III requires that public accommodations, businesses, and services be accessible to individuals with disabilities. Public accommodations are broadly defined to include places such as hotels and motels, theatres, museums, schools, shopping centers and stores, banks, restaurants, and professional service providers' offices. Effective January 26, 1993, most new construction for public accommodations must be accessible to individuals with disabilities.

• Requires that bus and railroad transportation systems address the needs of individuals with disabilities by purchasing adapted equipment, modifying facilities, and providing special transportation services that are comparable to regular transportation services.

• Title IV mandates that telephone companies provide relay services 24 hours a day, 7 days a week for individuals with hearing or speech impairments. Relay services enable individuals who have text telephones (TT) or another computer device that is capable of communicating across telephone lines to communicate with individuals who do not have such devices.

Copies of the ADA and all federal laws are available from Senators and Representatives. Agencies charged with formulating regulations and standards include the Architectural and Transportation Barriers Compliance Board, the Department of Transportation, the Equal Employment Opportunity Commission, the Federal Communications Commission, and the Attorney General. Regulations for enforcing individual sections of the ADA are available from the federal agencies charged with promulgating them and in the "Federal Register" (see "PUBLICATIONS" section below). In addition, many private agencies that work with individuals with disabilities have copies of the ADA available for distribution to the public.

Other major laws affecting people with disabilities include the *Rehabilitation Act of 1973* (P.L. 93-112) and its amendments, which are the centerpieces of federal law related to rehabilitation. States must submit a vocational rehabilitation plan to the Rehabilitation Services Administration indicating how the designated state agency will provide vocational training, counseling, and diagnostic and evaluation services required by the law. Subsequent reauthorizations of and amendments to the Rehabilitation Act expanded the services provided under this law. For example, the "Client Assistance Program" authorizes states to inform clients and other persons with disabilities about all available benefits under the Act and to assist them in obtaining all remedies due under the law (P.L. 98-221). "Comprehensive Services for Independent Living" (P.L. 95-602) expands rehabilitation services to individuals with severe disabilities, regardless of their vocational potential, making services available to many people who are no longer in the work force. The Act broadly defines services as any "service that will enhance the ability of a handicapped individual to live independently or function within his family and community..." These services may include counseling, job placement, housing, funds to make the home accessible, funds for prosthetic devices, attendant care, and recreational activities. The Rehabilitation Act Amendments of 1992 (P.L. 102-569) establish state rehabilitation advisory councils composed of representatives of independent living councils, parents of children with disabilities, vocational rehabilitation professionals, and business; the role of these councils is to advise state vocational rehabilitation agencies and to prepare an annual report for the governor. Each state agency was required to establish performance and evaluation standards by September 30, 1994. The amendments also establish a National Commission on Rehabilitation Services to study the quality and adequacy of rehabilitation services provided by the states. The Rehabilitation Act Amendments of 1998 (P.L. 105-220, part of the Workforce Investment Partnership Act) aim to bring more Americans with disabilities into the mainstream workforce and require federal agencies to adopt accessible electronic information systems, so that individuals with disabilities have comparable access as those without disabilities.

Section 503 of the Rehabilitation Act requires any contractor that receives more than $2,500 in contracts from the federal government to take affirmative action to employ individuals with disabilities. The Office of Federal Contract Compliance Programs within the Department of Labor is responsible for enforcing this provision (see "ORGANIZATIONS" section below). *Section 504* prohibits any program that receives federal financial assistance from discriminating against individuals with disabilities who are otherwise eligible to benefit from their programs. Virtually all educational institutions are affected by this law, including private postsecondary institutions which receive federal financial assistance under a wide variety of programs. Programs must be physically accessible to individuals with disabilities, and construction begun after implementation of the regulations (June 3, 1977) must be designed so that it is in compliance with standard specifications for accessibility. Federal agencies must have an affirmative action plan for hiring, placing, and promoting individuals with disabilities and for making their facilities accessible. The Civil Rights Division of the Department of Justice is responsible for enforcing this section.

Supplementary Security Income (SSI) is a federal minimum income maintenance program for elders and individuals who are blind or disabled and who meet a test of financial need. Monthly *Social Security Disability Insurance* (SSDI) benefits are available to individuals who are disabled and their dependents. To be eligible, individuals must have paid Social Security taxes for a specified number of years (dependent upon the applicant's age); must not be working; and must be declared medically disabled by the state disability determination service or through an appeals process. The disability must be expected to last at least 12 months or to result in death. Individuals who are blind and age 55 to 65 may receive monthly benefits if they are unable to carry out the work (or similar work) that they did before age 55 or becoming blind, whichever is later. Individuals who apply for disability insurance from the Social Security Administration must undergo an evaluation carried out by a state disability evaluation team, composed of physicians, psychologists, and other health care professionals. Social Security disability benefits are not retroactive, so it is important to apply for them immediately after becoming disabled.

Individuals who have received SSDI for two consecutive years are eligible for *Medicare*, a federal health insurance program, which may cover some of the necessary outpatient therapy or supplies discussed in this book. However, Medicare does not cover eyeglasses (except for recipients who have undergone cataract surgery), low vision aids, or hearing aids. *Medicaid* is a health insurance plan for individuals who are considered financially needy (i.e., recipients of financial benefits from governmental assistance programs such as Aid to Families with Dependent Children or Supplemental Security Income).

Medicaid is a joint federal/state program. While federal law requires that each state cover hospital services, skilled nursing facility services, physician and home health care services, and diagnostic and screening services, states have great discretion in other areas. Payments for prosthetics and rehabilitation equipment vary greatly from state to state.

The *Consolidated Omnibus Budget Reconciliation Act of 1985* (P.L. 99-272), more commonly known as COBRA, provides group health insurance continuation to individuals whose work or family status changes due to unemployment, divorce, or a spouse's death or retirement. COBRA requires that employers of 20 or more workers, including local and state governments, provide employees and their families with the option of continuing their group health insurance coverage for 18 months (longer under certain circumstances). This protection was later extended to federal employees and their families. Under COBRA, the individual must pay the entire monthly premium (both the employee and employer portions) and may be charged an administrative fee.

The *Health Insurance Portability and Accountability Act of 1996* (P.L. 104-191), also known as the Kennedy-Kassebaum law, protects individuals from being denied health insurance due to a pre-existing medical condition when they move from one job to another or if they become unemployed. "Portability" means that once individuals have been covered by health insurance, they are credited with having medical coverage when they enter a new plan. Group health plans, health insurance plans such as HMOs, Medicare, Medicaid, military health plans, Indian Health Service medical care, and public, state, or federal health benefits are considered creditable coverage (Fuch et al.: 1997). Coverage of a pre-existing medical condition may not be limited for more than 12 months for individuals who enroll in the health plan as soon as they are eligible (18 months for those who delay enrollment). Although the Act creates federal standards, the states have considerable flexibility in their requirements for insurers. The Departments of Treasury, Health and Human Services, and Labor are responsible for enforcing the provisions of the Act.

The *Family and Medical Leave Act of 1993* (P.L.103-3) requires employers with 50 or more employees at a worksite or within 75 miles of a worksite to permit eligible employees 12 workweeks of unpaid leave during a 12 month period in order to care for themselves, a spouse, son or daughter, or parent who has a serious health condition. During this period of leave, the employer must continue to provide group health benefits for the employee under the same conditions as the employee would have received while working. Upon return from leave, the employee must be restored to the same position he or she had prior to the leave or to a position with equivalent pay, benefits, and conditions of employment. Special regulations apply to employees of school systems and private schools and employees of the federal civil service.

The medical and social service benefits available from organizations receiving federal assistance are guaranteed by federal laws and protected by the Office of Civil Rights of the Department of Health and Human Services (HHS). When an individual feels that his or her rights have been violated, a complaint should be filed with the regional office of HHS (see "ORGANIZATIONS" section below).

The *Telecommunications Act of 1996* (P.L. 104-104) has several sections that apply to individuals with disabilities. Section 254 redefines "universal service" to include schools, health facilities, and libraries and requires that the Federal Communications Commission (FCC) work with state governments to determine what services must be made universally available and what is considered "affordable." Section 255 of the Act requires that manufacturers of telecommunications equipment and providers of telecommunications services ensure that equipment and services are accessible to and usable by individuals with disabilities. If these provisions are not "readily achievable," manufacturers and service providers must ensure that their equipment and services are compatible with the special equipment used by individuals with disabilities to make them accessible. Section 713 requires that video services be accessible to individuals with hearing impairments via closed captioning and to individuals with visual impairments via descriptive video services. Section 706 requires that the FCC encourage the development of advanced telecommunications technology that provides equal access for individuals with disabilities, especially school children. The FCC is authorized to establish regulations and time tables for implementing these sections. The Architectural and Transportation Barriers Compliance Board (ATBCB) was required to issue guidelines within 18 months of the Act's passage on January 31, 1996.

The *Technology-Related Assistance for Individuals with Disabilities Act Amendments of 1994* (P.L. 103-218) strengthens the original Act, passed in 1988. The Act mandates state-wide programs for technology-related assistance to determine needs and resources; to provide technical assistance and information; and to develop demonstration and innovation projects, training programs, and public awareness programs. The amendments set priorities for consumer responsiveness, advocacy, systems change, and outreach to underrepresented populations such as the poor, individuals in rural areas, and minorities.

The federal government allows special tax credits for people who are totally disabled and additional standard deductions for those who are legally blind. Legal blindness is defined as acuity of 20/200 or less in the better eye with the best possible correction or a field of 20 degrees or less diameter in the better eye. Tax deductions for business expenses include disability related expenditures, and deductions for medical expenses include special equipment such as wheelchairs, text telephones (formerly called telecommunications devices for the deaf), and the like. Contact the Internal Revenue Service (see "ORGANIZATIONS" section below) to obtain publications that explain these benefits, including Publication 501, "Exemptions, Standard Deduction, and Filing Information," and Publication 524, "Credit for the Elderly or the Disabled."

All states and many local governments have adopted their own laws regarding accessibility. Information about these laws may be obtained from the state or local office serving people with disabilities. In many areas, special legal services for people with disabilities are available, often with fees on a sliding scale. Check with the local bar association or with a law school. Some lawyers specialize in the legal needs of people with disabilities.

It is possible to locate the text of federal laws and information about federal programs on many sites on the Internet. The Library of Congress provides information on the status of proposed legislation, Congressional reports, and how to contact members of Congress at http://thomas.loc.gov.

ORGANIZATIONS

Architectural and Transportation Barriers Compliance Board (ATBCB)
1331 F Street, NW, Suite 1000
Washington, DC 20004-1111
(800) 872-2253   (800) 993-2822 (TT)   (202) 272-5434
(202) 272-5449 (TT)   FAX (202) 272-5447
e-mail: info@access-board.gov   http://www.access-board.gov

A federal agency charged with developing standards for accessibility in federal facilities, public accommodations, and transportation facilities as required by the Americans with Disabilities Act and other federal laws. Publishes the "Uniform Federal Accessibility Standards," which describes accessibility standards for buildings and dwelling units developed for four federal agencies. Provides technical assistance, sponsors research, and distributes publications. Publishes a free quarterly newsletter, "Access America." Publications available in standard print, large print, braille, audiocassette, computer disk, and on the web site.

Clearinghouse on Disability Information
Office of Special Education and Rehabilitative Services (OSERS)
Department of Education
Room 3132, Switzer Building
Washington, DC 20202-2524
(202) 205-8241   (202) 205-4208 (TT)
http://www.ed.gov/OFFICES/OSERS

Responds to inquiries about federal legislation and programs for people with disabilities and makes referrals.

Commission on Mental and Physical Disability Law
American Bar Association
740 15th Street, NW, 9th Floor
Washington, DC 20005-1009
(202) 662-1575   (202) 662-1012 (TT)   FAX (202) 662-1032
e-mail: cmpdl@abanet.org   http://www.abanet.org/disability

Operates a Disability Legal Support Center, which provides searches of databases of laws, legal cases, and recent developments in the field of disability. Provides technical consultations on rights, enforcement, and other issues related to the Americans with Disabilities Act.

Compliance/Disability Rights Support Division
Department of Housing and Urban Development (HUD)
451 7th Street, SW, Room 5240
Washington, DC 20410
(202) 708-0404   FAX (202) 708-1251   http://www.hud.gov
HUD Discrimination Hotline: (800) 669-9777   (800) 927-9275 (TT)

Operates programs to make housing accessible, including loans for developers of independent living and group homes and loan and mortgage insurance for rehabilitation of single or multifamily units. Individuals who feel their rights have been violated may file a complaint with one of the ten regional offices located throughout the country.

Disability Issues Task Force
Federal Communications Commission (FCC)
1919 M Street, NW
Washington, DC 20554
(888) 835-5322 (TT)   (202) 418-0190   (202) 418-2555 (TT)
e-mail: access@fcc.gov   http://www.fcc.gov/dtf/welcome.html

Responsible for developing regulations for telecommunication issues related to federal laws, including the ADA and the Telecommunications Act of 1996.

Disability Rights Education and Defense Fund (DREDF)
2212 6th Street
Berkeley, CA 94710
(510) 644-2555   (510) 644-2626 (TT)   FAX (510) 841-8645
e-mail: dredf@dredf.org   http://www.dredf.org

Provides technical assistance, information, and referrals on laws and rights; provides legal representation to people with disabilities in both individual and class action cases; trains law students, parents, and legislators. ADA Hotline [(800)-466-4232 (V/TT)] provides information on the Americans with Disabilities Act.

Disability Rights Section
Department of Justice, Civil Rights Division
PO Box 66738
Washington, DC 20035-6738
(800) 514-0301   (800) 514-0383 (TT)
FAX (202) 307-1198   http://www.usdoj.gov/crt/ada/adahom1.htm

Responsible for enforcing Titles II and III of the Americans with Disabilities Act. Copies of its regulations are available in standard print, large print, braille, audiocassette, computer disk, and braille and on the web site. Callers may request publications, obtain technical assistance, and speak to an ADA specialist.

Equal Employment Opportunity Commission (EEOC)
1801 L Street, NW, 10th floor
Washington, DC 20507
(800) 669-3362 to order publications
(800) 669-4000 to speak to an investigator
(800) 800-3302 (TT)
In the Washington, DC metropolitan area, (202) 275-7377
(202) 275-7518 (TT)   http://www.eeoc.gov

Responsible for promulgating and enforcing regulations for the employment section of the ADA. Copies of its regulations are available in standard print, large print, braille, computer disk, and audiocassette.

Internal Revenue Service (IRS)
(800) 829-1040   (800) 829-4059 (TT)
http://www.irs.ustreas.gov

The IRS provides technical assistance about tax credits and deductions related to accommodations for disabilities. To receive Publication 554, "Older Americans Tax Guide," Publication 501, "Exemptions, Standard Deduction, and Filing Information;" Publication 907, "Tax Highlights for Persons with Disabilities;" and Publication 524, "Credit for the Elderly or the Disabled," call (800) 829-3676; (800) 829-4059 (TT). These publications are available on the web site.

National Council on Disability (NCD)
1331 F Street, NW, Suite 1050
Washington, DC 20004-1107
(202) 272-2004   (202) 272-2074 (TT)   FAX (202) 272-2022
e-mail: mquigley@ncd.gov   http://www.ncd.gov

An independent federal agency mandated to study and make recommendations about public policy for people with disabilities. Holds regular meetings and hearings in various locations around the country. Publishes monthly newsletter, "NCD Bulletin," available in standard print, large print, braille, and computer disk. Free

Nolo Press Self-Help Law Center
Nolo Press
950 Parker Street
Berkeley, CA 94710
(800) 992-6656 (orders)   (800) 800-728-3555 (customer service)
FAX (510) 548-5902   e-mail: nolotec@nolo.com
http://www.nolo.com

This online service provides information on legal topics, updates legislation and court decisions, and features articles from "Nolo News."

Office for Civil Rights, Department of Health and Human Services

200 Independence Avenue, SW
Washington, DC 20201
(202) 619-0700   (202) 863-0101 (TT)   FAX (202) 619-3818
http://www.hhs.gov/progorg/ocrhmpg.html

Responsible for enforcing laws and regulations that protect the rights of individuals seeking medical and social services in institutions that receive federal financial assistance. Individuals who feel their rights have been violated may file a complaint with one of the ten regional offices located throughout the country.

Office of Civil Rights, Department of Education

300 C Street, SW
Washington, DC 20202
(800) 421-3481   (202) 205-5166 (TT)   (202) 205-5413
FAX (202) 205-9862   e-mail: OCR@ed.gov
http://www.ed.gov/offices/OCR

Responsible for enforcing laws and regulations designed to protect the rights of individuals in educational institutions that receive federal financial assistance. Individuals who feel their rights have been violated may file a complaint with one of the ten regional offices located throughout the country.

Office of Civil Rights, Federal Transit Administration

400 7th Street, NW
Washington, DC 20590
(888) 446-4511   (202) 366-4018   (202) 366-0153 (TT)

Responsible for investigating complaints covered by regulations set forth in the Americans with Disabilities Act regarding the transportation of individuals with disabilities.

Office of Federal Contract Compliance Programs (OFCCP)

Department of Labor, Employment Standards Administration
200 Constitution Avenue, NW, Room C-3325
Washington, DC 20210
(202) 219-9475   FAX (202) 219-6195   FAX (202) 219-6195

Reviews contractors' affirmative action plans; provides technical assistance to contractors; investigates complaints; and resolves issues between contractors and employees. Ten regional offices throughout the country serve as liaisons with the national office and with district offices under their jurisdiction.

Office of General Counsel, Department of Transportation
Department of Transportation
400 7th Street, SW
Washington, DC 20590
(202) 366-9306   (202) 755-7687 (TT)   FAX (202) 366-9313
http://www.dot.gov

Responsible for providing information and interpretation of the regulations for transportation of individuals with disabilities required by the Rehabilitation Act and the Americans with Disabilities Act. Regulations available in standard print or on audiocassette.

Social Security Administration
6401 Security Boulevard
Baltimore, MD 21235
(800) 772-1213   (800) 325-0778 (TT)
http://www.ssa.gov

To apply for Social Security benefits based on disability, phone the number above to set up an appointment with a Social Security representative, or visit the local Social Security office.

Thomas
Library of Congress
http://thomas.loc.gov

This online service provides a database of recent laws and pending legislation, as well as information about the committees of Congress and the text of the "Congressional Record." Searches for legislation and laws may be done by topic or public law number.

Americans with Disabilities Act: Questions and Answers
Department of Justice, Civil Rights Division, Disability Rights Section
PO Box 66738
Washington, DC 20035-6738
(800) 514-0301 Information Line
(800) 514-0383 (TT) Information Line
FAX (202) 307-1198   http://www.usdoj.gov/crt/ada/adahom1.htm

This booklet's question and answer format provides explanations of the ADA's effects on employment, state and local governments, and public accommodations. Available in standard print, large print, audiocassette, braille, disk, automated fax system, and on the web site. Free

Directory of Legal Aid and Defender Offices
National Legal Aid and Defender Association
1625 K Street, NW, 8th Floor
Washington, DC 20006
(202) 452-0620   FAX (202) 872-1031   http://www.nlads.org

A directory of legal aid offices throughout the U.S. Includes chapters on disability protection/advocacy, health law, and senior citizens. Updated biennially. $70.00

Federal Benefits for Veterans and Dependents
Consumer Information Center
PO Box 100
Pueblo, CO 81002
Order Line (888) 878-3256   FAX (719) 948-9724
e-mail: cic.info@pueblo.gsa.gov   http://www.pueblo.gsa.gov

This booklet describes the benefits available under federal laws. $3.75. Also available on the web site.

Federal Register
New Orders, Superintendent of Documents
PO Box 371954
Pittsburgh, PA 15250-7954
(202) 512-1800   FAX (202) 512-2250
e-mail: gpoaccess@gpo.gov   http://www.access.gpo.gov/su_docs/aces/aces140.html

A federal publication printed every weekday with notices of all regulations and legal notices issued by federal agencies. Domestic subscriptions, $607.00 annually for second class mailing of paper format; $220.00 annually for microfiche. Also available on the web site at no charge.

A Guide to Disability Rights Laws
Department of Justice, Civil Rights Division, Disability Rights Section
PO Box 66738
Washington, DC 20035-6738
(800) 514-0301   (800) 514-0383 (TT)
(202) 514-0301   (202) 514-0383 (TT)
http://www.usdoj.gov/crt/ada/adahom1.htm

This booklet provides an overview of the Americans with Disabilities Act, Fair Housing Act, Air Carrier Access Act, Civil Rights of Institutionalized Persons Act, Individuals with Disabilities Education Act, Rehabilitation Act, and the Architectural Barriers Act. Available in standard print, large print, audiocassette, braille, disk, automated fax system, and on the web site. Free

A Guide to Legal Rights for People with Disabilities
by Marc D. Stolman
Demos Vermande
386 Park Avenue South, Suite 201
New York, NY 10016
(800) 532-8663   (212) 683-0072   FAX (212) 683-0118

This book discusses civil rights, insurance, benefits, and legal issues faced by individuals with disabilities. Also available on audiocassette and disk (DOS or Mac). $24.95 plus $4.00 shipping and handling

Health Benefits Under COBRA
Consumer Information Center
PO Box 100
Pueblo, CO 81002
Order Line (888) 878-3256   FAX (719) 948-9724
e-mail: cic.info@pueblo.gsa.gov   http://www.pueblo.gsa.gov

This booklet describes the coverage provided by the Consolidated Omnibus Budget Reconciliation Act (COBRA). $.50 Also available on the web site.

How to File an Unfair Treatment Complaint
How Social Security Can Help with Vocational Rehabilitation
How We Decide If You Are Still Disabled
Social Security Disability Programs Can Help
Social Security: What You Need to Know When You Get Disability Benefits
Working While Disabled... How We Can Help
Social Security Administration
(800) 772-1213   (800) 325-0778 (TT)
http://www.ssa.gov

97

These booklets provide basic information about Social Security programs for individuals with disabilities. The Social Security Administration distributes many other titles, including many that are available in large print, braille, or audiocassette. Publications are available on the web site and at local Social Security offices, free.

Know Your Rights
National Technical Information Service (NTIS)
5285 Port Royal Road
Springfield, VA 22151
(800) 553-6847   (703) 487-4639   FAX (703) 605-6900
e-mail: orders@ntis.fedworld.gov   http://www.ntis.gov

This videotape explains the legal rights of residents in nursing homes, using actual examples. 9 minutes. $50.00 plus $5.00 shipping and handling

Laws Enforced by the U.S. Equal Employment Opportunity Commission
Equal Employment Opportunity Commission (EEOC)
1801 L Street, NW, 10th floor
Washington, DC 20507
(800) 669-3362 to order publications
(800) 669-4000 to speak to an investigator
(800) 800-3302 (TT)
In the Washington, DC metropolitan area, (202) 275-7377
(202) 275-7518 (TT)   http://www.eeoc.gov

Included in this booklet are Title VII of the Civil Rights Act of 1964, Equal Pay Act, Age Discrimination in Employment Act, Rehabilitation Act of 1973, Title I of the Americans with Disabilities, and the Civil Rights Act of 1991.

The Medicare Handbook
Social Security Administration
(800) 772-1213   (800) 325-0778 (TT)
http://www.ssa.gov

or

Health Care Finance Administration (HCFA)
7500 Security Boulevard
Baltimore, MD 21244
(800) 638-6833   (800) 820-1202 (TT)
(410) 786-3000   http://www.hcfa.gov   http://www.medicare.gov

Published annually, this book helps consumers understand their rights under Medicare, including what it pays for, appeal rights, and where to get additional information. Available in English and Spanish, free. Available in alternate formats, such as large print, braille, audiocassette, and computer disk. Also available at local Social Security offices and on the web site.

Meeting the Needs of Employees with Disabilities
Resources for Rehabilitation
33 Bedford Street, Suite 19A
Lexington, MA 02420
(781) 862-6455   FAX (781) 861-7517
e-mail: info@rfr.org   http://www.rfr.org

This book provides information to help people with disabilities retain or obtain employment. Information on government programs and laws, supported employment, training programs, environmental adaptations, and the transition from school to work are included. Chapters on mobility, vision, and hearing and speech impairments include information on organizations, products, and services that enable employers to accommodate the needs of employees with disabilities. $42.95 plus $5.00 shipping and handling (See order form on last page of this book.)

Mental and Physical Disability Law Reporter
Commission on Mental and Physical Disability Law
American Bar Association
740 15th Street, NW, 9th Floor
Washington, DC 20005
(202) 662-1570   (202) 662-1581   FAX (202) 662-1032
e-mail: cmpdl@abanet.org   http://www.abanet.org

A bimonthly journal with court decisions, legislative and regulatory news, and articles on treatment, accessibility, employment, education, federal programs, etc. Individual subscription, $229.00; organizational subscription, $289.00. Reprints of articles from back issues available.

The National Partnership for Women and Families Guide to the Family and Medical Leave Act
National Partnership for Women and Families
1875 Connecticut Avenue, NW, Suite 710
Washington, DC 20009
(202) 986-2600   FAX (202) 986-2539
e-mail: info@nationalpartnership.org
http://www.nationalpartnership.org

This booklet answers the most frequently asked questions about the law. Available in English and Spanish. Also available on the web site. Free

Pocket Guide to Federal Help for Individuals with Disabilities
Clearinghouse on Disability Information
Department of Education
Office of Special Education and Rehabilitative Services (OSERS)
Room 3132, Switzer Building
Washington, DC 20202-2524
(202) 205-8241   (202) 205-4208 (TT)
http://www.ed.gov/OFFICES/OSERS

A summary of benefits and services available from the federal government. Free

Report on Disability Programs
Business Publishers
951 Pershing Drive
Silver Spring, MD 20910
(800) 274-0122   (301) 587-6300   FAX (301) 589-8493
e-mail: bpinews@bpinews.com   http://www.bpinews.com

A biweekly newsletter with information on policies promulgated by federal agencies, laws, and
funding sources. $297.00

A Summary of Department of Veterans Affairs Benefits
(800) 827-1000   http://www.va.gov

This booklet is available from any VA regional office. Free

Tax Options and Strategies: A State-by-State Guide for Persons with Disabilities, Senior
Citizens, Veterans, and Their Families
by Bruce E. Bondo
Demos Vermande
386 Park Avenue South, Suite 201
New York, NY 10016
(800) 532-8663   (212) 683-0072   FAX (212) 683-0118

This book provides information that enables individuals to benefit from federal, state, and local
tax provisions such as tax exemptions, credits, and deductions. $29.95 plus $4.00 shipping
and handling

Tax Options and Strategies for People with Disabilities
by Steven Mendelsohn
Demos Vermande
386 Park Avenue South, Suite 201
New York, NY 10016
(800) 532-8663   (212) 683-0072   FAX (212) 683-0118

This book describes provisions in the tax laws that affect individuals with disabilities, including access to retirement funds to defray disability related expenses, deductions available for assistive technology, incentives for employers to hire individuals with disabilities, and dependent care. Also available on audiocassette and disk (DOS or Mac). $29.95 plus $4.00 shipping and handling

Chapter 4

CORONARY HEART DISEASE

Coronary heart disease (CHD), also called ischemic heart disease or coronary artery disease, is the result of arteriosclerosis or "hardening of the arteries," a generic term that describes narrowing of the arteries. The walls of the arteries thicken and lose elasticity, due to the formation of plaque. Atherosclerosis, a type of arteriosclerosis, affects larger arteries and is an underlying cause of most heart disease. One-third of men age 60 or over have coronary heart disease (Agency for Health Care Policy and Research: 1996). Severely narrowed coronary arteries may lead to angina pectoris (recurring chest pain), myocardial infarction (heart attack or MI), or congestive heart failure. In 1995, coronary heart disease was responsible for 481,287 deaths; this represents a decline of 28.7% in deaths from heart attacks from 1985 to 1995 (American Heart Association: 1998).

Men with family members who developed heart disease before age 55 and those with diabetes are at greater risk for heart disease (Texas Heart Institute: 1996). Other risk factors associated with the development of coronary heart disease in men are smoking, hypertension, obesity, elevated cholesterol levels, stress, and lack of exercise; all are amenable to treatment.

Men's higher rate of smoking places them at greater risk of myocardial infarction, sudden coronary death, and atherosclerosis (Waldron: 1983). Smoking increases the heart rate and raises blood pressure, which in turn damages the arteries, increasing the build-up of plaque on artery walls. The nicotine in cigarettes contributes to the formation of blood clots and the decrease of oxygen in the cells. An individual who resumes smoking after a heart attack doubles his chances of having a second attack (American Heart Association: 1990).

Type A behavior, characterized by competitiveness, aggressive behavior, and hostility, is another risk factor that contributes to the greater incidence of coronary heart disease in men (Waldron: 1983). Men who are intensely focused on their jobs are less likely to heed warning signs of heart disease such as fatigue, shortness of breath, and intermittent chest pain. Some men may recover faster after a heart attack by changing their focus from work to recovery (Helgeson: 1995).

Hypertension or high blood pressure accelerates the development of coronary heart disease because it damages the inner walls of the arteries. It may also affect the peripheral blood vessels. Blood pressure is the force exerted by the heart pumping blood through the body. High blood pressure may lead to damage to the heart (myocardial infarction), brain (stroke), eyes, and kidneys. The two types of high blood pressure are essential, or primary, hypertension and secondary hypertension. Essential hypertension accounts for about 90% of all cases of high blood pressure (Horowitz: 1988). The development of essential hypertension is affected by heredity, salt consumption, obesity, and stress. It may be treated with medication, diet, exercise, and stress reduction. Medications include diuretics, alpha-blockers, beta blockers, angiotensin-converting enzyme (ACE) inhibitors, calcium channel blockers, and antiadrenergic agents or centrally acting drugs that open arteries and slow heart beat. Secondary hypertension is high blood pressure that arises from other medical conditions, such as chronic kidney disease or adrenal gland disorders.

Too much cholesterol in the blood leads to a build-up of fatty deposits in the arteries, increasing the risk of heart attack. Cholesterol levels in the blood may be lowered by limiting saturated fat in the diet and substituting polyunsaturated fats from vegetable sources. Some individuals require medication to lower blood cholesterol levels satisfactorily.

Individuals with diabetes have an increased risk of coronary heart disease and an increased rate of heart attack. About four-fifths of individuals with diabetes die of premature cardiovascular disease, usually myocardial infarction (National Institutes of Health: 1989). To reduce the risk of heart disease, individuals with diabetes should maintain good control of their blood glucose (see Chapter 5, "Diabetes"), stop smoking, reduce high blood pressure and high cholesterol, and if necessary, lose weight.

Individuals who are overweight increase their risk for high blood pressure and diabetes. Losing weight helps to decrease cholesterol levels in the blood, lower blood pressure, and improve blood glucose tolerance. A low fat diet accompanied by aerobic exercise will help individuals lose weight and reduce their risk of heart disease.

TYPES OF CORONARY HEART DISEASE

Angina pectoris is caused by a lack of oxygen-rich blood to the heart; its symptoms are chest, arm, back, neck, or jaw pain. Eighty-five percent of angina is caused by coronary heart disease; the remaining 15% may be attributed to heart valve disease, spasms in artery walls, or abnormalities in the heart chamber (Texas Heart Institute: 1996). About 70% of all individuals with angina are men (Selwyn and Braunwald: 1994). Stable angina may occur with exertion, but the pain subsides quickly with rest. Unstable angina is characterized by frequent episodes and severe discomfort. Unstable angina is diagnosed through physical examination, electrocardiogram (ECG), exercise stress tests, and thallium stress tests. Exercise stress tests measure heart function but do not indicate where or how badly arteries are blocked; they are helpful in determining treatment options. In an exercise stress test, electrodes are placed on the chest, and the individual walks on a motor-driven treadmill, as the speed and incline are increased at regular intervals. The ECG is monitored carefully, and blood pressure is checked regularly. Exercise requires the heart to work harder; if there are blockages in the arteries, the ECG will show changes to its normal wave patterns. The thallium scan is used to determine the location of the blockage. Thallium, a radioactive isotope, is injected into a vein while the individual is walking on the treadmill; it travels through the bloodstream to the heart. With the individual lying flat, an imaging scan is performed to show the movement of the thallium throughout the heart muscle; areas that do not receive blood appear as "holes." It has recently been suggested that exercise-thallium testing of individuals who are symptom-free after coronary artery bypass grafts may predict subsequent myocardial infarction or death. Routine screening of these individuals has been discouraged in the past (Lauer et al.: 1998).

Unstable angina may be treated with medication, angioplasty (a procedure that is used to reduce arterial blockage), or coronary bypass surgery. Medications include aspirin, nitroglycerin, and beta-blockers. Aspirin prevents the formation of blood clots; side effects are usually avoided by taking buffered or coated aspirin. Nitroglycerin dilates blood vessels, increases blood flow, and lowers blood pressure, reducing the work of the heart. It may be taken orally, in ointments, or through a patch placed on the arm. When taken as a tablet, nitroglycerin is placed under the tongue and allowed to dissolve so that it enters the bloodstream rapidly. Relief is usually felt within a minute or two. Side effects include dizziness and tingling. Beta-blockers slow the heart rate and reduce the amount of oxygen it needs. Side effects include fatigue and dizziness, impotence, depression, diarrhea, or skin rashes; these conditions are relieved by reducing the dose or discontinuing the medication. Beta-blockers should be discontinued slowly over time to avoid complications. Calcium channel blockers help increase the blood supply to the heart and reduce its need for oxygen. They are effective in treating stable angina and have few side effects.

Cardiac catheterization is a test used to assess blood flow and the extent of blockage; a catheter is inserted into an artery in the arm or groin, threaded up through the artery to the heart, and a dye is injected. The procedure is monitored by x-ray which allows the physician to visualize the blockage. The resulting pictures are called arteriograms.

A *myocardial infarction* occurs when the blood cannot reach the heart muscle due to a partial or total blockage of the coronary arteries. The damage is irreversible. Common symptoms are intense chest pain, a cold sweat, dizziness, and shortness of breath. Individuals experiencing these symptoms should seek medical attention immediately. Two tests are used to determine the diagnosis of myocardial infarction, the electrocardiogram (ECG) and blood tests, which reveal the presence of cardiac enzymes released when heart muscle cells are injured. Electrodes, connected to the electrocardiograph, are placed on the individual's chest, arms, and legs. The electrocardiogram measures the electrical activity within the heart and records it as a tracing on a strip of moving paper; abnormalities are detected by comparing the tracing with recordings of normal heart activity.

Myocardial infarction is usually first treated in the hospital emergency room. Morphine may be administered to relieve chest pain. If an electrocardiogram detects abnormal heartbeat rhythms, known as arrhythmias, they are treated with medications such as lidocaine, or defibrillation (shock therapy) is used to interrupt the abnormal rhythm and return the heartbeat to normal. A pacemaker, a mechanical device that provides regular electrical stimulation to the heart, may be attached temporarily or permanently implanted. Once the physician has confirmed that a myocardial infarction has occurred, the drugs streptokinase or tissue plasminogen activator (tPA) are used to dissolve the blood clot that precipitated the heart attack. Streptokinase or tPA must be given, through a catheter or direct injection, soon after the attack in order to dissolve the clot. Some individuals develop blood clots in the heart after myocardial infarction; these clots may enter the bloodstream and cause damage to other organs. To counter clot formation, anticoagulants or blood thinners such as warfarin (Coumadin) are prescribed. Individuals taking anticoagulants are prone to excessive bleeding and must be carefully monitored. Aspirin should be avoided when taking anticoagulants, because it is also an anticoagulant, but acetaminophen may be taken. Individuals spend several days in an intensive care unit (ICU) for careful monitoring by ECG. Medications are administered through an intravenous line in a vein in the arm, and oxygen is usually administered. Following the stay in the ICU, the individual will be transferred to a less intensively monitored unit for additional care and initial cardiac rehabilitation services.

There are two interventions that may improve blood flow to the heart in individuals with angina or myocardial infarction. *Percutaneous transluminal coronary angioplasty* (PTCA) is a nonsurgical procedure used to open blocked arteries. A catheter is inserted into an artery in the arm or groin and carefully threaded through the aorta to the site of the blocked artery. This procedure is performed with the guidance of a fluoroscope, an x-ray camera. A tiny balloon, attached to the tip of another catheter, is passed through the first catheter. It is inflated to compress the plaque on the artery, opening the blocked area, then deflated, and removed. When it is successful, the benefits of angioplasty include pain reduction, a return to normal activity level, and a decrease in the need for medication. About 419,000 PTCA procedures were performed in the United States in 1995 (American Heart Association: 1998). Angioplasty is not without risk; the procedure may damage the artery or increase angina. According to the Agency for Health Care Policy and Research (1994), about 40% of arteries become blocked again within six months. An individual may then require emergency bypass surgery, have a heart attack, or die.

Coronary stenting is an alternative when arteries become blocked (restenosis) after an initial balloon angiography. A stent is a tiny tube that is implanted in the blood vessel in order to keep it open and clear. More than two-thirds of individuals undergoing procedures to open blocked arteries have had stents implanted since the procedure was approved in 1994 (Topol: 1998). When researchers compared individuals with restenosis who had had either a second balloon angioplasty or coronary stenting, they found that the rate of restenosis was less in those who had had the stenting procedure (Erbel et al.:1998).

Coronary artery bypass grafts (CABG) may be recommended for the individual who has severe blockages in the left coronary artery or in several blood vessels. Cardiac catheterization and angioplasty procedures are used to determine the degree and location of coronary artery blockage and its effect on heart function. A vein removed from the individual's leg or a mammary artery removed from the chest, is transplanted between the aorta and the coronary artery above the blockage. Grafts using mammary arteries remain open longer than those using veins (Selwyn and Braunwald: 1994). Coronary artery bypass graft surgery is "open-heart" surgery; a heart-lung machine is used to maintain blood flow and respiration while surgery takes place. By improving blood flow to the heart, coronary artery bypass grafts have been found to relieve anginal pain fully in about 70% of individuals and partially in another 20% (Texas Heart Institute: 1996), but they do not halt atherosclerosis. Other arteries may become clogged, angina may return, or the individual may have a heart attack.

Lange and Hillis (1998) claim that many patients undergo angiography and bypass surgery despite the fact that these procedures do not reduce the incidence of subsequent myocardial infarction or death. Four large, randomized studies that compared aggressive treatment (angiography followed by surgery) with conservative management (medical therapy or noninvasive testing) showed that although aggressive management is chosen by most physicians, the results do not justify their choices. In a study conducted for the Department of Veterans Affairs (Boden et al.: 1998), patients who were treated aggressively had poorer outcomes during hospitalization, one month, and one year following a myocardial infarction. Factors influencing physicians' choices include insistence on aggressive management by the patient and family; skepticism regarding the trials' results; habit; and the availability of facilities, trained personnel, and reimbursement (Lange and Hillis: 1998).

Two individuals with the same clinical symptoms may opt for different treatments. For example, individuals with chronic, stable angina may react differently to the same severity of pain. Those affected should be aware that surgery to perform coronary artery bypass graft may not result in increased survival time, but it may result in relief of symptoms. Nease and colleagues (1995) studied 220 individuals with angina and found that individuals with the same level of pain opted for different outcomes. While some opted for symptom relief through surgery with the knowledge that their survival time would be shorter, others chose to live longer and endure their pain.

The recovery period before a return to work is usually four to six weeks, longer if a job requires strenuous physical exertion. During recovery, individuals are encouraged to alternate light physical exercise, such as walking, with periods of rest. Leg swelling that occurs when a vein is removed may be relieved by wearing an elastic stocking, elevating the leg, avoiding prolonged sitting, and walking. Individuals will be advised to make lifestyle changes such as giving up smoking; reducing cholesterol, saturated fats, and sodium in their diet; reducing stress; losing weight; and engaging in aerobic exercise.

In *congestive heart failure*, the heart cannot pump enough blood to maintain normal circulation. Blood backs up into the lungs, causing congestion in the lungs and body tissues, and excess water and salt are retained in the kidneys. Congestive heart failure may be caused by chronic hypertension, damage to the heart muscle (myocardial infarction), defective or damaged heart valves, or congenital heart disease. Common symptoms of congestive heart failure are edema (swelling in the ankles, legs or feet), shortness of breath, and fatigue. Chest x-rays, which detect the presence of fluid in the lungs, and echocardiograms, which provide information on heart function, are used to diagnose the condition. The physician uses the echocardiogram to determine whether the symptoms are due to valve, muscle, or artery damage or a congenital heart defect. Cardiac catheterization and coronary angiography may also be used to confirm a diagnosis.

The goals for treating congestive heart failure are to increase the pumping function of the heart, decrease the work load on the heart, and control retention of salt and water. Digitalis strengthens heart muscle function; individuals taking digitalis must be monitored carefully for cardiac rhythm disorders. Side effects may include ringing in the ears, blurred vision, and nausea. Both angiotensin-converting enzyme (ACE) inhibitors and calcium channel blockers dilate blood vessels, lowering blood pressure and reducing the heart's workload. Diuretics are used to eliminate salt and water from the body. Potassium levels are monitored in individuals taking diuretics, since low levels may cause fatigue, weakness, or cardiac rhythm disorders. Individuals may be advised to supplement their diet with foods rich in potassium, such as bananas, broccoli, and potatoes. Rest, moderate restriction of physical activity, and mild sedation to reduce anxiety are helpful in decreasing cardiac work load (Braunwald: 1994).

SEXUAL FUNCTIONING

Most individuals with cardiac disease may resume sexual activity within a month or two after heart attack or heart surgery. Many reports indicate that the energy expended in sexual intercourse is equivalent to climbing two flights of stairs. The individual's ability to withstand this amount of activity can be measured by a treadmill test or the use of a Holter recorder (a portable ECG monitor). Despite these readiness tests, nearly a quarter of individuals do not become sexually active after myocardial infarction and about a third of those who have coronary artery bypass grafts engage in less sexual activity than prior to their surgery (Papadopoulos: 1991).

In many men, psychological responses to heart surgery or heart attack affect sexual activity more than the physiological aspects. Anxiety, fear, and depression may affect libido; a man or his partner may fear precipitating another heart attack or anginal chest pain. A man whose self-esteem is affected by invalidism and a partner who is also the caregiver may find it difficult to return to the role of lovers.

Men who experience erectile dysfunction as a result of blood vessel deterioration in the penis may find that the use of a vacuum pump, penile injections, or a penile prosthesis enables them to achieve an erection. Sexual function is improved by giving up smoking and drinking less alcohol. A small number of men have benefited from vascular surgery to improve the blood flow to the penis. While some cardiovascular medications, such as those taken for high blood pressure, affect desire, erection, and ejaculation, others, such as nitroglycerin, taken before sexual activity, reduce the risk of anginal chest pain.

Some couples find that using different positions for coitus, such as the healthy partner on top or a side-by-side position, requires less energy and causes less muscle fatigue. Since digestion places strain on the heart, it is recommended that couples wait several hours after a heavy meal before engaging in sexual activity. To avoid fatigue, couples might plan to have sex in the morning, when energy levels are higher. Cardiac exercise programs help men increase physical strength and provide a sense of well-being that boosts their self-image and confidence in performing sexually.

Sexual counseling should be a part of cardiac rehabilitation programs. Physicians and other health care professionals should be willing and prepared to initiate conversations with individuals during follow-up office visits. Referrals may also be made to sex therapists.

PSYCHOLOGICAL ASPECTS OF CORONARY HEART DISEASE

Once the immediate threat to life caused by a heart attack has been overcome, the man with heart disease often experiences anxiety due to fears for his future health, employment, and family relationships. He may become depressed due to a combination of physical weakness, dependence on others, and fatigue. Medications used to treat the acute symptoms of heart attack may affect his memory, and he may refuse necessary medication for fear of becoming addicted to the drugs. These fears may become worse upon discharge from the hospital. A man who has spent time in a coronary care or surgical intensive care unit may miss the security of close monitoring and observation and feel defenseless at home. Minor chest pain or indigestion may be misinterpreted as precursors of another heart attack. In many cases, these pains may be attributed to the muscle aches that accompany a cardiac exercise regimen.

Men who are accustomed to physical activity chafe at the enforced six to eight week rest period that is prescribed to allow the heart to heal and form scar tissue. Gradually, they are allowed to resume moderate exercise; fatigue and lack of energy decrease with time.

Although anxiety, fear, and feelings of uselessness are common in the weeks following a heart attack, they should abate in time; however, if the individual becomes apathetic, has trouble concentrating, takes no interest in his appearance or formerly pleasurable activities, tires easily, has difficulty sleeping, or expresses feelings of inadequacy, he may be seriously depressed. Changes in medication may be required, or the individual may be referred for counseling.

Family members may fear that their actions will precipitate another attack, or they may feel guilty about causing the attack in the first place. Family members may be overprotective, interfering with recommended timelines for resumption of activity. Both the man and his family may have concerns about medical bills, return to work, and lifestyle changes to diet, daily routine, and physical activities.

It is important that health care professionals provide opportunities for men and their families to discuss their fears and ask questions. Cardiac rehabilitation programs offer individual and group counseling for participants and their families. Men who might otherwise refuse referral to support programs often find that they receive encouragement and practical advice from other participants in exercise programs. Mended Hearts is a support program for individuals with heart disease (see "ORGANIZATIONS" section below). Nutrition classes offer counseling and instruction in "heart-healthy" meal preparation, providing information and motivation to follow dietary recommendations.

After a two to three months recovery period, between 80 and 90% of individuals return to work after heart attack (American Heart Association: 1990). Shorter work hours and rest periods are advisable in the early weeks. If the physical requirements of the job are deemed to be too strenuous, a job change is recommended. Vocational rehabilitation agencies, available in every state, will provide counseling, training, and placement services (see Chapter 1, p. 18).

The effects of stress in employment and everyday activities may be ameliorated by engaging in routine exercise and learning relaxation techniques. In addition to cardiac rehabilitation services, community organizations such as YMCA's, local recreation programs, and adult education centers offer aerobics training and stress reduction classes. Stress management or relaxation audiotapes use visual imagery and meditation to help individuals cope with stress.

PROFESSIONAL SERVICE PROVIDERS

Primary care physicians, who are often internists, oversee the individual's general health. Internists are physicians who specialize in the diagnosis and treatment of the body's internal organs, such as the heart, lungs, and kidneys. Internists make referrals to specialists such as cardiologists for further tests and treatment. *Cardiologists* are physicians who specialize in diagnosing and treating heart disease. They perform diagnostic tests such as exercise stress tests and angiograms and procedures such as coronary angioplasty. *Cardiovascular surgeons* are physicians who perform operations such as coronary artery bypass surgery, heart valve replacements, and heart transplants.

The *cardiac rehabilitation team* is a multidisciplinary group of health care professionals made up of physicians, nurses, physical and occupational therapists, dietitians, and psychologists or social workers.

Cardiac rehabilitation programs have several goals: exercise training, risk factor modification, and psychological well-being. Candidates for cardiac rehabilitation services are those who have had heart attacks or heart surgery and those with congestive heart failure. A physician's referral is required for cardiac rehabilitation services. Of the 13.5 million Americans affected by coronary heart disease, only 11 to 20% have enrolled in cardiac rehabilitation programs (Wenger et al.: 1995). Nearly 4.7 million individuals with congestive heart failure may also benefit from cardiac rehabilitation. Benefits from cardiac rehabilitation are increased exercise tolerance, symptom modification, blood lipid level reduction, lowered blood pressure, weight loss, and smoking cessation.

Although cardiac rehabilitation usually starts prior to hospital discharge, the bulk of the program takes place in outpatient settings in the hospital or medical center, community center, or, in some cases, in the workplace. After an initial medical evaluation, an individualized plan is designed. Exercise training is the key ingredient of cardiac rehabilitation programs. Individuals who participate in three 20 to 40 minute sessions of aerobic exercise per week are reported to receive the most benefit (Wenger et al.: 1995). Elders, who often receive fewer services due to age bias, also gain functional improvement when enrolled in exercise programs (Hellman: 1994).

While some individuals will discontinue smoking on their own after a heart attack, most require a program that combines education, behavior modification, and counseling. Nutrition education and training, behavior modification, and physical exercise may help most individuals lower their blood lipid levels, but some will require medication. Weight reduction is best accomplished with nutrition education and exercise training; exercise alone is not sufficient. In order to reduce blood pressure, individuals must employ a combined strategy of sodium restriction, weight reduction, and exercise training along with medication. The combination of diet, weight loss, and exercise may lead to reduced need for medication.

Wenger and her colleagues (1995) reported that although exercise training alone provides improvement in the individual's sense of well-being, the added components of education, counseling, and psychosocial interventions result in even greater benefits, such as social adjustment and stress reduction.

In choosing a cardiac rehabilitation program, individuals should consider its location, schedule, service options, and cost. Distance and availability of private or public transportation and parking may affect the individual's ability to participate in a program that meets three or more times per week. On-the-job sites offer advantages to the individual who has returned to work. Some people prefer group services rather than individual exercise plans; group interaction and social supports provide motivation for adherence to an exercise schedule. Medical insurance may cover the cost of cardiac rehabilitation. Less expensive programs may be found in a community setting such as a YMCA or other community organization. The American Association of Cardiovascular and Pulmonary Rehabilitation offers a national directory of cardiac rehabilitation programs (see "ORGANIZATIONS" section below).

Heart disease was the most common reason that men utilized home health services in 1991-92 (Dey: 1995). Skilled nursing services, physical therapy, occupational therapy, and homemaker services may be provided by public and private clinics; local hospitals; home

109

health agencies such as visiting nurse associations; state, federal, and private agencies which serve elders; Veterans Affairs Medical Centers; and therapists in private practice. Meals on Wheels provides nutritious meals to those who are unable to prepare meals themselves or who are alone for long periods of time.

References

Agency for Health Care Policy and Research
1996 "Ischemic Heart Disease PORT Examines In-Hospital Death Rates for CABG Patients" Research Activities 194 (June):1-2
1994 Managing Unstable Angina Rockville, MD: Agency for Health Care Policy and Research

American Heart Association
1998 1998 Heart and Stroke Statistical Update Dallas, TX: American Heart Association
1990 After a Heart Attack Dallas, TX: American Heart Association

Boden, William E. et al.
1998 "Outcomes in Patients with Acute Non-Q-Wave Myocardial Infarction Randomly Assigned to an Invasive as Compared with a Conservative Management Strategy" New England Journal of Medicine 338(June 18):25:1785-1792

Braunwald, Eugene
1994 "Heart Failure" pp. 998-1009 in Kurt J. Isselbacher et al. (eds.) Harrison's Principles of Internal Medicine New York, NY: McGraw Hill, Inc.

Dey, A. N.
1995 "Characteristics of Elderly Men and Women Discharged from Home Health Care Services 1991-92" Advance Data from Vital and Health Statistics No. 259 Hyattsville, MD: National Center for Health Statistics

Erbel, Raimund et al.
1998 "Coronary-Artery Stenting Compared with Balloon Angioplasty for Restenosis After Initial Balloon Angioplasty" New England Journal of Medicine 339:23(December):1678

Helgeson, Vicki S.
1995 "Masculinity, Men's Roles, and Coronary Heart Disease" pp. 68-104 in Donald Sabo and David Frederick Gordon (eds.) Men's Health and Illness: Gender, Power, and the Body Newbury Park, CA: Sage Publications

Hellman, E. A. and M. A. Williams
1994 "Outpatient Cardiac Rehabilitation in Elderly Patients" Heart-Lung 23:(6):506-12

Horowitz, Emmanuel
1988 Heartbeat: A Complete Guide to Understanding and Preventing Heart Disease Los Angeles, CA: Health Trend Publishing

Lange, Richard A. and L. David Hillis
1998 "Use and Overuse of Angiography and Revascularization for Acute Coronary Syndromes" New England Journal of Medicine 338(June 18):25:1838-39

Lauer, M. S. et al.
1998 "Prediction of Death and Myocardial Infarction By Screening with Exercise-thallium Testing After Coronary-Artery-Bypass Grafting" Lancet 351(9103):615-22

National Institutes of Health

1989 Heart Attacks Washington, DC: National Institutes of Health Clinical Center

Nease, Robert F. Jr. et al.

1995 "Variation in Patient Utilities for Outcome of the Management of Chronic Stable Angina: Implications for Clinical Practice Guidelines" Journal of the American Medical Association 273(15):1185-1190

Papadopoulos, Chris

1991 "Sex and the Cardiac Patient" Medical Aspects of Human Sexuality August:18-21

Selwyn, Andrew P. and Eugene Braunwald

1994 "Ischemic Heart Disease" pp. 1077-1085 in Kurt J. Isselbacher et al. (eds.) Harrison's Principles of Internal Medicine New York, NY: McGraw Hill, Inc.

Texas Heart Institute

1996 Heart Owner's Handbook New York, NY: John Wiley & Sons, Inc.

Topol, Eric J.

1998 "Coronary-Artery Stents--Gauging, Gorging, and Gouging" New England Journal of Medicine 339:23(December):1704

Waldron, Ingrid

1983 "Sex Differences in Illness Incidence, Prognosis and Mortality: Issues and Evidence" Social Science and Medicine 17:16:1107-1123

Wenger, N. K. et al.

1995 Cardiac Rehabilitation as Secondary Prevention Clinical Practice Guideline. Quick Reference Guide for Clinicians, No. 17 Rockville, MD: Agency for Health Care Policy and Research Pub. No. 96-0673

ORGANIZATIONS

American Association of Cardiovascular and Pulmonary Rehabilitation
7611 Elmwood Avenue, Suite 201
Middletown, WI 53562
(608) 831-6989   FAX (608) 831-5122
http://www.aacvpr.org

Will make referrals to cardiac rehabilitation programs in the caller's area.

American Heart Association
7272 Greenville Avenue
Dallas, TX 75231-4596
(800) 242-8721   (214) 373-6300   FAX (214) 706-1341
http://www.americanheart.org

Promotes research and education and publishes professional and public education brochures. Local affiliates. Membership fees vary.

Mended Hearts
7272 Greenville Avenue
Dallas, TX 75231
(214) 706-1442   FAX (214) 706-5231
http://www.mendedhearts.org

This affiliate of the American Heart Association has chapters in many states. It offers support to individuals with heart disease through monthly meetings, raises funds for medical equipment and scholarships, and trains volunteers to visit individuals who have undergone heart surgery. Membership, individuals, $17.00; family, $24.00; includes quarterly newsletter, "Heartbeat."

National Heart, Lung, and Blood Institute (NHLBI)
31 Center Drive, MSC 2480
Bethesda, MD 20892-2480
(301) 496-5166   http://www.nhlbi.nih.gov

Conducts research and national education programs and issues clinical guidelines on topics such as high blood pressure and high cholesterol.

National Heart, Lung, and Blood Institute Information Center
PO Box 30105
Bethesda, MD 20824-0105
(301) 251-1222   FAX (301) 251-1223
http://www.nhlbi.nih.gov/nhlbi

A federal information center which distributes publications about cardiovascular disease. NHLBI Information Line provides recorded messages in English and Spanish about prevention and treatment of high blood pressure; [(800) 575-9355]. Free publications list. Many publications and publication list are available on web site.

National Hypertension Association
324 East 30th Street
New York, NY 10016
(212) 889-3557   FAX (212) 447-7032

Conducts research, promotes public and professional education, and provides hypertension work-site detection programs. General information packet, free, plus $2.00 shipping and handling. Also available, "Week by Week to a Strong Heart," $8.50; "Lower Your Blood Pressure and Live Longer," $8.50; and "High Blood Pressure & What You Can Do About It," $2.50.

Advances in Cardiac Surgery
Aquarius Health Care Videos
5 Powderhouse Lane
PO Box 1159
Sherborn, MA 01770
(508) 651-2963   FAX (508) 650-4216
e-mail: aqvideos@tiac.net   http://www.aquariusproductions.com

In this videotape, cardiac surgeons describe new, minimally invasive techniques and which patients qualify for them. 28 minutes. $150.00 plus $9.00 shipping and handling

American Heart Association Cookbook
Random House, Order Department
400 Hahn Road, PO Box 100
Westminster, MD 21157
(800) 793-2665   http://www.randomhouse.com

This cookbook provides low fat, low cholesterol recipes. $29.50 plus $4.00 shipping and handling

American Heart Association Guide to Heart Attack
American Heart Association Fulfillment Center
200 State Road
South Deerfield, MA 01373-0200
(800) 611-6083   FAX (800) 499-6464

This book describes medical and surgical treatment for heart attack and the recovery process as well as controlling risk factors. Hardcover, $23.00; softcover, $15.00; plus $5.75 shipping and handling.

Angioplasty
Cardiac Catheterization and Coronary Angiography
Coronary Bypass Surgery
Exercise Testing
Radioisotope with Exercise Testing
Transesophageal Echocardiography
American Heart Association Fulfillment Center
200 State Road
South Deerfield, MA 01373-0200
(800) 611-6083   FAX (800) 499-6464

These videotapes describe diagnostic and surgical procedures. Available in English and Spanish. $29.00 plus $5.75 shipping and handling for each title May also be available through local affiliates' videotape lending libraries; call (800) 242-8721.

Cardiac Comeback 1, 2, 3
Info Vision
102 North Hazel Street
Glenwood, IA 51534
(800) 237-1808   FAX (888) 735-2622

This series of three videotapes provides beginning, intermediate, and advanced exercise programs for individuals with heart disease. $59.00 plus $5.00 shipping and handling

Cleveland Clinic Heart Advisor
PO Box 420235
Palm Coast, FL 32142-0235
(800) 829-2506

This monthly newsletter discusses coronary care, including information on surgical techniques, medications, risk factors, and research. $30.00

Congestive Heart Failure
American Heart Association Fulfillment Center
200 State Road
South Deerfield, MA 01373-0200
(800) 611-6083   FAX (800) 499-6464

This videotape provides information about the causes and symptoms of congestive heart failure and describes diagnostic methods and treatments. Available in English and Spanish. $29.00 plus $5.75 shipping and handling. May also be available through local affiliates' videotape lending libraries; call (800) 242-8721.

Congestive Heart Failure: What You Should Know
American Heart Association
7272 Greenville Avenue
Dallas, TX 75231-4596
(800) 242-8721   (214) 373-6300   FAX (214) 706-1341
http://www.americanheart.org

This brochure discusses the causes and signs of congestive heart failure. Describes treatment with medications, lifestyle changes, and surgery. Free

Coping with Heart Illness
by Wayne M. Sotile
Human Kinetics
1607 North Market Street
PO Box 5076
Champaign, IL 61825-5076
(800) 747-4457   (217) 351-5076   FAX (217) 351-2674
http://www.humankinetics.com

This series of three videotapes features physicians and patients discussing psychosocial aspects of cardiac rehabilitation such as depression, sexuality, lifestyle changes, and family issues. $49.95 plus $4.50 shipping and handling

Coronary Artery Bypass Graft Surgery
American Heart Association
7272 Greenville Avenue
Dallas, TX 75231-4596
(800) 242-8721   (214) 373-6300   FAX (214) 706-1341
http://www.americanheart.org

This brochure discusses treatment of coronary artery disease using bypass graft surgery. Describes pre-surgical preparation and post-surgical care and makes suggestions for recuperating at home.   Free

Diabetes and Heart Disease
American Heart Association Fulfillment Center
200 State Road
South Deerfield, MA 01373-0200
(800) 611-6083   FAX (800) 499-6464

This videotape discusses the increased risk of cardiovascular disease in people with diabetes and how diabetes management techniques may help reduce these risks. Available in English and Spanish. $29.00 plus $5.75 shipping and handling. May also be available through local affiliates' videotape lending libraries; call (800) 242-8721.

Facts About How to Prevent High Blood Pressure
National Heart, Lung, and Blood Institute Information Center
PO Box 30105
Bethesda, MD 20824-0105
(301) 251-1222   FAX (301) 251-1223
http://www.nhlbi.nih.gov/nhlbi

116

This booklet discusses high blood pressure and the problems it can lead to if undetected and untreated. Describes prevention strategies, provides charts listing sodium content of foods and calories burned during exercise, and provides a sample walking program. Free

Heart Attack and Recovery
by Kevin Waite
Coffey Communications, Inc.
1505 Business One Circle
Walla Walla, WA 99362
(800) 952-9089   (509) 525-0101   FAX (509) 525-0281
e-mail: coffey@coffeycomm.com   http://www.life-and-health.com

This booklet discusses the risk factors for heart attack, diagnosis and treatment, and strategies for prevention of another attack. $1.25 plus 7% shipping and handling (minimum order, $5.00).

Heart Illness and Intimacy: How Caring Relationships Aid Recovery
by Wayne M. Sotile
Johns Hopkins University Press
2715 North Charles Street
Baltimore, MD 21218
(800) 537-5487   FAX (410) 516-6998
http://muse.jhu.edu/press

This book describes the psychological effects of heart disease on the individual, spouse, and family. Includes discussions of personality, attitude, sexuality, and stress reduction. $36.00 plus $4.50 shipping and handling

Heartmates
PO Box 16202
Minneapolis, MN 55416
(800) 946-3331   FAX (612) 929-6395
e-mail: heartmates@outtech.com   http://www.heartmates.com

Developed by a social worker whose husband has heart disease, this web site includes resources for the emotional needs of spouses and family members of individuals who have had a heart attack.

Heart Owner's Handbook
by the Texas Heart Institute
John Wiley & Sons, Inc.
1 Wiley Drive
Somerset, NJ 08875
(800) 225-5945   (908) 469-4400   FAX (908) 302-2300
http://www.wiley.com

This book provides information on the cardiovascular system, symptoms and treatment of heart disease, and cardiac rehabilitation. Also describes the risk factors for heart disease and how to control them. Includes recipes for "heart-smart" cooking. $16.95 plus $2.50 shipping and handling

Learning About Heart Attacks: The Patient and the Family
AIMS Media
9710 DeSoto Avenue
Chatsworth, CA 91311-4409
(800) 367-2467   (818) 773-4300   FAX (818) 341-6700
http://www.aims-multimedia.com

This videotape enables families to discuss reactions such as fear and guilt when a member has a heart attack. 16 minutes. $49.95 plus $8.95 shipping and handling

Living with Heart Disease: Is It Heart Failure?
Agency for Health Care Policy and Research (AHCPR)
Publications Clearinghouse
PO Box 8547
Silver Spring, MD 20907
(800) 358-9295   e-mail: info@ahcpr.gov   http://www.ahcpr.gov

This brochure discusses the causes, symptoms, diagnosis, and treatment of congestive heart failure. Makes suggestions for lifestyle changes and daily activities. Includes a sample medication record. Free

Managing Unstable Angina
Agency for Health Care Policy and Research (AHCPR)
Publications Clearinghouse
PO Box 8547
Silver Spring, MD 20907
(800) 358-9295   e-mail: info@ahcpr.gov   http://www.ahcpr.gov

This booklet describes unstable angina and its relationship to other heart conditions. Describes diagnostic tests and medical and surgical treatments. Available in English and Spanish. Free

Men and Heart Disease
by Michael Lancaster
Coffey Communications, Inc.
1505 Business One Circle
Walla Walla, WA 99362
(800) 952-9089   (509) 525-0101   FAX (509) 525-0281
e-mail: coffey@coffeycomm.com   http://www.life-and-health.com

This booklet describes risk factors, diagnostic tests, and treatment options. $1.25 plus 7% shipping and handling (minimum order, $5.00).

The New Living Heart
by Michael E. DeBakey and Antonio M. Gotto, Jr.
Adams Media Corporation
260 Center Street
Holbrook, MA 02343
(800) 872-5627   (508) 767-8100
http://www.adamsmedia.com

This book discusses heart conditions such as coronary heart disease, coronary artery disease, atherosclerosis, congestive heart failure, and stroke. Includes information on surgical and medical treatment and rehabilitation. $17.95 plus $4.50 shipping and handling

Open Heart Surgery: A Personal Experience
Open Heart Surgery: Going Home
Sacred Heart Medical Center
PO Box 2555
Spokane, WA 99220-2555
(509) 458-5236   FAX (509) 626-4475
e-mail: mediaservices@shmc.org
http://www.spokanehealth.org/shmc/mediaservices

These videotapes provide an overview of surgical preparation, surgery, post-operative care, and recovery from both physical and emotional perspectives. 9 minutes each. Available in English and Spanish. Purchase, institutions, $150.00 each; for home use, $19.95 each; one week rental, $45.00 each; plus $5.00 shipping and handling for each tape.

Psychosocial Interventions for Cardiopulmonary Patients: A Guide for Health Professionals
by Wayne M. Sotile
Human Kinetics
1607 North Market Street
PO Box 5076
Champaign, IL 61825-5076
(800) 747-4457   (217) 351-5076   FAX (217) 351-2674
http://www.humankinetics.com

This book provides practical strategies for teaching patients how to manage the emotional stress of heart and lung disease. $36.00 plus $4.50 shipping and handling

Recovering From A Heart Attack
American Heart Association Fulfillment Center
200 State Road
South Deerfield, MA 01373-0200
(800) 611-6083   FAX (800) 499-6464

This videotape discusses issues such as management of medications, diet and exercise, emotions, sexuality, and returning to work. Available in English and Spanish. $29.00 plus $5.75 shipping and handling. May also be available through local affiliates' videotape lending libraries; call (800) 242-8721.

Recovering From Heart Problems Through Cardiac Rehabilitation
Agency for Health Care Policy and Research (AHCPR)
Publications Clearinghouse
PO Box 8547
Silver Spring, MD 20907
(800) 358-9295   e-mail: info@ahcpr.gov   http://www.ahcpr.gov

This booklet discusses the goals of cardiac rehabilitation and how to choose a cardiac rehabilitation program. Includes sample recordkeeping guide. Available in English and Spanish. Free

The Sensuous Heart: Sex After a Heart Attack or Heart Surgery
by Suzanne Cambre
Pritchett and Hull Associates
3440 Oakcliff Road, NE, Suite 110
Atlanta, GA 30340-3079
(800) 241-4925   http://www.ph.com

This booklet answers questions about the resumption of sexual activity after heart attack or heart surgery. Includes information about comfortable positions and the effects of medications. $5.75 plus $1.24 shipping and handling

Sex and Heart Disease
American Heart Association
7272 Greenville Avenue
Dallas, TX 75231-4596
(800) 242-8721   (214) 373-6300   FAX (214) 706-1341
http://www.americanheart.org

This brochure provides guidelines for resuming sexual activity after heart attack or heart surgery. Discusses the effects of age, medications, and psychological factors on sexual interest and activity. Free

A User's Guide to Bypass Surgery
by Ted Klein
University of Chicago Press
11030 South Langley Avenue
Chicago, IL 60628
(800) 621-2736   FAX (800) 621-8476
http://www.press.uchicago.edu

Written by a man who had bypass surgery, this book makes recommendations for finding a cardiologist and discusses alternatives to bypass surgery; describes the operation and recovery; and provides information about post-surgical diet and exercise. Includes a chapter of frequently asked questions and answers. $14.95 plus $3.50 shipping and handling

What You Should Know About P.T.C.A.
American Heart Association
7272 Greenville Avenue
Dallas, TX 75231-4596
(800) 242-8721   (214) 373-6300   FAX (214) 706-1341
http://www.americanheart.org

This brochure describes percutaneous transluminal coronary angioplasty (P.T.C.A.) treatment for coronary artery disease. Free

Chapter 5

DIABETES

Diabetes mellitus is a term that applies to a variety of disorders related to the production or utilization of insulin, a substance that is necessary to metabolize the glucose (a sugar) that the body needs for energy. As a result of diabetes, the body is unable to maintain normal glucose levels. *Hypoglycemia* is a condition where the level of glucose is too low. It occurs when the individual does not eat soon enough or eats too little, uses too much insulin, or engages in overactivity. Hypoglycemia may lead to an insulin reaction; symptoms may include feeling shaky or sweaty, headache, hunger, irritability, and dizziness. Insulin shock sometimes occurs if an insulin reaction is not treated quickly; in these cases individuals may lose consciousness. *Hyperglycemia* is a condition where the level of glucose in the blood is too high. Symptoms include extreme thirst, a dry mouth, excessive urination, blurred vision, and lethargy. Sometimes when an individual who has had an insulin reaction takes food high in sugar to replace glucose in the body, too much glucose is released, resulting in high blood glucose levels (hyperglycemia). The combination of too much sugar without enough insulin to use it properly may gradually lead to diabetic coma if warning signs are not monitored; diabetic coma usually occurs only in individuals with insulin-dependent diabetes.

As the prevalence of diabetes has increased, it has become a major health problem in the United States and an important contributor to the cost of health care. From 1980 to 1994, the number of individuals with diagnosed diabetes increased 39% (Centers for Disease Control and Prevention: 1997). Over 10 million Americans age 20 or older, or 5.1% of the population, have been diagnosed with diabetes; an additional 5.4 million have the disease but have not been diagnosed (Harris et al.: 1998). African-American males have higher rates of diabetes than white males; the overall rates are 35.9 and 28.4 per thousand respectively. Men with diabetes experience high rates of limitations in activity due to diabetes; approximately half of all men with diabetes report such limitations (Centers for Disease Control and Prevention: 1997).

Diabetes was the third most frequent primary diagnosis for individuals who visited outpatient departments in non-federal hospitals in 1994 (Lipkind: 1996). Diabetes and its complications are responsible for many hospital stays and have a large economic impact on society. Direct medical expenses for diabetes care totaled 44.1 billion dollars in 1997. Factoring in the cost of lost work productivity and premature mortality increased the cost of the disease by an additional 54 billion dollars. On a per capita basis, individuals with diabetes spent on average $10,071 in 1997 for medical care compared to $2,669 for individuals without diabetes (American Diabetes Association: 1998).

Currently, there is no cure for diabetes; however, there are means to control the disease and to decrease the risk of the numerous associated complications. Early diagnosis and intervention are crucial steps in maintaining proper control of diabetes.

Transplantations of the pancreas (the gland responsible for secreting insulin), although no longer considered experimental, are performed only in a select group of patients. Currently, transplantations are performed on patients who have end-stage renal disease, have had or plan to have a kidney transplant as well, have serious clinical difficulty with insulin injections, and do not present an excessive risk for this type of surgery (American Diabetes Association: 1996). When successful, pancreas transplantation results in the elimination of insulin injections. Rejection of transplanted tissue and the need for large amounts of immunosuppressive drugs are important factors that have prevented this type of transplantation from becoming standard procedure. Because people with diabetes are especially prone to infection, transplantation involves more risks for this population than for other individuals. Research to improve the management of diabetes through innovative administration of insulin and drugs that improve the body's use of insulin are ongoing. Transplantation of islet cells in the pancreas that are responsible for insulin production is also under investigation.

TYPES OF DIABETES

The two major types of diabetes mellitus are referred to as type 1 and type 2. In *type 1*, the pancreas does not produce insulin. Individuals with type 1 diabetes must take regular injections of insulin. For this reason, type 1 is also referred to as insulin-dependent diabetes mellitus (IDDM). This variant of the disease was formerly called juvenile-onset diabetes, because it is usually diagnosed at a young age. Symptoms of type 1 diabetes include extreme thirst, weight loss despite increased appetite, weakness and fatigue, and blurred vision.

Approximately five to ten percent of Americans who have diabetes have type 1 (Centers for Disease Control and Prevention: 1997). In addition to daily insulin injections, individuals with IDDM must carefully watch their diet and coordinate meals with insulin doses to maintain a balanced glucose level. Insulin may be injected by syringe or by "jet injectors" that do not use actual needles. Some individuals, especially those who are on erratic schedules that prevent them from eating on a regular schedule, use insulin pumps that automatically provide insulin throughout the day. The use of insulin pumps often results in improved control of blood glucose levels over other methods. Prior to eating, pump users determine the amount of insulin they need and program the pump to release that amount.

In *type 2* diabetes, the body produces some insulin but does not produce enough or does not utilize it properly. Because type 2 diabetes usually does not require insulin injections, it is also referred to as noninsulin-dependent diabetes mellitus (NIDDM). This type of the disease is often called adult-onset or maturity-onset diabetes, because it is most frequently diagnosed after age forty. It is estimated that over 90% of the cases of diabetes in the United States are type 2 (National Center for Health Statistics: 1987).

Although the causes of type 2 diabetes are not known, obesity (80 to 90% of all individuals with type 2 diabetes are obese) and a family history of diabetes are predisposing factors. Symptoms of type 2 diabetes include fatigue, frequent urination, and excessive thirst. Individuals who have these symptoms should make an appointment for a physical examination. However, diabetes is sometimes present when no symptoms are evident (Williams: 1983). Tests for glucose in urine or a blood glucose test conducted during a routine physical examination are often the first indications of diabetes.

In many cases, type 2 diabetes can be controlled through both diet and exercise. For obese individuals who have diabetes, a change in diet and reduction of caloric intake may make a dramatic difference in blood glucose levels. Research suggests that individuals with type 2 diabetes may lower their blood glucose and insulin levels throughout the day by increasing the frequency and decreasing the size of their meals. This strategy slows the rate of carbohydrate absorption. A possible disadvantage is that obese individuals who use this dietary plan may have a tendency to gain weight (Jenkins: 1995).

A subtype of diabetes caused by a defect in the mitochondrial DNA has recently been discovered. Called maternally inherited diabetes and deafness (MIDD) because the mitochondrial DNA is inherited only from the mother, this type of diabetes is associated with deafness and may be either type 1 or type 2 diabetes (Kobayashi et al.: 1997). In most cases, individuals with this type of diabetes are not obese. If they have type 2 diabetes, they usually do not need insulin in the early stages of the disease, although they may need it as the disease progresses. Protein in the urine, a sign of kidney disease, is sometimes diagnosed in individuals with MIDD; this clinical symptom is caused by the mutation, not the diabetes (Jansen et al.: 1997). A recent study of individuals with MIDD found that subjects treated with a dietary supplement, coenzyme Q10, had better outcomes in terms of beta cell production (the cells produced by the pancreas that are responsible for insulin production) and hearing than members of a control group (Suzuki et al.: 1998).

Diet and exercise for people with either type of diabetes should be planned with a physician's advice to ensure that all medical conditions are taken into account. The goals of dietary restrictions are to control the intake of glucose (carbohydrates) and to reduce total body weight for those with type 2 diabetes. Recent policy recommendations from the American Diabetes Association (1994) indicate that the use of simple sugars such as sucrose (table sugar) is not off limits and that they do not cause greater or more rapid rises in blood glucose than other carbohydrates. Scientific evidence suggests that sucrose has a similar effect on blood glucose as bread, rice, and potatoes. It is important to keep in mind the total amount of carbohydrates consumed; simple sugars must be used in place of other carbohydrates in the diet. With the new food labeling laws mandated by the federal government, this calculation becomes much easier, as the amount of carbohydrates per serving must be indicated on the food label. In order to control the amount of carbohydrates, many foods, including desserts and candies, are sweetened with artificial sweeteners. The American Diabetes Association has produced many publications about diet for people with diabetes, including "Exchange Lists" (developed jointly with the American Dietetic Association), which list foods with similar caloric and nutrient contents (see "PUBLICATIONS AND TAPES" section below).

Exercise helps the body to burn off the glucose and thus is an important part of the plan to control diabetes. In some individuals with type 2 diabetes, the muscle cells that are receptors for glucose do not work efficiently; exercise enables muscle cells to use the glucose efficiently without requiring more insulin (Cantu: 1982). Exercise also reduces fat, which is known to reduce the body's sensitivity to insulin. After consulting with a physician, even individuals who have been sedentary can begin a gradual exercise program by starting to take brief daily walks. A regular exercise regimen has been shown to be useful in reducing the required levels of daily insulin injections. Men who exercise regularly may also derive the benefits of reduced tension and increased interactions with others who join them in sports such as tennis or as jogging companions.

When diet and exercise are insufficient to control type 2 diabetes, oral medications are prescribed. Sulfonylureas are a type of medication that causes the pancreas to produce increased amounts of insulin. Side effects of this type of medication include hypoglycemia

124

and hyperinsulinemia, a condition in which too much insulin is in the bloodstream. Hyperinsulinemia is a risk factor for vascular disease and heart attack. In addition, sulfonylureas often fail to work after a number of years, as the pancreas can no longer produce sufficient insulin. When this occurs, individuals must begin injecting insulin.

Several drugs that use different mechanisms to control diabetes have recently been approved by the Food and Drug Administration (FDA). One drug that has been available throughout much of the world since the late 1950's, metformin (Glucophage), has been distributed in the United States since 1995. Although it is not clear exactly how metformin works, it is effective in lowering blood glucose levels and has no serious side effects, unless the individual has kidney disease at the outset. Another drug recently approved by the Food and Drug Administration is acarbose, a carbohydrase inhibitor. Carbohydrases are the enzymes that break down carbohydrates and turn them into glucose. The side effects of acarbose are bloating, gas, and diarrhea, which may subside after six months of taking the drug (American Diabetes Association: 1995). Troglitazone (Rezulin), another recent addition to the drug therapies available for people with type 2 diabetes, has recently been implicated in a small number of liver problems and fatalities. Although it has not been recalled, warnings have been issued so that patients on this drug have regular liver function assessments prior to and while taking the drug. Repaglinide (Prandin) was approved by the FDA in 1997 and is a fast acting drug taken anywhere from 30 minutes before until the start of a meal. It is metabolized and leaves the bloodstream after about three to four hours and is eliminated through the liver. In contrast, many other medications are eliminated through the kidneys and therefore are inappropriate for people with diabetes who have kidney disease.

Although testing urine for sugar was previously used to monitor blood glucose levels, this method is not as accurate as testing the blood directly. People with both types of diabetes use home blood glucose monitoring equipment to measure glucose levels; this involves putting a drop of blood from the fingertip on a specially treated strip designed to react to the glucose. The color of the strip indicates the level of glucose that is present. A digital display or speech output indicates the blood glucose level, and some monitors even record the date and time of the reading. Illness, even a simple cold, can affect how the body uses insulin; glucose monitoring is even more important at these times. Log booklets enable individuals to keep a record of their blood glucose levels and to analyze their diets and schedules to determine what causes them to have varying levels of blood glucose. Home blood glucose monitors are inexpensive and are quite compact, making them suitable for travel and to take to work or school.

Both types of diabetes have the same potential long term health effects. It is essential that everyone with diabetes be aware of the proper management of the disease and all of the potential complications. Complications of diabetes include greater risks of heart disease, stroke, infections, and kidney disease; circulatory problems that can be especially problematic for legs and feet (resulting in amputation in extreme cases); neuropathy or nerve disease which may cause tingling, numbness, double vision, pain, or dizziness; and vision problems. Good control of blood glucose levels can help to prevent these long term complications.

Among the leading vision problems caused by diabetes is diabetic retinopathy. Visual impairment occurs when the small blood vessels in the retina are damaged and fail to nourish the retina adequately. One consequence of this process is bleeding inside the eye. If detected early, diabetic retinopathy can sometimes be treated successfully by laser therapy. In other cases, complex surgical procedures are performed in the attempt to restore useful vision. To manage their diabetes, many people with visual impairments use a wide range of adapted equipment such as glucometers, scales, and thermometers with speech output; syringe magnifiers; special insulin gauges; and special syringes that automatically measure insulin doses.

The Diabetes Control and Complications Trial (1993) reported the results of a study which monitored 1,441 individuals with type 1 diabetes who were assigned to receive either conventional therapy (one or two injections of insulin daily) or intensive therapy (three or more injections of insulin daily). Results indicate that the intensive therapy group had a significantly lower incidence of retinopathy, nephropathy, and neuropathy. The chief adverse effect of intensive therapy was increased episodes of severe hypoglycemia. A British study carried out over a period of 20 years (UK Prospective Diabetes Study Group: 1998a) found that intensive control had similar benefits for individuals with type 2 diabetes. Individuals whose diabetes was controlled by sulfonylureas or insulin also had increased episodes of hypoglycemia. Obese individuals treated with metformin had lower risks for diabetes complications and fewer episodes of hypoglycemia than individuals treated with sulfonylureas or insulin (UK Prospective Diabetes Study Group: 1998b).

Currently, the National Institute of Diabetes and Digestive and Kidney Diseases is conducting a national study to see if type 1 diabetes can be prevented. Close relatives of individuals who have type 1 diabetes and who have a greater than 50% risk of developing the disease will be randomly assigned to an experimental group that receives two daily doses of insulin injections plus a four day hospital stay each year to receive intravenous insulin. Those who have a 25 to 50% risk of developing the disease will be randomly assigned to an experimental group that receives oral medication such as insulin and other beta cell materials. Each trial includes a control group that does not receive treatment (Diabetes Dateline: 1994). Individuals with impaired glucose tolerance are subjects in a study to learn how to prevent type 2 diabetes. Members of minority groups with high rates of type 2 diabetes, obese individuals, and women who have had gestational diabetes are assigned to test groups that undergo behavioral modification of diet and exercise or receive oral anti-diabetes medications (Diabetes Dateline: 1996).

SEXUAL FUNCTIONING

One of the many potential complications of diabetes is erectile dysfunction, a problem that may occur with either type 1 or type 2 diabetes. It has been estimated that 50% of men with diabetes experience impotence and that age is a major contributing factor (Baum: 1995; Sandowski: 1989). However, a recent population based study of men who had type 1 diabetes for at least 10 years found that only 20% reported erectile dysfunction (Klein et al.: 1996). The authors suggest that differing rates of impotence reported by other studies may be caused by the populations that they studied; in many cases, the data were derived from patients who visit clinics that specialize in diabetes and therefore attract patients with more severe disease.

There is empirical evidence to support the belief that maintaining good control of blood glucose lowers the risk of impotence (Fedele et al.: 1998; Klein et al.: 1996; Schiavi et al.:

1993). Both neuropathy, which may prevent normal transmission of nerve impulses to the blood vessels in the penis, and vascular damage, which may restrict blood flow to the penis, have been suggested as causes of impotence. A study by Benvenuti et al. (1993) found that both neurological and vascular damage can occur as soon as one year after diagnosis of diabetes, suggesting the need for early screening, even in asymptomatic patients. According to Baum (1995), it is not unusual for men who seek treatment for impotence to learn that they have diabetes, which is the cause of their impotence.

Some observers have suggested that physicians may cause psychogenic impotence in men who have diabetes by telling them that impotence is inevitable (Schover and Jensen: 1988). Depression following the diagnosis of diabetes or poor control of the disease may result in decreased interest in sexual activity. Men with poor control of their diabetes may have transient impotence due to a lack of energy; if their control improves and their energy returns, their potency also may return (Lodewick et al.: 1991). A study carried out at an impotence clinic in Britain (Veves et al.: 1995) found organic causes in the majority of diabetic subjects (65%); psychological factors were the only (11%) or the main (24%) cause in over a third of the cases and a contributing factor in 17% of the cases. Psychological counseling proved successful in 60% of the cases where it was used.

Men are often hesitant to discuss sexual problems with health care providers. They should understand that most cases of impotence can be resolved, once the cause is determined. As in all cases of impotence, a history of sexual functioning should be conducted and, if necessary, a sex counselor should provide therapy. To determine if the cause of the impotence is organic, several tests may be performed by the urologist in the office, including tests of nerve function and blood pressure in the penis and possible blockages in the blood vessels. If the results of these tests are normal, then the cause of impotence is likely to be psychological and should be treated with psychotherapy with an experienced counselor. If the cause is organic, the man has several options.

One option involves injecting drugs directly into the base of the penis; these drugs dilate the arteries and increase the blood flow to the penis. This method is relatively inexpensive and has minimal side effects if used properly. However, men with diabetes often do not succeed with this treatment because of the damage to their vascular system (Ryder et al.: 1992). Older men are less likely to succeed with this treatment than younger men (Bell et al.: 1992). When urologists test men to determine the cause of their impotence, they often use penile injections to determine if vascular problems exist. Therefore, a test in the urologist's office should determine immediately whether this treatment will work.

Vacuum pump devices create a partial vacuum around the penis, drawing blood into the penis and causing an erection. The device consists of a plastic cylinder placed over the penis; a pump which draws air out of the cylinder; and an elastic band placed at the base of the penis to maintain the erection. The vacuum pump does not have any side effects and works satisfactorily in most cases (Nadig: 1994).

Penile implants should be considered only when other treatments have failed. Penile implants may be semi-rigid or inflatable. Possible complications include infection and mechanical malfunction, requiring replacement. Men with diabetes are at high risk for implant failure due to infection, especially those men whose diabetes is not in good control (Bishop et al.: 1992). If penile implants must be removed due to recurrent infection, the man permanently loses the ability to have an erection.

The introduction of oral drugs to overcome erectile dysfunction offers another option for men with diabetes. Sildenafil, more commonly known as Viagra, has recently been approved for use in the United States. A study of men with diabetes in Britain (Price et al.: 1998) found that Viagra resulted in improved erections in half of the subjects and was well tolerated with only minor side effects.

Men with diabetes may have difficulty ejaculating, or their semen volume may be decreased (Schover and Jensen: 1988). Electroejaculation, a procedure in which an electric probe is inserted in the rectum, stimulating the prostate and enabling the collection of semen for artificial insemination, may solve the problem for these men. The procedure is done under anesthesia because of the pain involved. Couples considering this method should understand that the procedure may need to be repeated several times and that a successful pregnancy is not guaranteed.

PSYCHOLOGICAL ASPECTS OF DIABETES

Although shock, fear, and depression are normal reactions to diabetes at first, these emotions may subside once the individual understands how to control the disease. Many men feel a loss of control over their bodies. Because diabetes affects so many parts of the body, it also affects many aspects of daily life. In addition to prescribed changes in diet and exercise, men with diabetes must always be aware of the symptoms that indicate hyperglycemia or hypoglycemia. Individuals who must take daily injections of insulin may have to overcome a fear of needles. According to one diabetologist, often men who appear to be physically strong are the most afraid of needles, affecting their ability to monitor blood glucose and inject insulin (Lodewick et al.: 1996). Talking with others who have experienced this fear and overcome it may prove extremely valuable.

Unlike many disabling illnesses, diabetes can be controlled by a change in lifestyle; eating an appropriate diet, exercising, and cessation of smoking are all important aspects of self-management. Since diabetes is sometimes asymptomatic in the short run, especially with adult onset type 2 diabetes, some men may resist making these changes, while their wives may view the disease more seriously and prod them to change. In some cases, wives may view the disease less seriously and be unwilling to adhere to the restrictions imposed by good self-management. The threat of disability or even death may provoke one spouse to focus energy on imminent disability and fail to make an emotional investment in the current status of the marriage. No matter which spouse holds the perspective that the disease is serious, differences between spouses' perspectives may cause friction in the marital relationship (Peyrot et al.: 1988).

For men with diabetes, changes in lifestyle and the need to monitor glucose may cause great stress. Some men may keep their diabetes a secret for fear of appearing weak or losing their jobs. A more positive approach is to plan daily activities, social events, and travel carefully to ensure that meals will comply with special diets. Selecting exercise that is enjoyable ensures that it will be carried out.

The diagnosis of diabetes may result in the fear that most food is off limits and that it will be impossible to enjoy eating. The knowledge that people with diabetes should eat what is considered a healthy diet for the general public as long as they keep track of their carbohydrate intake may prove comforting to men who have recently been diagnosed with diabetes. In addition, a number of food manufacturers cater to the dietary needs of individuals with diabetes by producing foods that are low in carbohydrates; their products are often available in the dietetic food section of supermarkets. Perseverance in tracking down the right foods will allow for an interesting and varied diet; however, the shock and depression that follow the diagnosis of diabetes may limit the man's emotional endurance. Support from a family member or close friend can help the man with diabetes to carry out this endeavor.

Public libraries are a good source for the myriad cookbooks that have been written specially for people with diabetes. Discovering the variety of interesting recipes, including those for dessert and candies, should prove to be a psychological boost for the man who fears being restricted to bland meals.

Diabetes in adolescent boys and teenagers may be especially difficult to deal with. The youth culture places a strong emphasis on physical appearance and conformity. Having a restricted diet and taking insulin injections make boys with diabetes feel different and have a low sense of self-esteem. As they are developing sexually, boys do not want to appear sickly or weak. It is not uncommon for teenagers to deny their diabetes, falsify their blood glucose levels, and eat inappropriate foods (Weissberg-Benchell et al.: 1995). Such behavior may result in stunting their growth and their sexual development. Parents should make sure that their sons with diabetes understand the consequences of these actions and monitor their diets as well as their blood glucose. Teenage boys should understand that while impotence is a potential complication, good control lowers the risk.

Diligent efforts to control glucose by following the recommended dosages of insulin or diets do not always result in the desired response. Individuals whose glucose is out of control should learn not to feel guilty; they may need to have their dosage and diet modified on the advice of a health care professional.

A common response to adult-onset or type 2 diabetes is that "It's just a touch of diabetes." This response is a form of denial and can be extremely dangerous when the individual fails to properly monitor and control the disease. Men with diabetes and their family members must discuss the disease and its potential effects so that they understand the importance of the prescribed dietary regimen, exercise, and blood glucose monitoring.

PROFESSIONAL SERVICE PROVIDERS

Because diabetes is a systemic disease, it has a wide range of effects. As a result, many types of health care professionals are involved in caring for people with diabetes.

Family physicians and *internists* are the physicians in charge of coordinating the various aspects of care for individuals with diabetes. *Diabetologists* (endocrinologists) are physicians who specialize in the treatment of individuals with diabetes. *Nephrologists* are physicians who treat people with kidney disease, which is a common complication of diabetes. *Ophthalmologists* are physicians who specialize in diseases of the eye. If diabetic retinopathy is detected, individuals are often referred to subspecialists called retina and vitreous specialists.

Urologists specialize in treatment of kidneys, the bladder, the ureter, and the urethra. Urologists treat men with sexual dysfunction by performing diagnostic tests to determine the cause of the impotence, prescribing vacuum devices or pharmacologic treatment, and performing surgery to implant penile prostheses.

Certified diabetes educators (CDE) are health care professionals certified by the American Association of Diabetes Educators to teach individuals with diabetes how to effectively manage their disease. Certified diabetes educators may be physicians or nurses. Many are dietitians or nutritionists who help people with diabetes plan a diet to control their blood glucose levels.

Psychologists, *social workers*, and other counselors help people with diabetes and their family members adjust to the regimen prescribed to control the diabetes and deal with complications, including sexual function.

WHERE TO FIND SERVICES

In some areas, special treatment centers for diabetes and dialysis centers for people with kidney disease are available. Some of these centers have special divisions for the treatment of impotence and sexual problems. The special physicians listed above practice in hospitals or have private practices. Affiliates of the American Diabetes Association (ADA) exist in every state. These affiliates may provide publications, educational programs, sponsor camps for children with diabetes, and make referrals to local resources. The national office (described in the "ORGANIZATIONS" section below) can provide the address and phone number of local affiliates. The ADA also has information about support groups that individuals can join. Understanding that others with diabetes continue to live fulfilling lives can be an extremely important benefit of attending support groups.

ASSISTIVE DEVICES

Individuals with type 1 diabetes use a variety of devices to administer their insulin, such as syringes; insulin pens which combine the insulin dose and injector; needle-free jet injectors; and insulin pumps, which automatically deliver insulin slowly throughout the day and night through a plastic tube attached to a needle. Equipment to measure blood glucose is necessary for both type 1 and type 2 diabetes. Some health insurance policies will pay some of the costs for glucose monitors and test strips. It is wise to check with the insurance carrier before purchasing such equipment.

Supplies and equipment to help individuals with diabetes to monitor and manage their disease are usually available at pharmacies or medical supply stores. Mail order catalogues also sell these supplies.

HOW TO RECOGNIZE AN INSULIN REACTION AND GIVE FIRST AID

Individuals experiencing an insulin reaction may feel shaky or dizzy, sweat profusely, complain of a headache, or act irritable. Suggestions for giving first aid to individuals who have had an insulin reaction are:

- Give the individual some food, such as orange juice, milk, or even sugar itself, to replace the low blood sugar level. Many individuals with diabetes carry sugar packets, glucose tablets, or candy with them for use in emergencies.
- If the individual is unconscious, rub honey or another sugary substance into the mouth, between the teeth and cheek.

Frequent insulin reactions should be reported to the physician. It is recommended that individuals with diabetes wear a medical identification bracelet so that emergency care personnel will know that they have diabetes.

References

American Diabetes Association
1998 "Economic Consequences of Diabetes Mellitus in the U.S. in 1997" Diabetes Care 21:2(February):296-309
1996 "Pancreas Transplantation for Patients with Diabetes Mellitus" Diabetes Care 19(January):Supplement 1:S39
1995 "Surge Protector" Diabetes Forecast 48(May)5:23-24
1994 "Nutrition Recommendations and Principles for People with Diabetes Mellitus" Diabetes Care 17(May)5:519-522
Baum, Neil
1995 "Overcoming Impotence" Diabetes Self-Management 12(July/August)4:29-34
Bell, D. S. et al.
1992 "Factors Predicting Efficacy of Phentolamine-Papaverine Intracorporeal Injection for Treatment of Erectile Dysfunction in Diabetic Male" Urology 40:1(July):36-40
Benvenuti, F. et al.
1993 "Male Sexual Impotence in Diabetes Mellitus: Vasculogenic versus Neurogenic Factors" Neurologic Urodynamics 12:2:145-151
Bishop, J. R. et al.
1992 "Use of Glycosylated Hemoglobin to Identify Diabetics at High Risk for Penile Periprosthetic Infections" Journal of Urology 147:2(February):386-388
Cantu, Robert C.
1982 Diabetes and Exercise New York, NY: E.P. Dutton
Centers for Disease Control and Prevention
1997 Diabetes Surveillance 1997 Atlanta, GA: Public Health Service
Diabetes Control and Complications Trial Research Group
1993 "The Effect of Intensive Treatment of Diabetes on the Development and Progression of Long-Term Complications in Insulin-Dependent Diabetes Mellitus" New England Journal of Medicine 329(September 30):14:977-986
Diabetes Dateline
1996 "Volunteers Sought for NIDDK Studies" Diabetes Dateline Fall p. 4
1994 "NIDDK Launches Study to Prevent Insulin-Dependent Diabetes" Diabetes Dateline May pp. 1-2

Fedele, Domenico et al.

1998 "Erectile Dysfunction in Diabetic Subjects in Italy" <u>Diabetes Care</u> 21:11(November):1973-1977

Harris, Maureen I. et al.

1998 "Prevalence of Diabetes, Impaired Fasting Glucose, and Impaired Glucose Tolerance in U.S. Adults" <u>Diabetes Care</u> 21:4(April):518-524

Jansen, J. J. et al.

1997 "Mutation in Mitochondrial tRNA (Leu(UUR)) Gene Associated with Progressive Kidney Disease" <u>Journal of the American Society of Nephrology</u> 8:7(July):1118-1124

Jenkins, David J. A.

1995 "Nutritional Principles and Diabetes" <u>Diabetes Care</u> 18(November)11:1491-1498

Klein, Ronald et al.

1996 "Prevalence of Self-Reported Erectile Dysfunction in People with Long-Term IDDM" <u>Diabetes Care</u> 19(February):2:135-140

Kobayashi, Tetsuro et al.

1997 "In Situ Characterization of Islets in Diabetes with a Mitochondrial DNA Mutation at Nucleotide Position 3243" <u>Diabetes</u> 46:1-(October):1567-15710

Lipkind, Karen L.

1996 "National Hospital Ambulatory Medical Care Survey: 1994 Outpatient Department Summary" <u>Advance Data from Vital and Health Statistics</u>, No. 276, Hyattsville, MD: National Center for Health Statistics, June 11

Lodewick, Peter, June Biermann, and Barbara Toohey

1996 <u>The Diabetic Man</u> Los Angeles, CA: Lowell House

Nadig, Perry W.

1994 "Vacuum Constriction Devices in Patients with Neurogenic Impotence" <u>Sexuality and Disability</u> 12:1:99-105

National Center for Health Statistics

1987 "Health Practices and Perceptions of U.S. Adults with Noninsulin-Dependent Diabetes. Data from the 1985 National Health Interview Survey of Health Promotion and Disease Prevention" <u>Advance Data from Vital and Health Statistics</u>, No. 141, DHHS Pub. No. (PHS) 87-1250. Public Health Service, Hyattsville, MD September 23

Peyrot, Mark, James F. McMurry, Jr. and Richard Hedges

1988 "Marital Adjustment to Adult Diabetes: Interpersonal Congruence and Spouse Satisfaction" <u>Journal of Marriage and the Family</u> 50(May):363-376

Price, D. E. et al.

1998 "Sildenafil: Study of a Novel Oral Treatment for Erectile Dysfunction in Diabetic Men" <u>Diabetic Medicine</u> 15:10(October):821-825

Ryder, R. E.

1992 "Impotence in Diabetes: Aetiology, Implications for Treatment and Preferred Vacuum Device" <u>Diabetic Medicine</u> 9:10(December):893-898

Sandowski, Carol L.

1989 <u>Sexual Concerns When Illness or Disability Strikes</u> Springfield, IL: Charles C. Thomas Publishers

Schiavi, R. C. et al.

1993 "Diabetes Mellitus and Male Sexual Function: A Controlled Study" <u>Diabetologia</u> 36:8(August):745-51

Schover, Leslie and Soren Buus Jensen

1988 <u>Sexuality and Chronic Illness: A Comprehensive Approach</u> New York, NY: Guilford Press

Suzuki, S. et al.

1998 "The Effects of Coenzyme Q10 Treatment on Maternally Inherited Diabetes and Deafness and Mitochondrial DNA 3243 (A to G) Mutation" <u>Diabetologia</u> 41:5(May):584-588

UK Prospective Diabetes Study Group

1998a "Intensive Blood-Glucose Control with Sulphonylureas or Insulin Compared with Conventional Treatment and Risk of Complications in Patients with Type 2 Diabetes" <u>The Lancet</u> 352(September 12):837-853

1998b "Effect of Intensive Blood-Glucose Control with Metformin on Complications in Overweight Patients with Type 2 Diabetes" <u>The Lancet</u> 352(September 12):854-865

Veves, A. et al.

1995 "Aetopathogenesis and Management of Impotence in Diabetes Males: Four Years Experience from a Combined Clinic" <u>Diabetic Medicine</u> 12:1(January):77-82

Weissberg-Benchell, Jill et al.

1995 "Adolescent Diabetes Management and Mismanagement" <u>Diabetes Care</u> 18(January)1:77-82

Williams, T. Franklin

1983 "Diabetes Mellitus in Older People" pp. 411-415 in William Reichel (ed.) <u>Clinical Aspects of Aging</u> Baltimore, MD: Williams and Wilkins

ORGANIZATIONS

American Amputee Foundation
PO Box 250218
Little Rock, AR 72225
(501) 666-2523   FAX (501) 666-8367

A national information clearinghouse and referral center. Provides technical assistance in starting self-help groups and sponsors self-help groups across the country. Membership, $25.00, includes newsletter and "AAF National Resource Directory."

American Association of Diabetes Educators (AADE)
100 West Monroe, Suite 400
Chicago, IL 60603-1901
(800) 338-3633   (312) 644-2233   FAX (312) 424-2427
http://www.aadenet.org

Membership organization for health care professionals who work with people with diabetes. Holds annual meeting. Membership, $85.00, includes a bimonthly journal, "The Diabetes Educator," $45.00. Journal only, $45.00.

American Association of Kidney Patients
100 South Ashley Drive, Suite 280
Tampa, FL 33602
(800) 749-2257   (813) 223-7099   FAX (813) 223-0001
e-mail: AAKPnat@aol.com   http://www.aakp.org

Advocates on behalf of patients with kidney disease; sponsors local patient and family support groups; holds conferences and seminars. Membership, patients/families, $25.00; professionals, $35.00; includes quarterly newsletter, "aakpRENALIFE."

American Diabetes Association (ADA)
1660 Duke Street
Alexandria, VA 22314
(800) 232-3472   In the Washington, DC, (703) 549-1500
FAX (703) 836-7439   http://www.diabetes.org

National membership organization with local affiliates. Publications for both professionals and consumers, including cookbooks and guides for the management of diabetes (see "PUBLIC-ATIONS AND TAPES" section below). Membership, $24.00, includes discounts on publications, a subscription to "Diabetes Forecast" (Also available on disc from the National Library Service. Many local affiliates offer their own publications, sponsor support groups, and conduct professional training programs. The web site includes featured articles from "Diabetes Forecast" and the medical journal "Diabetes Care."

American Kidney Fund
6110 Executive Boulevard, Suite 1010
Rockville, MD 20852
(800) 638-8299   (301) 881-3052   FAX (301) 881-0898
e-mail:clhpe@akfinc.org   http://www.arbon.com/kidney/home.htm

Provides public and professional education and financial aid to individuals who have chronic kidney problems.

Amputee Coalition of America (ACA)
National Limb Loss Information Center
900 East Hill Avenue, Suite 285
Knoxville, TN 37915-2568
(888) 267-5669   (423) 524-8772   FAX (423) 525-7917
e-mail: ACAONE@aol.com   http://www.amputee-coalition.org

Provides education and support services to individuals with amputations through a network of peer support groups, educational programs for health professionals, and a database of resources. Membership, individuals, $25.00; professionals, $50.00; amputee support groups, $75.00; includes magazine, "In-Motion." Guides for organizing peer support groups and peer visitation programs also available.

Centers for Disease Control and Prevention (CDC)
1600 Clifton Road, NE
Atlanta, GA 30333
(770) 488-5024   http://www.cdc.gov

The Division of Diabetes Translation conducts research related to the prevalence of diabetes; assesses clinical practices in order to develop optimal treatment; and works with state health departments to develop diabetes control programs.

Diabetes Action Network, National Federation of the Blind
811 Cherry Street, Suite 309
Columbia, MD 65201
(573) 875-8911 (V/FAX)   http://www.nfb.org/diabetes.htm

A national support and information network. Regular membership, $10.00. Publishes a quarterly magazine, "Voice of the Diabetic," which includes personal experiences, medical information, recipes, and resources. Available in standard print, four-track audiocassette, and on the web site. Free for members; nonmembers may also obtain free subscriptions but are encouraged to donate $20.00. Also available, "Resource Guide to Aids and Appliances," a list of adaptive equipment; large print, audiocassette, and braille, $2.00.

Impotence Information Center
PO Box 9
Minneapolis, MN 55440
(800) 843-4315   http://www.ammedsys.com

Sponsored by American Medical Systems, Inc., a subsidiary of Pfizer, Inc., this center provides free information and physician referrals. Pfizer is the manufacturer of Viagra.

Impotence World Institute (IWI)
PO Box 410
Bowie, MD 20718-0410
(800) 669-1603   (301) 262-2400   FAX (301) 262-6825
e-mail: IWABOWIE@aol.com   http://www.impotenceworld.org

A membership organization with support groups throughout the country, including Impotents Anonymous (IA) and I-ANON (for partners). Produces a variety of fact sheets, books, videotapes, and audiotapes that address the various causes and treatments for impotence. Operates a help line and makes referrals to physicians. Membership, $25.00, includes quarterly newsletter, "Impotence Worldwide."

International Diabetic Athletes Association (IDAA)
1647-B West Bethany Home Road
Phoenix, AZ 85015
(800) 898-4322   (602) 433-2113   FAX (602) 433-9331
e-mail: idaa@diabetes-exercise.org
http://www.diabetes-exercise.org

An organization that provides education for individuals with diabetes who participate in sports and fitness activities, family members, and service providers through conferences, workshops, and publications. Membership, individual, $20.00; corporate, $150.00; includes quarterly newsletter, "The Challenge."

Juvenile Diabetes Foundation International (JDF)
The Diabetes Research Foundation
120 Wall Street, 19th Floor
New York, NY 10005-4001
(800) 223-1138   (212) 785-9500   FAX (212) 785-9595
e-mail: info@jdfcure.com   http://www.jdfcure.com

Supports research and provides information to individuals with diabetes and their families. Chapters in many states and affiliates in other countries. Membership, $25.00, includes quarterly magazine, "Countdown" and discounts on books.

National Center for Nutrition and Dietetics
American Dietetic Association
216 West Jackson Boulevard
Chicago, IL 60606
Consumer Nutrition Hot-line (800) 366-1655
(312) 899-0040   FAX (312) 899-1758
http://www.eatright.org

Callers may receive a referral to a registered dietitian or listen to recorded nutrition messages in English and Spanish. Customized food and nutrition information from a registered dietitian is available by calling (900) 225-5267; the cost of a call is $1.95 for the first minute, $.95 for each minute thereafter. Free publications.

National Institute of Diabetes and Digestive and Kidney Diseases (NIDDK)
National Institutes of Health
31 Center Drive, MSC 2560
Building 31, Room 9A-04
Bethesda, MD 20892-2560
(301) 496-3583   http://www.niddk.nih.gov/

Funds basic and clinical research in the causes, prevention, and treatment of diabetes. Free list of publications. The web site contains fact sheets and patient education materials.

National Kidney and Urologic Diseases Information Clearinghouse (NKUDIC)
3 Information Way
Bethesda, MD 20892-3580
(301) 654-4415   FAX (301) 907-8906
e-mail: nddic@info.niddk.nih.gov   http://www.niddk.nih.gov

Responds to individual requests from the public and professionals about diseases of the kidneys and urologic system. Publishes quarterly newsletter, "KU Notes," free. Free list of publications.

National Kidney Foundation (NKF)
30 East 33rd Street
New York, NY 10016
(800) 622-9010   (212) 889-2210   FAX (212) 689-9261
http://www.kidney.org

A professional membership organization that provides professional and public education; produces literature on kidney disease; and promotes kidney transplantation and organ donation.

<u>Neuropathy Association</u>
PO Box 2055
Lenox Hill Station
New York, NY 10021
(800) 247-6968   (212) 692-0662
e-mail: info@neuropathy.org   http://www.neuropathy.org

This organization serves individuals who experience neuropathy and their family members through the support of research into the causes and treatments of neuropathy, education, and dissemination of information.

Buyer's Guide to Diabetes Products
American Diabetes Association (ADA)
Order Fulfillment
PO Box 930850
Atlanta, GA 31193-0850
(800) 232-6733   FAX (404) 442-9742

This guide compares prices and features for a wide variety of products for people with diabetes. $4.95 plus $4.99 shipping and handling

Carbohydrate Gram Counter
by Corinne T. Netzer
Distribution Service
Bantam Doubleday Dell Books
2451 South Wolf Road
Des Plaines, IL 60018
(800) 223-5780   FAX (800) 233-3294   http://www.bantam.com

A comprehensive listing of the carbohydrates in fresh foods as well as packaged foods. $5.99 plus $2.50 shipping and handling

Coping with Kidney Failure
by Robert H. Phillips
Avery Publishing Group
120 Old Broadway
Garden City Park, NY 11040
(800) 548-5757   (516) 741-2155   FAX (516) 742-1892
e-mail: averypubg@aol.com

This book provides information on kidney dialysis and transplants for individuals with end-stage renal failure. $12.95 plus $3.50 shipping and handling

Coping with Limb Loss
by Ellen Winchell
Avery Publishing Group
120 Old Broadway
Garden City Park, NY 11040
(800) 548-5757   (516) 741-2155   FAX (516) 742-1892
e-mail: averypubg@aol.com

Written by a woman who had a limb amputated, this book provides information about surgery, prosthetics, and rehabilitation as well as practical coping strategies. $14.95 plus $3.50 shipping and handling

Diabetes and the Kidneys
American Kidney Fund
6110 Executive Boulevard, Suite 1010
Rockville, MD 20852
(800) 638-8299   (301) 881-3052   FAX (301) 881-0898
e-mail: clhpe@akfinc.org   http://www.arbon.com/kidney/home.htm

A booklet that describes how diabetes affects the kidneys' function and measures that may be taken to slow down the course of kidney disease. Available in standard print and large print. Free

Diabetes: Caring for Your Emotions As Well as Your Health
by Jerry Edelwich and Archie Brodsky
Harper Collins
PO Box 588
Scranton, PA 18512
(800) 331-3761   http://www.harpercollins.com

In addition to describing diabetes and its treatment, this book discusses the many effects diabetes has on social and psychological aspects of life. Practical suggestions for adaptation and relationships with medical personnel and family are provided. Information about sexual function, employment, technology, and support groups is also included. $15.00 plus $2.75 shipping and handling

Diabetes Self-Management
PO Box 52890
Boulder, CO 80321
(800) 234-0923

A bimonthly magazine that helps people with diabetes manage their disease. Tips on diet, foot care, medical news, etc. 1 year, $18.00; 2 years, $36.00

Diabetes: The Role of Insulin
AIMS Media
9710 DeSoto Avenue
Chatsworth, CA 91311
(800) 367-2467   (818) 773-4300   FAX (818) 341-6700
http://www.aims-multimedia.com

This videotape describes how body cells use insulin and the causes and treatments for hypoglycemia and hyperglycemia. 18 minutes. $49.95 plus $8.95 shipping and handling

Diabetes Treated with Insulin: A Short Guide
Joslin Diabetes Center
Publications Department
One Joslin Place
Boston, MA 02215
(800) 344-4501   (617) 732-2429   FAX (617) 732-2562
http://www.joslin.org

Written for individuals with diabetes who read at a fourth grade level or those who speak English as a second language. $10.50 plus $3.50 shipping and handling

Diabetes, Visual Impairment, and Group Support: A Guidebook
by Judith Caditz
The Center for the Partially Sighted
720 Wilshire Boulevard, Suite 200
Santa Monica, CA 90401-1713
(310) 458-3501   FAX (310) 458-8179
e-mail: lowvision@compuserve.com

Written by a woman with type 1 diabetes, this guidebook is designed for individuals with diabetes and vision loss, their families, and professionals. Discusses diabetes mellitus, how it affects vision, psychosocial aspects, diet, assistive devices, and organizing education/support groups. Available in standard print and large print. $12.95 plus $2.50 shipping and handling

The Diabetic Man
by Peter Lodewick, June Biermann, and Barbara Toohey
NTC/Contemporary Publishing Group
4255 West Touhy Avenue
Lincolnwood, IL 60646-1975
(800) 323-4900   FAX (847) 679-2494

Written in question and answer format, this book addresses the effects that diabetes has on men, including information on diet, sports, exercise, psychological aspects, and sex. Many case examples are presented throughout the book. Peter Lodewick is a diabetologist who has diabetes himself, as does June Biermann. $16.00 plus $5.00 shipping and handling

Diabetic Retinopathy: Information for Patients
National Eye Institute (NEI)
Building 31, Room 6A32
Bethesda, MD 20892
(301) 496-5248   http://www.nei.nih.gov

This booklet discusses the symptoms of diabetic retinopathy; treatment; vitrectomy; and research. Available free in large print from NEI and on audiocassette ($2.00) from VISION Community Services, 818 Mt. Auburn Street, Watertown, MA 02472.

The Diabetic's Book
by June Biermann and Barbara Toohey
Penguin Putnam
PO Box 12289
Newark, NJ 07101-5289
(800) 253-6476   FAX (201) 896-8569
http://www.penguin.com

This book answers basic questions about diabetes, including diet, exercise, management of the disease, emotional responses, and other aspects of daily life. June Biermann has had type 2 diabetes since 1965. $13.95 plus $2.50 shipping and handling

The Diabetic Traveler
PO Box 8223 RW
Stamford, CT 06905
(203) 327-5832

Quarterly newsletter that focuses on safe and secure travel; special articles on popular travel destinations. $18.95

Don't Lose Sight of Diabetic Eye Disease: Information for People at Risk
National Eye Institute (NEI)
Building 31, Room 6A32
Bethesda, MD 20892
(301) 496-5248   http://www.nei.nih.gov

This booklet describes how diabetes affects the eyes and problems such as cataract, glaucoma, and diabetic retinopathy. Discusses symptoms, diagnosis, and treatment of diabetic retinopathy. Free in large print from NEI; on audiocassette ($2.00) from VISION Community Services, 818 Mt. Auburn Street, Watertown, MA 02472.

Exchange Lists for Meal Planning
American Diabetes Association (ADA)
Order Fulfillment
PO Box 930850
Atlanta, GA 31193-0850
(800) 232-6733   FAX (404) 442-9742

This guide lists foods based on carbohydrate, protein, and fat content. Members, $1.20;
nonmembers, $1.50; plus $4.99 shipping and handling.

The Fitness Book: For People with Diabetes
American Diabetes Association (ADA)
Order Fulfillment
PO Box 930850
Atlanta, GA 31193-0850
(800) 232-6733   FAX (404) 442-9742

This book discusses the benefits of exercise as well as specific exercise programs to control
diabetes. $18.95 plus $4.99 shipping and handling

The Johns Hopkins Guide to Diabetes for Today and Tomorrow
by Christopher D. Saudek, Richard R. Rubin, and Cynthia Shump
Johns Hopkins University Press
2715 North Charles Street
Baltimore, MD 21218
(800) 537-5487   FAX (410) 516-6998
http://muse.jhu.edu/press

Written by a physician, a psychologist, and a nurse who specialize in treating individuals with
diabetes, this book provides basic information on diabetes and its treatment, emotional and
social aspects of the disease, complications, and sexuality and reproduction. $16.95 plus
$4.00 shipping and handling

Know Your Diabetes, Know Yourself
Joslin Diabetes Center, Publications Department
One Joslin Place
Boston, MA 02215
(800) 344-4501   (617) 732-2429   FAX (617) 732-2562
http://www.joslin.org

In this videotape, Joslin patients (not actors) talk about the daily issues of diabetes management: using a meal plan; the important roles exercise, monitoring, injections, and foot and eye
care play in their lives; and how they manage their disease when sick or traveling. Joslin

health professionals discuss the essentials of good diabetes care. 60 minutes. $39.50 plus $3.95 shipping and handling

Learning to Live Well with Diabetes
by Donnell D. Etzwiler et al.
International Diabetes Center
3800 Park Nicollet Boulevard
Minneapolis, MN 55123
(612) 993-3874   FAX (612) 993-1302
e-mail: idcpub@found.hsmnet.com http://www.idcdiabetes.com

This collection of articles written by experts addresses current medical treatments and research and how to live an active life with diabetes. $24.95 plus $4.00 shipping and handling

Living with Diabetes $1.75 per copy
Living with Diabetic Retinopathy $1.75 per copy
Resources for Rehabilitation
33 Bedford Street, Suite 19A
Lexington, MA 02420
(781) 862-6455   FAX (781) 861-7517
e-mail: info@rfr.org   http://www.rfr.org

Designed for distribution by professionals to people with diabetes, these large print (18 point bold type) publications describe the condition, service providers, organizations, devices, and publications. Minimum purchase 25 copies. (See order form on last page of this book.)

Living with Diabetes: A Winning Formula
Info Vision
102 North Hazel Street
Glenwood, IA 51534
(800) 237-1808   FAX (888) 735-2622

This videotape provides information about diet, weight loss, insulin, and self-monitoring of blood glucose and gives recipes. 35 minutes. $25.00 plus $5.00 shipping and handling

Living with Low Vision: A Resource Guide for People with Sight Loss
Resources for Rehabilitation
33 Bedford Street, Suite 19A
Lexington, MA 02420
(781) 862-6455   FAX (781) 861-7517
e-mail: info@rfr.org   http://www.rfr.org

A large print (18 point bold type) comprehensive directory that helps people with sight loss locate the services that they need to remain independent. Chapters describe products that

144

enable people to keep reading, working, and carrying out their daily activities. Information about resources on the Internet is included. $44.95 plus $5.00 shipping and handling (See order form on last page of this book.)

Managing Diabetes on a Budget
by Leslie Y. Dawson
American Diabetes Association (ADA)
Order Fulfillment
PO Box 930850
Atlanta, GA 31193-0850
(800) 232-6733   FAX (404) 442-9742

This book provides advice on finding the best buys on supplies and medications, cooking tips, and general diabetes management. $7.95 plus $4.99 shipping and handling

Monitoring Your Blood Sugar
Juvenile Diabetes Foundation
The Diabetes Research Foundation
120 Wall Street, 19th Floor, New York, NY 10005
(800) 223-1138   (212) 889-7575   FAX (212) 785-9595
e-mail: info@jdfcure.com   http://www.jdfcure.com

This brochure describes the process and benefits of blood glucose monitoring. Free

National Diabetes Information Clearinghouse (NDIC)
1 Information Way
Bethesda, MD 20892-3560
(301) 654-3327   FAX (301) 907-8906
e-mail: ndic@info.niddk.nih.gov   http://www.niddk.nih.gov/Brochures/NDIC.htm

Sponsored by the federal government, this clearinghouse publishes a variety of booklets related to diabetes. Titles include "The Diabetes Dictionary," a glossary of terms individuals with diabetes are likely to encounter; "Noninsulin-Dependent Diabetes" and "Insulin-Dependent Diabetes," two booklets that describe the prevalence, causes, and treatments for each type of diabetes; "Diabetes and Periodontal Disease," a brochure describing the nature of periodontal disease, its relation to diabetes, and proper care of teeth and gums for diabetics (free); and "Diabetic Neuropathy: The Nerve Damage of Diabetes;" free.

Take Charge of Your Diabetes
National Diabetes Information Clearinghouse (NDIC)
1 Information Way
Bethesda, MD 20892-3560
(301) 654-3327   FAX (301) 907-8906
e-mail: ndic@info.niddk.nih.gov   http://www.niddk.nih.gov/Brochures/NDIC.htm

A book written in simple language and printed in large type to help people with diabetes manage their disease. Information on blood sugar, dental, foot, vision, and kidney problems, and nerve damage. Includes forms for keeping records of visits with health care providers and sick days. Free

A Touch of Diabetes: A Straightforward Guide for People Who Have Type 2, Non-insulin Dependent Diabetes
by Lois Jovanovic-Peterson, Charles M. Peterson, and Morton Stone
John Wiley and Sons
1 John Wiley Drive
Somerset, NJ 08875
(800) 225-5945   (908) 469-4400   FAX (908) 302-2300
http://www.wiley.com

This guide to help people with type 2 diabetes manage their condition includes information about preventing complications and dietary advice. $13.95

Type 2 Diabetes: Your Healthy Living Guide
American Diabetes Association (ADA)
Order Fulfillment
PO Box 930850
Atlanta, GA 31193-0850
(800) 232-6733   FAX (404) 442-9742

A guidebook that helps people with type 2 diabetes manage their disease through proper diet, exercise, and the safe use of medications. $16.95 plus $4.99 shipping and handling

The Uncomplicated Guide to Diabetes Complications
by Marvin E. Levin and Michael A. Pfeifer
American Diabetes Association (ADA)
Order Fulfillment
PO Box 930850
Atlanta, GA 31193-0850
(800) 232-6733   FAX (404) 442-9742

This book covers the major complications that diabetes may cause, including nephropathy, heart disease, stroke, and neuropathy. Special issues such as obesity and hypoglycemia are also discussed. $18.95 plus $4.99 shipping and handling

<u>Weight Management for Type II Diabetes: An Action Plan</u>
by Jackier Labat and Annette Maggi
John Wiley and Sons
1 John Wiley Drive
Somerset, NJ 08875
(800) 225-5945   (908) 469-4400   FAX (908) 302-2300
http://www.wiley.com

This book provides recommendations for lifestyle changes for weight control and good diabetes management. $12.95

Chapter 6

HIV/AIDS

The human immunodeficiency virus (HIV) was discovered in 1981 and since that time has infected millions of people worldwide. People infected with the virus may remain asymptomatic for many years. When HIV has caused severe suppression of the immune system's ability to respond to disease, the individual is subject to a wide variety of opportunistic diseases that the healthy person's immune system is able to fend off. Individuals who experience these diseases are diagnosed as having acquired immunodeficiency syndrome (AIDS). AIDS is not a disease in and of itself but is the group of diseases that occur in association with the effects of HIV. As treatment for HIV/AIDS improves, people are living longer, although it is not uncommon for them to experience disabilities that impair their lifestyles. For this reason, HIV/AIDS should be viewed as a chronic condition that requires both medical and rehabilitation services to enhance the quality of life. HIV/AIDS affects men in far greater numbers than women. In 1997 in the United States, the rate of AIDS cases per 100,000 population was nearly four times as high for men (44.0) as for women (11.5) (Centers for Disease Control and Prevention: 1998).

At the end of 1997, the cumulative number of AIDS cases reported in the United States had surpassed 641,000. This figure does not include those individuals infected with HIV who have not developed AIDS, as some states do not collect statistics on HIV alone. The Centers for Disease Control and Prevention has recently told all states that they should collect data on HIV cases. Although the exact number of individuals with HIV is not known, it has been estimated at well over a million Americans.

From 1996 to 1997, the incidence of AIDS among all Americans dropped from just over 68,000 to just over 60,000, a decrease of 11.7%. For male adults/adolescents, the decrease was proportionately greater; the number of new cases dropped from 54,370 to 47,056 or 13.4%. The decrease in new cases over the past few years may be attributed to educational programs related to safe sex, which have been effective in the gay community, especially with older men (Hays: 1995).

The numbers of AIDS deaths dropped from 31,130 in 1996 to 16,685 in 1997, a decrease of 47% (National Center for Health Statistics: 1998). The decrease in deaths among people with AIDS is attributed largely to combination drug therapy, including protease inhibitors (see "Treatments" section below). A study by Palella et al. (1998) found that both morbidity, defined as the incidence of any of three opportunistic diseases (pneumocystis carinii pneumonia, mycobacterium avium complex, and cytomegalovirus retinitis), and mortality had declined significantly by 1997. The authors attributed these declines to the use of combination antiretroviral therapy, which is enhanced by the use of protease inhibitors.

HIV/AIDS is transmitted through the transfer of body fluids such as semen and blood. Sexual intercourse accounts for the greatest proportion of infections, especially among gay men who have anal intercourse with other men. The motion of intercourse may cause breaks in the lining of the rectum, which is thin and fragile, providing an entry for the infected fluid into the body. Male-to-male sexual contact accounted for just under half (45%) of the cases of AIDS reported in the United States in 1997, a decrease from the proportion of new cases in 1996

(Centers for Disease Control and Prevention: 1998). Infection via heterosexual intercourse is also possible, although the lining of the vagina is thicker than that of the anus and therefore is somewhat less likely to break during intercourse. Heterosexual contact accounted for 7% of AIDS cases in 1997 (Centers for Disease Control and Prevention: 1998). There are no known cases of HIV transmitted via saliva, tears, or sweat. Intravenous drug users who share needles and other drug paraphernalia are also susceptible to infection with HIV, as infected blood that remains on the needle is injected into the user's bloodstream. In 1997, intravenous drug use accounted for 22% of AIDS cases (Centers for Disease Control and Prevention: 1998). Blood transfusions for individuals with hemophilia and those requiring transfusions for surgery or other health reasons had been a source of transmission in the past; since 1985, however, the blood supply has been tested for HIV, and this method of transmission has been virtually eliminated.

In 1997, the incidence rate for African-American men, who account for a much smaller proportion of the population than whites, was the highest of any group at 163.4 per 100,000 population. Hispanic men had the second highest incidence rate at 78.5 per 100,000 population, and white men had an incidence rate of 22.5 (Centers for Disease Control and Prevention: 1998).

The mode of transmission among men varies by race/ethnic group. In 1997, most of the white men with AIDS (67%) had contracted the virus through homosexual contact. For African-American men, the transmission was equally divided between homosexual contact (30%) and intravenous drug use (29%). A third of Hispanic men (34%) contracted AIDS through homosexual contact, while 30% contracted the disease through intravenous drug use. The diagnosis of AIDS is most frequently made when individuals are in their 30's, whether they acquire it through homosexual contact, intravenous drug use, or a combination of the two methods (Centers for Disease Control and Prevention: 1998).

HIV is a retrovirus, which means that it has a protein called reverse transcriptase, enabling it to produce new virus cells. The HIV virus causes an extreme depression of the immune system by attaching to the CD4+ T cells, white blood cells that are found throughout the body; they are referred to as the helper cells as they coordinate the immune system's defense against infection. The virus spreads to all parts of the body, including the brain. The lymph nodes, which are collections of white blood cells found throughout the body, are the source of propagation of the HIV virus.

Some people infected with the HIV virus develop acute HIV syndrome shortly after exposure to the virus and prior to testing positive for HIV antibodies. Symptoms are similar to those of mononucleosis and include fever, fatigue, sore throat, achiness, and enlarged lymph nodes. These symptoms may last from three to six weeks. Three to ten weeks after this syndrome appears, blood tests for antibodies to HIV will be positive.

Responses to HIV infections progress by stage. In the first stage, the individual has tested positive for HIV but is asymptomatic. The length of this stage varies, although the reasons for this variance are not clear. The particular strain of the virus, the type of transmission, and age do contribute to this variance. Most people remain asymptomatic for eight to ten years (Bartlett and Finkbeiner: 1993). In homosexual and bisexual men, the median time from infection to clinical symptoms is 10 years; the disease is more aggressive in intravenous drug users (Fauci and Lane: 1994). In older men, the asymptomatic stage is usually shorter than in younger men, as aging makes the immune system less effective. As drug therapies become more effective in reducing the viral load in the bloodstream, the asymptomatic period is increasing.

The second stage is called AIDS related complex or ARC; many of the conditions that occur during this stage may also occur in individuals who are not infected with HIV. Symptoms include thrush, a yeast infection of the mouth that may be treated with drugs; oral hairy leukoplakia, an infection resembling thrush which requires no treatment unless the person is in pain; herpes zoster or shingles, a band of painful blisters that may be localized or disseminated throughout the body; idiopathic thrombocytopenic purpura, a state in which the body attacks its own blood platelets, resulting in bruises and bleeding; pneumococcal pneumonia of the lungs; and constitutional symptoms which become chronic, such as weight loss, weakness, diarrhea, fever, and fatigue. Generalized lymphadenopathy is a condition in which two or more sites of lymph nodes are swollen for at least three months and for which HIV is the only explanation.

The diagnosis of full AIDS is made when one or more opportunistic diseases associated with AIDS occur as a result of the CD4+ T cells falling to a critically low level, usually below 200 per microliter (Fauci and Lane: 1994). In 1993, the Centers for Disease Control and Prevention expanded the definition of AIDS to include asymptomatic individuals with a CD4+ T cell count of less than 200 cells per microliter and individuals infected with HIV who have pulmonary tuberculosis and those with recurrent episodes of pneumonia.

OPPORTUNISTIC DISEASES

When the CD4+ T cells decline to abnormally low levels, opportunistic diseases including infections and neoplasms occur. Virtually all organs and systems may be affected by the virus or the secondary diseases that occur. The most common diseases with the most serious effects are described briefly below.

Neurological problems may occur prior to decline of the T cells, although there is no known explanation for this development (Fauci and Lane: 1994). These problems are a result of opportunistic infections and neoplasms that affect the central nervous system. Many people with AIDS will encounter at least one neurological problem during the course of the disease. HIV associated dementia or **AIDS dementia complex** occurs in the latter stage of the disease and causes cognitive problems such as memory loss, inability to carry out complex tasks, and behavioral problems. As the disease continues to progress, individuals with dementia may become extremely withdrawn (Bartlett and Finkbeiner: 1993). Motor problems resulting from this condition include unsteady gait and poor balance. Depression and apathy often accompany these symptoms. Although no one yet understands how the HIV virus affects the brain, there is speculation that gaps may form in brain tissue and that the brain may shrink. Blood flow to the brain and metabolism in the brain are also affected. Some of the symptoms respond well to standard drugs prescribed for dementia and depression (McLaughlin: 1998).

Pneumocystis carinii pneumonia (PCP) is the most frequently reported opportunistic disease associated with AIDS (Moorman et al.: 1998); about four-fifths of individuals with HIV develop pneumocystis carinii pneumonia (PCP). This form of pneumonia begins with a dry cough that progresses slowly. Prophylactic treatment has reduced the incidence and

150

severity of the disease (Fauci and Lane: 1994). Individuals whose CD4+ T cell count is less than 200 are candidates for prophylactic treatment as are those individuals who have already had a bout of PCP. Antibiotics are the usual course of treatment; trimethoprim-sulfa-methoxazole is the preferred agent, as it also provides protection against toxoplasmosis and many bacterial infections. Some people are unable to take these drugs because of the serious side effects and must change drug regimens. A recent study (El-Sadr et al.: 1998) found that two other drugs, dapsone and atovaquone, are equally effective for patients who cannot tolerate trimethoprin-sulfamethoxazole.

Toxoplasmosis is an infection caused by the parasite toxoplasma gondii. The parasite is present in healthy individuals, where it does not pose a problem. The parasite is transmitted from cat excrement and raw or undercooked meat, especially lamb, pork, and venison. Individuals with a CD4+ T cell count of less than 100 should receive the same prophylactic treatment as noted above for PCP. This treatment must continue throughout life. Toxoplas-mosis encephalitis is the most common form of the disease, affecting the brain, and causing seizures and neurological impairment.

Tuberculosis is a disease that normally affects the lungs, but in individuals infected with HIV, it may spread to other parts of the body, including the lymph system. It causes cough, bloody sputum, difficulty breathing, fever, weight loss, and chest pain. Individuals who have AIDS and have inactive tuberculosis should be treated to prevent the onset of active tuberculosis. Unfortunately, the skin test for tuberculosis is often falsely negative in people with AIDS, preventing an accurate diagnosis.

Herpes simplex is a sexually transmitted virus that may become chronic in people with AIDS. Painful ulcers appear on the genitals, rectum, or lips and mouth. The use of latex condoms is recommended to reduce the risk of exposure to the herpes virus. Individuals with HIV/AIDS are subject to recurrent episodes of herpes simplex and may be treated with acyclovir.

Cytomegalovirus (CMV) is a herpes virus that is transmitted by kissing, sexual intercourse, and blood transfusions. It is very common among heterosexual men and women and even more prevalent among homosexual men. In healthy individuals, CMV poses no problem. In individuals with compromised immune systems, CMV may cause serious illness, including pneumonia and diseases of the intestinal and nervous systems. When it infects the retina, it can lead to severe visual impairment or blindness if untreated (Heinemann: 1992). The cause and prevalence of CMV are unknown, although it has been estimated that 20 to 25% of individuals with AIDS develop this virus (National Eye Institute: 1990). Three drugs, ganciclovir, foscarnet, and cidofovir, are currently available for the prevention and treatment of CMV retinitis. All three are effective in delaying the progression of the disease, but none is effective in curing it (Kuppermann: 1997).

Cryptosporidiosis is caused by a parasite and results in diarrhea. Healthy individuals may also have this condition, but in people with AIDS, the diarrhea can be severe and chronic. Since people with AIDS are prone to weight loss and malnutrition, cryptosporidiosis com-pounds the situation. There is no effective treatment other than replacing fluids.

A common form of malignancy in individuals with HIV/AIDS is *Kaposi's sarcoma*, which is most prevalent among homosexual men and initially presents as purple nodules or plaques on the skin. It may also affect the eyelids or conjunctiva, the mouth, lymph nodes, or gastrointestinal tract. Although there is no cure, combination chemotherapy may result in a regression of the tumors. The incidence of this disease has been decreasing. *Lymphoma* is another type of malignancy that appears in individuals with HIV/AIDS; in this disease, lymphocytes, white blood cells that play a role in immunological response, grow uncontrollably. Of the three lymphomas found in individuals with HIV/AIDS, non-Hodgkins lymphoma and Hodgkin's disease are treated with combination chemotherapy. Primary CNS (central nervous system) lymphoma is treated with radiation to the brain and corticosteroids.

People with AIDS are especially susceptible to bacterial infections of the respiratory system and the gastrointestinal system. *Mycobacterium avium complex* (MAC) is the most common bacterial infection in people with advanced disease, especially those with a CD4+ T cell level of less than 50. Symptoms are similar to those of the flu - fever, sweats, diarrhea, abdominal pain, fatigue, and weight loss. A combination of drugs is used to treat the condition.

Wasting or chronic, unintended, rapid, progressive weight loss may occur at any stage in the disease process; it may also be an indicator of an undiagnosed opportunistic disease. Some individuals have a more gradual weight loss, which cannot be explained (Beach and Thompson: 1995). Chronic diarrhea, a common symptom of HIV/AIDS, contributes to weight loss. Nutritional supplements may be recommended by a physician or dietitian.

TREATMENTS

Many health care providers believe that people with HIV who pay attention to "wellness" instead of dwelling on their illness slow down the progression of the disease, although there are no empirical data to prove this claim. Eating nutritious meals, exercising, and avoiding stress contribute to a sense of control over one's life and certainly cannot be detrimental. During the asymptomatic period, tests for the level of CD4+ T cells should be performed regularly to monitor the progress of the disease. Treatment for HIV/AIDS may begin early in an attempt to prevent the suppression of the immune system and the development of opportunistic diseases.

Recent guidelines put forth by the National Institutes of Health (Department of Health and Human Services: 1998) recommend that treatment be initiated for all symptomatic patients. Both viral load and immunological factors determine when treatment should begin for asymptomatic patients, but all patients should begin treatment within six months of seroconversion (presence of antibodies to the virus in the blood). Some experts recommend delaying treatment, based on variables such as stability of viral load and CD4+ T cell count. Yet others believe that individuals with any detectable viral load should be treated (HIV Frontline: 1998). As new research findings are made available and new treatments developed, the guidelines change, so it is important for health care providers and consumers to keep abreast of the medical literature.

Available treatments have serious side effects, and resistant strains of the virus may develop as a result of treatment. Effects of long term treatment are beginning to emerge (Carpenter et al.: 1998), suggesting the need for ongoing monitoring and the development of new types of treatment protocols. Examples of serious side effects include metabolic abnormalities, including occasional reports of diabetes, and changes in the distribution of body fat (Volberding and Deeks: 1998).   Drugs prescribed for individuals with HIV/AIDS are very expensive, although the manufacturers do have assistance programs for those in need. In the 18 years that HIV/AIDS has been recognized, pharmaceutical companies have developed a variety of drugs that have worked with varying degrees of success in halting the progression of the virus. As of December 1998, the Food and Drug Administration had approved 15 drug products for use in the treatment of HIV infections. These include protease inhibitors, reverse transcript inhibitors (nucleoside analogues), and non-nucleoside analogues. Researchers have been working on a vaccine to help the immune system combat HIV/AIDS, but to date, none has been effective.

Protease inhibitors, including indinavir, ritonavir, and saquinavir, work at a later stage in the viral life cycle than the reverse transcriptase inhibitors; they bind to the viral protease enzyme, preventing it from cleaving the protein elements of the virus, thereby preventing the virus from becoming infectious. Because they work at a different stage of the virus than the reverse transcriptase inhibitors, they provide an additive and possibly a synergistic effect (American Foundation for AIDS Research: 1996). Findings of recent studies indicate that treatment with protease inhibitors in combination with reverse transcript inhibitors has decreased the presence of the HIV virus in the blood to undetectable levels; the virus remains in the lymph nodes but has stopped reproducing significantly (James: 1996).

Reverse transcript inhibitors (nucleoside analogues) work by competing with the viral enzyme for binding to reverse transcriptase, and they may also be incorporated into newly formed DNA sequences, thereby terminating the chain (American Foundation for AIDS Research: 1996). The first drug approved for treatment of AIDS by the Food and Drug Administration was zidovudine (AZT; Retrovir), which decreases the rates of opportunistic infections and increases the levels of CD4+ T cells. Individuals who have been taking AZT for six months or more may develop strains of HIV that are resistant to the drug (Fauci and Lane: 1994). When this occurs, they are given didanosine (ddI; Videx) in addition to AZT. Zalcitabine (ddC; Hivid) has been approved for use only in combination with AZT. Stavudine (D4T; Zerit) is approved for use with individuals who are intolerant of the other drugs or who have deteriorated immunologically while taking these drugs. Non-nucleoside analogues, the newest class of anti-HIV drugs, directly combine with and block HIV's reverse transcriptase enzyme.

Studies indicate that treatment with a combination of drugs is effective in delaying progression from HIV to AIDS and decreasing the risk of death. An international study of 1,900 patients was ended ahead of time when it was discovered that those patients receiving a drug called lamivudine (3TC; Epivir) along with other standard anti-AIDS drugs, such as AZT, ddI, or ddC, fared much better than those in a control group who received only the standard anti-AIDS drugs (Knox: 1996).

Discontinuation of the combination therapy, however, may result in re-activation of the virus, according to a study by Chun and colleagues (1998), as these drugs do not completely eradicate the virus from the body. Researchers at the National Institute of Allergy and Infectious Diseases recently reported that they were able to eliminate the HIV virus from their "hiding places" in individuals who had no detectable virus in their bloodstreams. The virus, which remains in the inner structure of the CD4+ T cells even after it is eradicated from the bloodstream, is brought out of the these cells with interleukin-2 and then treated with antiretroviral drugs. This experimental treatment appears to have worked in three patients but failed in three others; why it works in some and not in others is not clear (National Institute of Allergy and Infectious Diseases: 1998).

A new therapeutic protocol has been developed for individuals who know they have been exposed to the HIV virus and seek immediate medical attention, such as health care workers. Postexposure prophylaxis, or PEP, consists of antiretroviral medications taken over a four week period. Administered within two hours of exposure, the treatment is effective in about four-fifths of the cases (Carpenter et al.: 1998; Emery: 1997).

Rehabilitation is necessary for men with AIDS as the disease progresses or the therapy causes side effects. The variety of infections and neoplasms may in turn cause a variety of impairments, including mobility, vision, hearing, speech, and cognitive impairments. The health care system has viewed HIV/AIDS as a terminal disease; for many men who continue on combination antiretroviral therapy, it is now more appropriate to consider AIDS a chronic illness. In order for men with the condition to receive optimal services, health care providers must realize that the quality of life will improve when men with HIV/AIDS receive rehabilitation services. For some men, rehabilitation may involve spending time in the rehabilitation unit of a hospital, where they learn to walk using a cane, a walker, or with the aid of an orthotic device or to use a wheelchair. Learning how to carry out activities of daily living while using assistive devices may also be part of the rehabilitation process. Men with AIDS who are too weak to actively participate in rehabilitation may require the services of home health agencies. Those who experience visual impairment or blindness may benefit from talking books, volunteer readers, radio reading services, or descriptive video services for television programs.

SEXUAL FUNCTIONING

The main concern of men with HIV/AIDS regarding sex should be the prevention of further spread of the virus. Local gay organizations have been conducting campaigns to prevent unsafe sexual conduct and to halt the spread of AIDS. According to many reports, these campaigns have been successful in decreasing the amount of unsafe sex in the homosexual community (Kimmel and Levine: 1989). Refraining from sexual contact with infected partners and using latex condoms are the two major methods of prevention. Latex condoms, which are less porous than other types of condoms and therefore are less likely to permit the virus to enter the partner's body, must be used from start to finish during each act of intercourse. The condom should be applied as soon as erection occurs, leaving space at the tip, but no trapped air. When withdrawing from the sexual partner, the condom should be held in place to keep it from slipping off. Many individuals believe that sex is less pleasurable when using condoms and reject them. When weighing the alternatives, it is easy to see that using condoms is beneficial to both partners, who will not be worried about transmitting the virus and therefore be able to enjoy themselves more. Some partners may need convincing that this is the case.

A recent study (Zhang et al.: 1998) found that men who are being treated aggressively with antiretroviral drug therapy and have no detectable virus in their blood plasma may still have virus in their semen and are capable of transmitting the virus through sexual contact.

The extreme fear and anxiety brought on by the possibility of spreading HIV/AIDS may result in sexual dysfunction or denial of sexual desire. If transmission of the disease was through sexual contact, the thought of sex may provoke great anxiety. The couple should openly discuss their fears and concerns in order to maintain their sexual relationship (Sandowski: 1989). Men who are not involved in long term relationships may have difficulty entering into new relationships because of the fear of revealing their diagnosis to potential sex partners. Some men remain celibate for a while before they adjust to the need for safe sex. (Bartlett and Finkbeiner: 1993).

Testosterone deficiency and hypogonadism, caused by either the disease or drug treatment, may affect libido and ability to have an erection. As HIV/AIDS progresses, the individual may experience fatigue, which diminishes his interest in sexual activity. His partner should be understanding of his or her mate's physical condition; sexual intercourse may take place less frequently, and other types of physical intimacy may replace it.

PSYCHOLOGICAL ASPECTS OF HIV/AIDS

When men are first diagnosed with HIV, they are overcome with fear and anxiety. They worry about the types of illnesses they will experience as a result of the virus, are anxious about their uncertain future, and are frightened about death. Depression generated by a sense of hopelessness; anger, especially in young men who feel unfairly shortchanged at the prospect of an early death; and guilt about the possibility of transmitting the virus to others are also common responses. The fears and anxieties associated with HIV/AIDS may become so extreme that men may contemplate suicide; according to the experiences of two health care providers, however, it is rare for suicide to occur among individuals with HIV/AIDS (O'Dowd and Zofnass: 1991).

Telling family members and friends about their diagnosis also may cause anxiety (Wolf: 1995). Because of society's fears and misconceptions about HIV/AIDS, many individuals with the infection justifiably fear rejection by relatives, friends, colleagues, and even health care providers. It is well documented that HIV/AIDS cannot be transmitted by casual contact; the only known means of transmission is through the transfer of body fluids. Many local agencies offer educational programs to enlighten the general public about the condition and its transmission. Despite this assurance, many individuals fear interacting with people with HIV/AIDS, causing social isolation for those with the virus. At a time when men with HIV/AIDS need social support, they may find themselves feeling vulnerable and alone. Fear of losing a job is not unrealistic; among men with HIV/AIDS, only 41% were employed either full- or part-time in 1991-1992. The proportion of men in the workplace declines with the progression of asymptomatic HIV to AIDS (Sebesta and LaPlante: 1996).

Since the HIV virus is latent for so many years, men may adjust to their diagnosis and continue with their lives. Some men may worry every time that they develop a cold or flu that AIDS has developed. Their fears and anxieties erupt once more when the first symptoms of AIDS appear. Their emotions may become stronger as the reality of the disease can no longer be denied. Fear of dying may play a large role in their response to the disease, affecting their willingness to adhere to medical treatment. The need to cope with crises occurs throughout the course of the disease (Wolf: 1995). Upon diagnosis and as the disease

155

progresses and opportunistic infections occur, men with HIV/AIDS must learn to handle the medical aspects of the situation as well as the effects on daily living and financial affairs. The fear of rejection is countered by the fear of dependence during these crises. As one man stated:

> ...in relationships, the balance tips quickly to dependency. In the barrage of unexplained symptoms, the unexplained headaches, the unexplained fevers, the unexplained skin eruptions, the constant and fearful change, I needed to find the path with the people I loved, and I wanted to be loved with AIDS as much as I'd been loved without it. (Maier: 1993, x)

When a partner or spouse begins to take over the roles that the man with HIV/AIDS previously carried out, he begins to feel that he is losing control (Bartlett and Finkbeiner: 1993). As the disease progresses, activities of daily living become more difficult, and men who valued their independence must utilize the assistance of others to bathe, dress, and eat. Men with homosexual partners who are also infected with HIV may worry about how they will care for each other as both deteriorate and become weak. Caregivers who are not infected with HIV also face great strains, wondering how they will cope with the next crisis and how to maintain the proper balance between allowing the man with HIV/AIDS to retain as much independence as possible while providing the care that he needs. Caregivers as well as the man with HIV/AIDS may find that support groups alleviate some of the fears and concerns and provide practical suggestions for dealing with the everyday problems of living with HIV/AIDS.

PROFESSIONAL SERVICE PROVIDERS

In most instances the *primary care physician* will be the case manager for the person with HIV/AIDS throughout the course of the disease. This physician may specialize in infectious diseases or specifically in HIV/AIDS. The primary care physician will be in charge of prescribing medications to delay the progression of the virus, treat opportunistic infections, and alleviate pain. Referrals to other physicians such as *ophthalmologists* (specialists in diseases of the eyes), *neurologists* (specialists in diseases of the nervous system), *oncologists* (cancer specialists), and *gastroenterologists* (specialists in the gastrointestinal system) are made as needed. *Physical therapists* help men with HIV/AIDS develop an exercise program designed to keep their bodies as strong as possible; *occupational therapists* adapt the home environment and provide assistive technology that contributes to independent living. *Psychologists* and *social workers* provide counseling to help men with HIV/AIDS work through their fears, anxieties, and grief. *Rehabilitation counselors* help men with AIDS plan a program that enables them to remain living independently and continue working. *Registered dietitians* may work with men with HIV/AIDS to ensure that they eat a well balanced, nutritious diet.

Special centers that treat people with HIV/AIDS are located in most urban areas; in addition to providing medical services, these centers often provide support groups and psychological counseling. Some participate in clinical trials of new experimental treatments. Both local and state health departments make referrals to these centers. The hotlines listed in the "ORGANIZATIONS" section below also make referrals to service providers. Directories of service providers are listed under the "PUBLICATIONS AND TAPES" section below. Local voluntary organizations offer counseling services, support groups, and information and referral. Vocational rehabilitation agencies offer assessments and assistance in the form of adapted equipment, job training and placement, and environmental adaptation of the home and the workplace. Special programs administered by pharmaceutical companies and state departments of health provide financial assistance to those in need. Each state department of health has a toll-free hotline for people with HIV/AIDS. In the end stage of HIV/AIDS, home health care agencies and hospices administer medications and provide services to make people more comfortable.

Individuals with HIV/AIDS are eligible for Social Security Disability Insurance and Supplemental Security Income when they meet specified criteria and are protected against discrimination by the Americans with Disabilities Act (see Chapter 3, "Laws that Affect Men with Disabilities"). The Ryan White Comprehensive AIDS Resources Emergency (CARE) Act was passed in 1990 and reauthorized in 1996; it enables communities to provide medical treatment to uninsured and underinsured individuals.

References

American Foundation for AIDS Research
1996   "Treatments for HIV Infection: Antiretroviral Therapy" AIDS/HIV Treatment Directory 8:2(June):16-55
Bartlett, John G. and Ann K. Finkbeiner
1993   The Guide to Living with HIV Infection Baltimore, MD: Johns Hopkins University Press
Beach, Richard and Cynthia A. Thomson
1995   "HIV and Nutrition" pp. 133-145 in Cynthia G. Carmichael et al. (eds.) HIV/AIDS Primary Care Handbook Norwalk, CT: Appleton & Lange
Carpenter, Charles C. et al.
1998   "Antiretroviral Therapy for HIV Infection in 1998" JAMA 280(July 2):78-86
Centers for Disease Control and Prevention
1998   HIV/AIDS Surveillance Report 9(2)
Chun, Tae-Wook
1998   "Induction of HIV-1 Replication in Latently Infected CD4+ T Cells Using a Combination of Cytokines" Journal of Experimental Medicine 188:1(July 6):83-91

Department of Health and Human Services
1998 <u>Guidelines for the Use of Antiretroviral Agents in HIV-Infected Adults and Adolescents</u>
December 1

El-Sadr, Wafaa M. et al.
1998 "Atovaquone Compared with Dapsone for the Prevention of Pneumocystis carinii
Pneumonia in Patients with HIV Infection Who Cannot Tolerate Trimethoprim,
Sulfonamides, or Both" <u>New England Journal of Medicine</u> 339(December 24):26:895

Emery, Theo
1997 "AIDS Drug Cocktail Finds Growing Role in Preventing Infection" <u>Boston Globe</u>
January 13

Fauci, Anthony and H. Clifford Lane
1994 "Human Immunodeficiency Virus (HIV) Disease: AIDS and Related Disorders" pp.
1566-1618 in Kurt J. Isselbacher et al. (eds) <u>Harrison's Principles of Internal Medicine</u>
New York, NY: McGraw Hill, Inc.

Hays, Robert B.
1995 "What Are Young Gay Men's HIV Prevention Needs?" <u>HIV Prevention: Looking Back,
Looking Ahead</u> Center for AIDS Prevention, University of California, San Francisco

Heinemann, M. H.
1992 "Ophthalmic Problems" <u>Medical Management of AIDS Patients, The Medical Clinics
of North America</u> 76(January)1:83-97

HIV Frontline
1998 "Long-term Treatment Strategies for HIV Disease" <u>HIV Frontline</u> Summer 33 pp. 1-
5

James, John S.
1996 "Vancouver in Perspective" <u>AIDS Treatment News</u> 251(July 19):1-3

Kimmel, Michael S. and Martin P. Levine
1989 "Men and AIDS" pp. 344-354 in Michael S. Kimmel and Michael A. Messner (eds.)
<u>Men's Lives</u> New York, NY: Macmillan Publishing Company

Knox, Richard A.
1996 "Success of a New AIDS Treatment Brings Study to Early End" <u>Boston Globe</u> July 24

Kupperman, B. D.
1997 "Therapeutic Options for Resistant Cytomegalovirus Retinitis" <u>Journal of Acquired
Immune Deficiency Syndrome Human Retrovirology</u> 14:Supplement 1:S13-21

Maier, Joseph
1993 "To People with HIV Infection and Their Caregivers" pp. vii-xiii in John G. Bartlett
and Ann K. Finkbeiner <u>The Guide to Living with HIV Infection</u> Baltimore, MD: Johns
Hopkins University Press

McLaughlin, Loretta
1998 "AIDS-Related Dementia" <u>Harvard AIDS Review</u> Winter 16-18

Moorman, A. C. et al.
1998 "Pneumoncystis Carinii Pneumonia Incidence and Chemoprophylaxis Failure in
Ambulatory HIV-Infected Patients" <u>Journal of Acquired Immune Deficiency Syndromes
and Human Retrovirology</u> 19:2(October 1):182-188

National Center for Health Statistics

1998 "Births and Deaths: Preliminary Data for 1997" <u>National Vital Statistics Report</u> 47:4(October 7)

National Eye Institute

1990 <u>Clinical Trials Supported by the National Eye Institute</u> Bethesda, MD: NIH Publication No. 90-2910, p. 55

National Institute of Allergy and Infectious Diseases

1998 <u>Treatment with IL-2 plus HAART Markedly Reduces HIV in Immune System 'Hiding Places'</u>" November 15

O'Dowd, Mary Alice and Joan S. Zofnass

1991 "Psychosocial Issues and HIV: Part II" <u>AIDS Clinical Care</u> 3:11(November):81-83

Palella, F. J., Jr. et al.

1998 "Declining Morbidity and Mortality Among Patients with Advanced Human Immunodeficiency Virus Infection" <u>New England Journal of Medicine</u> 338(March 26):853-860

Sandowski, Carol L.

1989 <u>Sexual Concerns When Illness or Disability Strikes</u> Springfield, IL: Charles C. Thomas Publishers

Sebesta, Douglas S. and Mitchell P. LaPlante

1996 <u>HIV/AIDS, Disability, and Employment</u> Washington, DC: U.S. Department of Education, National Institute on Disability and Rehabilitation Research

Volberding, Paul A. and Steven G. Deeks

1998 "Antiretroviral Therapy for HIV Infection" <u>JAMA</u> 279(May 8):1343-1344

Wolf, Maria

1995 "HIV/AIDS Means Disability" <u>Advance/Rehabilitation</u> v:6(January):12-17

Zhang, Hui, et al.

1998 "Human Innunodeficiency Virus Type 1 in the Semen of Men Receiving Highly Active Antiretroviral Therapy" <u>New England Journal of Medicine</u> 339:25(December 17):1803-1809

ORGANIZATIONS

AIDS Clinical Trials Information Service (ACTIS)
PO Box 6421
Rockville, MD 20849-6421
(800) 874-2572   (888) 480-3739 (TT)   (301) 519-0459
FAX (301) 519-6616   e-mail: actis@actis.org   http://www.actis.org

This information and referral service provides the latest information on eligibility criteria for participating in clinical trials for experimental drugs and other therapies as well as results of recently completed trials. A Spanish speaking specialist is available. AIDSTRIALS and AIDSDRUGS are available on the web site.

AIDS Treatment Data Network
611 Broadway, Suite 613
New York, NY 10012
(800) 734-7104   (212) 260-8868   FAX (212) 260-8868
e-mail: atdn@aidsnyc.org   http://www.aidsnyc.org/network

This organization provides AIDS and HIV treatment information, counseling, referrals, and case management support. Newsletter, "Treatment Review," is published eight or more times per year in English and Spanish; $16.00. There is no charge for Network membership, but contributions are encouraged.

American Bar Association AIDS Coordinating Committee
740 15th Street, NW
Washington, DC 20005-1009
(202) 662-1025   FAX (202) 662-1032
e-mail: powells@staff.abanet.org

Established to help lawyers provide pro bono assistance to people with AIDS, this organization serves as a clearinghouse, makes referrals, conducts workshops, provides consultation, and produces publications.

American Foundation for AIDS Research (AmFAR)
120 Wall Street, 13th floor
New York, NY 10005
(212) 806-1600   FAX (212) 806-1601
e-mail: amfar@amfar.org   http://www.amfar.org

Funds basic biomedical research; operates the Community-Based Clinical Trials Network which enables physicians across the country to enroll patients in trials of new drugs and new therapies; and funds education for AIDS prevention. Publishes "The AmFAR Report" and "The AmFAR Newsletter."

Bereavement and Hospice Support Netline
University of Baltimore
http://ube.ubalt.edu/www/bereavement

This web site lists bereavement groups by state, including special groups for parents and widows and widowers, and hospices by state throughout the country. Also provides links to related sites.

CDC National AIDS Hotline
(800) 342-2437   (800) 344-7432 (Spanish)   (800) 243-7889 (TT)

A 24 hour hotline that provides information about HIV transmission and prevention, HIV testing and treatment, referrals, and educational materials. Special resources are available for minorities. Spanish information specialists are available 8:00 a.m. to 2:00 a.m. EST and a Spanish recording is available from 2:00 a.m. to 8:00 a.m. EST. The Centers for Disease Control and Prevention (CDC) monitors the HIV/AIDS epidemic and promotes the public understanding of the disease as well as prevention of high risk behavior among students and adults.

CDC National Prevention Information Network (NPIN)
National Center for HIV, STD, and TB Prevention
PO Box 6003
Rockville, MD 20849-6003
(800) 458-5231   (800) 243-7012 (TT)   (301) 217-0023
FAX (888) 282-7681   e-mail: info@cdcnpin.org
http://www.cdcnpin.org

Answers questions and makes referrals. Produces a variety of reports, including statistics on the incidence of HIV/AIDS, information on current treatment options, and resources to help people with HIV/AIDS find services. Provides a daily news service on the web site and by e-mail subscription, "CDC HIV/STD/TB Prevention News Update," which has information about scientific articles related to HIV/AIDS, sexually transmitted diseases, and tuberculosis. Many publications are available in Spanish as well as English.

Center for AIDS Prevention Studies
University of California San Francisco
74 New Montgomery, Suite 600
San Francisco, CA 94105
(415) 597-9100   FAX (415) 597-9213
http://www.caps.ucsf.edu/capsweb/index.html

A research center that carries out projects and produces publications related to the prevention of AIDS.

Food and Drug Administration (FDA)
Office of Special Health Issues
5600 Fishers Lane, HF-12, Room 9-49
Rockville, MD 20857
(301) 827-4460   FAX (301) 443-4555
e-mail: OSHI@oc.fda.gov   http://www.fda.gov/oshi/aids/news.html

Provides information about drugs approved for the treatment of AIDS and problems encountered in the manufacturing process, etc. Provides Internet links to other web sites with information about therapy for AIDS.

Gay Men's Health Crisis
http://www.gmhc.org

This web site provides information on a variety of topics related to HIV/AIDS, including treatments, mental health issues, and insurance coverage.

Harvard AIDS Institute
651 Huntington Avenue
Boston, MA 02115
(617) 432-4400   FAX (617) 432-4545
e-mail: hai@hsph.harvard.edu   http://www.hsph.harvard.edu/hai

Sponsors multidisciplinary research, seminars, and conferences and produces special reports.

HIV/AIDS Education
American Red Cross National Headquarters
17th and D Streets, NW
Washington, DC 20006
(202) 728-6500   e-mail: info@usa.redcross.org
http://www.crossnet.org/hss/HIVAIDS/index.html

162

Conducts a number of educational programs to prevent the spread of HIV/AIDS, especially among youths. Special programs for African-American and Hispanic youths and for employers.

HIV/AIDS Treatment Information Service (ATIS)
(800) 448-0440   http://www.hivatis.org

The hotline provides information about treatments approved by the Food and Drug Administration. Information is available in English and Spanish. Hours: 9:00 a.m. to 7:00 p.m. EST. The web site provides information about treatment options approved by the federal government and links to other Internet sites. The Department of Health and Human Services' "Guidelines for the Use of Antiretroviral Agents in HIV-Infected Adults and Adolescents" is available on the site.

Housing Opportunities for Persons with AIDS, Office of HIV/AIDS Housing (HOPWA)
Department of Housing and Urban Development
451 Seventh Street, SW, Room 7154
Washington, DC 20410
(800) 998-9999   (800) 483-2209 (TT)   (202) 708-1934
(202) 708-2565 (TT)   FAX (202) 708-1744   http://www.comcon.org

This federal program provides funding for housing assistance and supportive services, including housing information services and counseling. Funds are available to enable individuals with AIDS and their families to remain in their homes.

National AIDS Fund
1400 I Street, NW, Suite 1220
Washington, DC 20005-2208
(202) 408-4848   FAX (202) 408-1818   http://www.aidsfund.org

Provides consulting, education, and publications related to HIV/AIDS in the workplace. Free publications list. Publications also available on the web site.

National AIDS Health Fraud Hotline
(888) 332-1820   http://www.flairs/tcrs/news.htm

This hotline accepts reports of suspected or known fraud in the treatment of HIV/AIDS. The web site also provides information about accepted treatments and links to other web sites.

National Association for People with AIDS (NAPWA)
1413 K Street, NW, Suite 700
Washington, DC 20006
(202) 898-0414   FAX (202) 898-0435
e-mail: napwa@napwa.org   http://www.napwa.org

Promotes public and private sector funding for AIDS. Serves as a national information resource. Holds an annual conference. Operates a mail order pharmacy. Publishes newsletters "The Active Voice," "NAPWA Notes," and "The Update," plus "Medical Alert." Newsletters plus information about pharmacy and daily medical alerts are available on the web site.

National Center for Nutrition and Dietetics
American Dietetic Association
216 West Jackson Boulevard
Chicago, IL 60606
Consumer Nutrition Hot-line   (800) 366-1655   (312) 899-0040
FAX (312) 899-1758   http://www.eatright.org

Callers may receive a referral to a registered dietitian or listen to recorded nutrition messages in English and Spanish. Customized food and nutrition information from a registered dietitian is available by calling (900) 225-5267; the cost of a call is $1.95 for the first minute, $.95 for each minute thereafter. Free publications.

National Hospice Organization (NHO)
1901 North Moore Street, Suite 901
Arlington, VA 22209
(800) 658-8898   (703) 243-5900   FAX (703) 525-5762
http://www.nho.org

A group that advocates for the rights of terminally ill patients and promotes hospice. Provides informational and educational materials and referrals. The web site enables users to locate hospices in their geographical area. For referral to a hospice, call NHO's toll-free Hospice Helpline at (800) 658-8898.

National Institute of Allergy and Infectious Diseases (NIAID)
National Institutes of Health
Building 31, Room 7A-50
31 Center Drive MSC 2520
Bethesda, MD 20892-2520
(301) 496-5717   http://www.niaid.nih.gov

Supports clinical and basic research related to AIDS and other infectious diseases. "NIAID AIDS Agenda" discusses new developments and the establishment of research centers, and "NIAID Dateline" summarizes recent research and developments. Free. The web site provides information on research findings, fact sheets, resources, and clinical trials.

Project Inform
205 13th Street, Suite 2001
San Francisco, CA 94103
(800) 822-7422   (415) 558-8669   FAX (415) 558-0684
http://www.projinf.org

This AIDS treatment hotline provides information about the latest treatments. Hours: Monday through Friday, 9:00 a.m. to 5:00 pm; Saturday, 10:00 a.m. to 4:00 p.m. PST. Publishes Fact Sheets on diseases, treatment, research, etc. Conducts town meetings at various locations around the country and operates the Treatment Action Network to advocate for the effective and accessible treatment of HIV.

Sexuality Information and Education Council of the United States (SIECUS)
130 West 42nd Street, Suite 350
New York, NY 10036-7802
(212) 819-9770   FAX (212) 819-9776
e-mail: siecus@siecus.org   http://www.siecus.org

Provides information and education about sexuality through publications, database, library, symposia, and advocacy. Bimonthly journal, "SIECUS Report," $65.00, has articles on HIV/AIDS prevention. Publications catalogue, free.

The Treatment Overview
http://www.thebody.com

This web site provides information about treatments for HIV/AIDS and links to other Internet sites. "POZ" magazine is available online.

AIDS Care at Home
by Judith Greif and Beth Ann Golden
John Wiley and Sons
1 John Wiley Drive
Somerset, NJ 08875
(800) 225-5945   (908) 469-4400   FAX (908) 302-2300
http://www.wiley.com

Written by two nurses who specialize in treating people with HIV/AIDS, this book provides practical information for caregivers on the daily needs of people with AIDS. Includes information on emotional stress, how to recognize the symptoms of diseases that affect people with AIDS, when to consult a physician, and resources for the various potential conditions. $17.95; phone for shipping and handling.

AIDS Clinical Care
Massachusetts Medical Society
PO Box 9085
Waltham, MA 02454-9085
(800) 843-6356   (781) 893-3800   FAX (781) 893-0413
e-mail: info@massmed.org   http://www.mms.org

A monthly newsletter written by physicians and other health care providers reporting on the latest clinical advances in the treatment of HIV/AIDS. $98.00

AIDSDRUGS, AIDSTRIALS, and AIDSLINE
National Library of Medicine
8600 Rockville Pike
Building 38, Room 2S-10
Bethesda, MD 20894
(888) 346-3656   (301) 594-5983   http://www.nlm.nih.gov

AIDSDRUGS is a dictionary about new drugs being evaluated to treat AIDS; AIDSTRIALS reports on clinical trials currently underway (including patient eligibility criteria) and those that have been completed; and AIDSLINE contains references to research and policy related to AIDS. Also available at the ACTIS web site (see listing above in "ORGANIZATIONS" section).

AIDS/HIV Treatment Directory
American Foundation for AIDS Research (AmFAR)
120 Wall Street, 13th floor
New York, NY 10005
(212) 806-1600   FAX (212) 806-1601
e-mail: amfar@amfar.org   http://www.amfar.org

This semi-annual publication includes information about the latest prevention strategies and treatments, drug assistance programs, drug trials that are actively seeking participants, and other resources such as hotlines and community based treatment programs. Individuals, $55.00; physicians/institutions, $125.00. Individuals with HIV/AIDS who cannot afford a subscription may obtain a free copy by calling CDC National Prevention Information Network at (800) 458-5231.

AIDS Treatment News
ATN Publications
PO Box 411256
San Francisco, CA 94141-9914
(800) 873-2812   (415) 255-0588   FAX (415) 255-4659
e-mail: aidsnews@aidsnews.org   http://www.aidsnews.org

A bimonthly newsletter that provides information on the latest treatment for AIDS and public policy regarding drug therapies. Individuals at home, $120.00; call for subsidized rates for individuals who cannot afford regular rates; institutions and professional offices, $270.00; nonprofit and community organizations, $135.00.

Directory of Legal Resources for People with AIDS and HIV
American Bar Association AIDS Coordinating Committee
740 15th Street, NW
Washington, DC 20005-1009
(202) 662-1025   FAX (202) 662-1032
e-mail: powells@staff.abanet.org

This publication provides information on national, state, and local organizations that provide legal services and make referrals. $15.00 plus $3.00 shipping and handling

Dying At Home: A Family Guide for Caregiving
by Andrea Sankar
Johns Hopkins University Press
2715 North Charles Street
Baltimore, MD 21218
(800) 537-5487   FAX (410) 516-6998
http://muse.jhu.edu/press

Using extensive interviews with individuals, family members, and professional caregivers, this book discusses the decision to die at home. Offers practical suggestions for health care including nutrition, mobility, medication, and pain control. $29.95 plus $3.00 shipping and handling

Glossary of HIV/AIDS-Related Terms
CDC National Prevention Information Network (NPIN)
PO Box 6003
Rockville, MD 20849-6003
(800) 458-5231   (800) 243-7012 (TT)   (301) 217-0023
FAX (888) 282-7681   e-mail: info@cdcnpin.org
http://www.cdcnpin.org

Glossary of terms commonly used in association with the diagnosis and treatment of HIV/AIDS and associated diseases. Single copy, free; multiple copies, $5.00 each.

A Guide to AIDS in the Workplace Resources
CDC National Prevention Information Network (NPIN)
PO Box 6003
Rockville, MD 20849-6003
(800) 458-5231   (800) 243-7012 (TT)   (301) 217-0023
FAX (888) 282-7681   e-mail: info@cdcnpin.org
http://www.cdcnpin.org

This publication provides information about organizations and publications that assist employers and employees to deal with AIDS in the workplace. Free

Guide to Selected HIV/AIDS-Related Internet Resources
CDC National Prevention Information Network (NPIN)
PO Box 6003
Rockville, MD 20849-6003
(800) 458-5231   (800) 243-7012 (TT)   (301) 217-0023
FAX (888) 282-7681   e-mail: info@cdcnpin.org
http://www.cdcnpin.org

This publication provides annotated listings of web sites and Listserv addresses for information about HIV/AIDS. Free

Harvard AIDS Review
Harvard AIDS Institute
651 Huntington Avenue
Boston, MA 02115
(617) 432-4400   FAX (617) 432-4545
e-mail: hai@hsph.harvard.edu   http://www.hsph.harvard.edu/hai

A semi-annual publication that reviews recent research findings and social issues. $20.00. Complimentary subscriptions available to people with AIDS and community based organizations serving people with AIDS.

HIV/AIDS Clinical Trials: Knowing Your Options
AIDS Clinical Trials Information Service (ACTIS)
PO Box 6421
Rockville, MD 20849-6421
(800) 874-2572   (888) 480-3739 (TT)   (301) 519-0459
FAX (301) 519-6616   e-mail: actis@actis.org   http://www.actis.org

This videotape provides information that helps people with HIV/AIDS decide whether to enroll in clinical trials. 19 minutes. Free

The HIV Drug Book
by Project Inform
Simon and Schuster
200 Old Tappan Road
Old Tappan, NJ 07675
(800) 223-2336   FAX (800) 445-6991
e-mail: ss cust serv@prenhall.com http://www.simonsays.com

This book describes 250 drugs used in treatment of HIV/AIDS and includes a chart of drug interactions. Also included are listings of buyers' clubs, mail order pharmacies, and state and pharmaceutical assistance programs. $18.00 plus $4.00 shipping and handling

HIV Frontline
World Health CME
41 Madison Avenue, 42nd floor
New York, NY 10010-2202

This newsletter provides information on the latest treatment options for patients with HIV/AIDS. Funded by Glaxo Wellcome, manufacturer of several antiviral drugs approved for treating AIDS. Free

HIV: How to Help Yourself
National Institute of Allergy and Infectious Diseases (NIAID)
NIAID Office of Communications
Building 31, Room 7A-50
31 Center Drive, MSC 2520
Bethesda, MD 20892-2520
(301) 496-5717   http://www.niaid.nih.gov

This set of eight booklets includes "Taking the HIV (AIDS) Test," "Testing Positive for HIV," "Infections Linked to AIDS," "The Lung Infection PCP," "The Brain Infection Toxo," "AIDS-Related CMV," "AIDS-Related MAC," and "HIV-Related TB." Single copy (full set or individual titles), free. Also available on the web site.

HIV Protease Inhibitors & You
CDC National Prevention Information Network (NPIN)
PO Box 6003
Rockville, MD 20849-6003
(800) 458-5231   (800) 243-7012 (TT)   (301) 217-0023
FAX (888) 282-7681   e-mail: info@cdcnpin.org
http://www.cdcnpin.org

This brochure describes the protease inhibitors that have been approved by the FDA for the treatment of AIDS. Available in English and in Spanish. $.10 per copy

Living with Life-Threatening Illness: A Guide for Patients, Their Families, & Caregivers
by Kenneth J. Doka
Jossey-Bass Inc.
350 Sansome Street, 5th Floor
San Francisco, CA 94104
(800) 956-7739   (415) 433-1767   FAX (800) 605-2665
http://josseybass.com

This book discusses individuals' responses to life-threatening illness and coping with various phases of illness, the possibility of recovery, and the terminal phase. Includes effects on the family and special populations and makes suggestions for health professionals and caregivers. $26.95 plus $5.50 shipping and handling

Living with Low Vision: A Resource Guide for People with Sight Loss
Resources for Rehabilitation
33 Bedford Street, Suite 19A
Lexington, MA 02420
(781) 862-6455   FAX (781) 861-7517
e-mail: info@rfr.org   http://www.rfr.org

A large print (18 point bold type) comprehensive directory that helps people with sight loss locate the services that they need to remain independent. Chapters describe products that enable people to keep reading, working, and carrying out their daily activities. Information about resources on the Internet is included. $44.95 plus $5.00 shipping and handling (See order form on last page of this book.)

Locating Basic Resources on HIV/AIDS and Nutrition
CDC National Prevention Information Network (NPIN)
PO Box 6003
Rockville, MD 20849-6003
(800) 458-5231   (800) 243-7012 (TT)   (301) 217-0023
FAX (888) 282-7681   e-mail: info@cdcnpin.org
http://www.cdcnpin.org

This publication provides information about organizations, newsletters, and books that help people with HIV/AIDS maintain their quality of life through good nutrition. Free

The Measure of Our Days
by Jerome Groopman
Penguin Putnam
PO Box 12289
Newark, NJ 07101-5289
(800) 253-6476   FAX (201) 896-8569
http://www.penguin.com

Written by a physician who cares for patients with AIDS and cancer, this book uses real cases to depict a humane type of medical care, where the physician is aware of the social aspects of his patients' lives. $23.95

Positive Options
Body Positive
19 Fulton Street, Room 308B
New York, NY 10038-2100
Helpline (800) 566-6599   (212) 566-7333   FAX (212) 566-4539
e-mail: bodypos@aol.com

Written for people who are newly diagnosed as HIV positive, this book covers a wide variety of issues, including feelings upon learning the diagnosis, discrimination, sources of support, sex, staying fit, and spirituality. $15.00

POZ
Old Chelsea Station
PO Box 1279
New York, NY 10013-1279
(212) 242-2163   FAX (212) 675-8505
e-mail: pozmag@aol.com

A monthly magazine that covers a wide variety of topics related to people with HIV/AIDS, including health, nutrition, sex, and politics. $24.95 Also available online at web site, The Treatment Overview (see "ORGANIZATIONS" section above).

Primer of Palliative Care
by Porter Storey
American Academy of Hospice and Palliative Medicine (AAHPM)
PO Box 14288
Gainesville, FL 32604-2288
(352) 377-8900   FAX (352) 371-2349
e-mail: aahpm@aahpm.org   http://www.aahpm.org

This booklet, written by the medical director of a hospice, provides information on pain management as well as psychological, social, and spiritual needs of patients. $4.95

To Choose No Harm
Fanlight Productions
47 Halifax Street
Boston, MA 02130
(800) 937-4113   (617) 524-0980   FAX (617) 524-8838
e-mail: fanlight@tiac.net   http://www.fanlight.com

This videotape presents discussions regarding medical decision-making at the end of life by professional caregivers, when conflict exists between the patients and professionals or patients and family members. The cases include a young man with AIDS and an older women with terminal cancer. 45 minutes. Purchase, $195.00; rental, $50.00 per day; plus $9.00 shipping and handling.

Workplace Profiles Project
National AIDS Fund
1400 I Street, NW, Suite 1220
Washington, DC 20005-2208
(202) 408-4848   FAX (202) 408-1818   http://www.aidsfund.org

This publication includes 13 case studies of businesses that have successfully managed employees with HIV/AIDS. $15.00

You Can Prevent Cytomegalovirus: A Guide for People with HIV Infection
CDC National Prevention Information Network (NPIN)
PO Box 6003
Rockville, MD 20849-6003
(800) 458-5231   (800) 243-7012 (TT)   (301) 217-0023
FAX (888) 282-7681   e-mail: info@cdcnpin.org
http://www.cdcnpin.org

This brochure describes cytomegalovirus, its relation to HIV, and how people can protect themselves. $.10 per copy

Chapter 7

MULTIPLE SCLEROSIS

Multiple sclerosis (MS) is a chronic central nervous system condition in which the nerve fibers of the brain and spinal cord are damaged. A fatty substance called myelin protects the nerve fibers and enables the smooth transmission of neurological impulses between the central nervous system and the rest of the body. If inflammation damages or destroys the myelin, it may heal with no loss of function. Later, however, scar (or plaque) may form and interfere with the transmission of neurological impulses. Function may be diminished or lost. The disease is called multiple sclerosis because there are multiple areas of scarring or sclerosis (Minden and Frankel: 1989).

Estimates of the number of individuals with multiple sclerosis vary from less than 200,000, based on hospital and physicians' records, to 500,000, based on public surveys and pathology records (National Institute of Neurological Disorders and Stroke: 1990). Age of onset ranges from mid to late adolescence to middle age. Although multiple sclerosis affects twice as many women as men (Scheinberg and Smith: 1989), the physical symptoms that affect sexual performance occur at an age when men are becoming sexually active. Erectile dysfunction and urinary symptoms occur in about 70% of men with multiple sclerosis (Betts: 1996).

Over three-quarters (77%) of individuals with multiple sclerosis have activity limitations (National Center for Health Statistics: 1988). The broad economic and social implications of multiple sclerosis include medical expenses, unemployment or underemployment, the cost of special services, and the emotional and physical effects on the individual as well as the family. Cognitive problems such as memory loss, forgetfulness, and the inability to maintain a train of thought have been reported by many individuals with multiple sclerosis (Sullivan et al.: 1990).

Each man with multiple sclerosis has unique symptoms based on the location of the damage to the nervous system. These symptoms may include blurred or double vision, numbness in the extremities, balance or coordination problems, fatigue, muscle spasticity or stiffness, slurred speech, muscle weakness, inability to have an erection, or loss of bladder or bowel control.

The cause of multiple sclerosis is unknown. Scientists who believe that multiple sclerosis is an autoimmune disease are investigating the role of a variety of viruses in triggering damage to the immune system, which in turn may lead to the development of multiple sclerosis. Other investigators are studying the role of heredity. Their studies suggest that certain genetic factors may predispose some individuals to acquire multiple sclerosis, but there is no known pattern of direct inheritance.

DIAGNOSIS OF MULTIPLE SCLEROSIS

In the past, positive diagnosis of multiple sclerosis often took months or years. Physicians would verify loss of function in more than one area of the central nervous system and confirm that these losses had occurred at least twice over an interval of at least a month. Individuals with multiple sclerosis were often frustrated by the length of time and the multiple procedures required to diagnose their symptoms.

The development of magnetic resonance imaging (MRI), which provides a recorded image of central nervous system lesions, led to the modification of these criteria. A diagnosis of multiple sclerosis is now made if there is evidence of two episodes of functional loss at least a month apart; clinical evidence of at least one lesion; and another separate lesion confirmed by laboratory evidence (Calvano: 1991). The MRIs images are produced by the interaction between its magnetic field and the hydrogen atoms in body cells. Nearly 90% of individuals with multiple sclerosis have abnormal brain scans (Kalb: 1996). Because MRIs are so accurate, diagnostic procedures used in the past, such as CT scans (which use x-rays to scan the central nervous system for signs of demyelination), lumbar punctures, and myelography (an x-ray procedure), are now used infrequently. However, since MRI abnormalities may be present in other diseases, additional diagnostic tools, such as evoked potentials, are used to confirm a diagnosis.

Evoked potentials (EP) studies measure how fast electrical impulses travel through the central nervous system to the brain and are used in conjunction with the MRI. The physician may use one of three evoked potentials to assess various losses of function. The visual evoked potential assesses the visual pathway to the optic nerve; the somatosensory evoked potential studies sensory reactions and limb and spinal cord nerve function; and the brainstem auditory evoked potential may reveal the cause of hearing and balance problems. Evoked potentials are performed on an outpatient basis. Electrodes are placed on the skin, using a conducting ointment. A mild electrical stimulus is administered by the technician, and a computer records the brain's response to the stimulus. The physician studies the computer recordings to determine the site of neurological damage.

TYPES OF MULTIPLE SCLEROSIS

The National Multiple Sclerosis Society describes four courses of the condition, including benign sensory, relapsing-remitting, secondary progressive, and primary progressive. Men with the *benign sensory* form of multiple sclerosis experience little or no progression of the disease after the initial attack. The benign sensory form affects about 20% of individuals with multiple sclerosis (Frankel: 1994). The most common symptoms are optic neuritis (inflammation of the optic nerve) and numbness of a limb. Individuals have no long term disability.

Relapsing-remitting describes a course of multiple sclerosis in which the individual experiences sudden deterioration followed by almost complete remission of symptoms. These attacks may be referred to as exacerbations, flares, or relapses. This pattern continues for months or years with few physical restrictions. About 25% of individuals have this form of multiple sclerosis (Frankel: 1994).

Some individuals with the relapsing-remitting form have remissions after exacerbations of the disease, but the cumulative effects of the symptoms slowly lead to disability. This course is called *secondary progressive*. About 40% of individuals with multiple sclerosis experience this form of the disease (Frankel: 1994).

The most severely disabling form of the disease is *primary progressive* multiple sclerosis, which occurs in about 15% of the population with multiple sclerosis (Frankel: 1994). In these individuals, the disease progresses without remission and may result in disability very quickly. These forms of multiple sclerosis are not exclusive; some individuals may experience progression of one form to another. Smith and Scheinberg (1985) report that there is a more favorable prognosis for individuals with early onset (before age 35); acute onset rather than gradual onset; complete remission after the first attack; and sensory rather than motor symptoms.

TREATMENT OF MULTIPLE SCLEROSIS

There is no cure for multiple sclerosis; however, physicians can treat the symptoms of multiple sclerosis and try to control its progress with anti-inflammatory medication.

Interferon beta-1b (Betaseron) is one of the medications used to treat ambulatory individuals ages 18 to 50 with relapsing-remitting multiple sclerosis. Clinical studies have shown that Betaseron reduces the frequency and severity of exacerbations. MRI studies have shown reduced number and size of brain lesions (Goodkin: 1995). Betaseron is injected by the individual subcutaneously every other day. The most common side effects reported are reactions at the injection site such as swelling, redness, and rashes, and flu-like symptoms, including chills, fatigue, fever, and muscle aches. Individuals using Betaseron must learn to inject the drug and determine an injection schedule that works best for them, minimizing side effects. Betaseron is expensive, nearly $10,000 per year. The Betaseron Foundation aids underinsured individuals to obtain the medication (see "ORGANIZATIONS" section below).

Interferon beta-1a (Avonex) has been shown to reduce disease activity in individuals with relapsing-remitting multiple sclerosis and to slow the progression of disability. Avonex is administered in a once-a-week intramuscular injection into the thigh, hip, or upper arm. Many individuals self-inject or receive treatments from a caregiver. In clinical trials, the major side effect was initial flu-like symptoms which diminished over the course of treatment. Biogen, the manufacturer of Avonex, offers a toll-free support line and literature to individuals (see "ORGANIZATIONS" section below).

Copolymer I or glatiramer acetate (Copaxone) also slows the rate of relapse in individuals with relapsing-remitting multiple sclerosis. It is injected subcutaneously on a daily basis. It does not produce the flu-like symptoms or depression associated with Betaseron and Avonex.

In 1998, the Medical Advisory Board of the National Multiple Sclerosis Society released a consensus statement on the use of interferon beta-1a, interferon beta-1b, and glatiramer acetate therapy in the treatment of multiple sclerosis. The Board recommends that:
- therapy be initiated as soon as possible following a definite diagnosis of multiple sclerosis and determination of a relapsing course
- access to therapy not be limited by age, level of disability, or frequency of relapses
- treatment should be continued unless there is a clear lack of benefit, intolerable side effects, new data which reveal other reasons for cessation, or better therapy is available
- these drugs be covered by third party payers
- the choice of drugs be decided upon jointly by the patient and physician

• movement from one drug to another should be permitted (National Multiple Sclerosis Society: 1998)

Prednisone, adrenocorticotropic hormone (ACTH), prednisolone, and other anti-inflammatory drugs have been effective in reducing the severity and duration of multiple sclerosis flare-ups. These medications are not recommended for long term use because of side effects such as nausea, drowsiness, changes in blood pressure and blood glucose levels, lowered resistance to infection, and thinning of bones (Lechtenberg: 1995). Medication may also be used to treat multiple sclerosis symptoms such as spasticity, dizziness, fatigue, bladder problems, tremors, depression, and sensory problems (a "pins and needles" feeling). The man with multiple sclerosis and the physician must carefully consider each medication and its possible side effects, which may appear to be symptoms of the disease itself.

Optic neuritis, *double vision*, and *nystagmus* are common visual symptoms of multiple sclerosis. Inflammation of the optic nerve (neuritis) causes loss of vision. If the muscles of the eye are weakened by nerve demyelination, the individual cannot focus and experiences double vision (diplopia). Double vision may occur during an exacerbation and disappear during remission of multiple sclerosis symptoms. Cortisone is often used to treat optic neuritis and double vision. Nystagmus is an involuntary rapid eye movement; it interferes with focusing and may cause dizziness.

Some men with multiple sclerosis experience *problems with gait* including weakness, spasticity, and lack of coordination (ataxia). Antispastic medications, stretching exercises, and swimming relieve symptoms such as a stiff gait, foot drop, and toe dragging. Tizanidine (Zanaflex) was approved by the Food and Drug Administration (FDA) in 1997 for the treatment of spasticity (Kalb et al.: 1997). It may be used alone or in combination with baclofen, another antispastic drug. Orthoses are assistive devices used to support weakened areas, provide proper alignment, and improve function. An ankle foot orthosis worn inside the shoe may relieve the symptoms of spasticity. Ataxia is treated with a sequential exercise program in which the man performs repetitive movements, often watching himself in a mirror, to increase sensory feedback and restore coordination.

About 80% of individuals with multiple sclerosis experience *urinary dysfunction* (Holland: 1996). Urinary tract infections, formation of bladder stones, and kidney damage may occur if the bladder is not completely emptied during voiding. Symptoms of urinary dysfunction include urgency, frequency, hesitancy, nocturia (waking up to urinate during the night), and incontinence. Although some men with occasional incontinence rely on absorbent undergarments, medications and catheterization are used when symptoms are more severe. Anticholinergic drugs may be used to control bladder dysfunction by regulating bladder contractions (Lechtenberg: 1995). In intermittent self-catheterization, a flexible catheter is inserted through the penis to the urethra, urine is emptied from the bladder, and the catheter is removed. Many individuals find that self-catheterization allows the bladder to regain normal function (Holland: 1996).

Bowel dysfunction; *weakness of upper extremities*; *fatigue*; and *speech problems* (dysarthria) are other disabling symptoms of multiple sclerosis. Individuals with severe multiple sclerosis may also have difficulty swallowing. Treatment options for these symptoms include medication, exercise, adaptations in everyday living, and counseling.

SEXUAL FUNCTIONING

Neurological impairments to a man's sexual functioning may include changes in sexual response, loss of sensation, difficulty in achieving an erection, or problems in ejaculation. The psychosocial aspects of multiple sclerosis on a man's self-image also affects sexual activity. Since multiple sclerosis is usually first diagnosed in young adulthood, many young men fear that they will not be able to develop intimate relationships. The unpredictable course of physical symptoms makes the man uncertain about his sexual performance.

A man with multiple sclerosis described his feelings about impotence:

> I was deeply ashamed and embarrassed about being impotent. It related to my manhood--not just to being macho or who can beat up who--or being gung-ho on sports--but about my being a male. It goes very deep mentally and is very hard to admit to yourself, let alone other people (Frames: 1992, 5).

According to Lechtenberg (1995), between one-quarter and one-half of men with multiple sclerosis age 18 to 50 are unable to have an erection or sustain it long enough to satisfy their partners. Alternatives are genital stimulation through oral sex or the use of a vibrator or a manual technique called "stuffing," in which the female partner manipulates the flaccid penis into her vagina. This contact may satisfy both partners.

Treatments for impotence include oral medication, injections into the penis, external vacuum pump devices, and penile implants. In March, 1998, the FDA approved sildenafil citrate (Viagra), an oral medication which enables many men to have an erection in response to sexual arousal. In clinical trials, men with mild erectile dysfunction had better results with Viagra than those with more severe cases. Clinical trials of men with multiple sclerosis and erectile dysfunction are being conducted in the U.S. and Europe; results are expected in 1999.

Injections directly into the base of the penis have resulted in satisfactory erections that last from one to two hours and enable men to have intercourse. It is important to carefully monitor these injections to avoid priapism, a prolonged erection. Men with multiple sclerosis are at greater risk for priapism due to their youth and healthy penile arteries (Opsomer: 1996). A man with limited hand dexterity may use an auto injector rather than a conventional syringe or may ask his partner to administer the injection. Vacuum pump devices create a partial vacuum around the penis, drawing blood into the penis and causing an erection. The device consists of a plastic cylinder placed over the penis; a pump which draws air out of the cylinder; and an elastic band placed at the base of the penis to maintain the erection. The vacuum pump works satisfactorily in most cases, with no serious side effects (Nadig: 1994). Penile implants should be considered only when other treatments have failed. Penile implants may be semi-rigid or inflatable. For men with multiple sclerosis, inflatable implants may be difficult to use because spasticity affects their manual dexterity.

If faulty muscle coordination affects ejaculation, the semen will flow back into the bladder instead of through the penis. Called retrograde ejaculation or "dry" ejaculation, this will affect a man's fertility but does not cause impotence. Muscle spasms in the thighs, which make intercourse extremely difficult, may respond to medications. Changing positions, with the woman on top, for example, may make intercourse more comfortable.

Worries about a partner's reactions to symptoms such as bowel or bladder incontinence or spasticity may affect men as well. Betts (1996) reports that it is common for impotence to be accompanied by incontinence. The parts of the spinal cord that control sexual function also control bladder and bowel function. It is not uncommon for worry about a bladder accident to affect the ability to have an erection. Men find that restricting fluids and emptying the bladder before sexual activity reduce the possibility of leakage or accidents. Varying positions for intercourse will reduce pressure on the bladder. Men who use catheters can fold the end of the tube over the penis and secure it with a condom drawn over both.

It is usually unnecessary to restrict sexual activity due to fatigue. Men who encounter problems with fatigue may find that they have more sexual energy in the morning and may plan sexual activities accordingly. They and their partners should not mistake post-coital drowsiness for exhaustion.

PSYCHOLOGICAL ASPECTS OF MULTIPLE SCLEROSIS

From the onset of symptoms of multiple sclerosis, the course of the disease is fraught with uncertainty and unpredictability. Individuals with the disease have a near normal life expectancy (Scheinberg: 1983) and must continually adjust to the exacerbations that may occur at any time. Men may encounter a variety of physical and cognitive symptoms, affecting their ability to work and remain independent. The necessary changes in lifestyle may decrease the man's sense of masculinity and self-esteem.

Men must plan their daily living and work schedules to accommodate the effects of the condition. For example, exacerbations often cause fatigue, which interferes with normal activities, including employment. Individuals must find a balance between activity and rest periods. Not surprisingly, individuals who are experiencing exacerbations express higher levels of emotional disturbances than individuals who are in remission (Warren et al.: 1991).

Fears about the future are to be expected, given the unpredictable course of the disease and the serious consequences that may ensue. Family members may often find that they are taking on additional responsibilities for running the household and making important decisions. Role reversal is not an uncommon phenomenon and men who are the chief breadwinners in their family may find this role threatened. Guilt and depression may ensue.

It may be difficult for the man's partner to move back and forth between the roles of nurse and lover (Vermote and Peuskens: 1996). Men in well adjusted relationships often find the relationship a source of strength and support to help them cope with the condition (Rodgers and Calder: 1990). Counseling for both the man with multiple sclerosis and other family members is often beneficial. Often ignored by health care professionals, the caregiving partner should receive advice on respite care and supportive counseling (White et al.: 1993). However, professional counselors themselves sometimes have fears about the disease that must be addressed in order to provide counseling that meets their clients' psychological needs (Segal: 1991).

About half of all individuals with multiple sclerosis experience cognitive problems (Mahler: 1992; Rao et al.: 1991) and must take measures to overcome these difficulties.

178

Among these difficulties are memory problems, concept formation, and depression. Rao and colleagues (1991) found that individuals with multiple sclerosis who had cognitive problems were less likely to be employed and to engage in social activities than individuals without cognitive impairments, even though the severity of physical problems and the duration of the disease were similar for both groups. A study by Sullivan and his colleagues (1990) found that most individuals who experienced memory loss and forgetfulness used simple aids such as notepads or daily agendas to enable them to keep abreast of their daily needs and schedules. If there are vision problems, large print or a tape recorder may be used to record information.

Symptoms such as stumbling, dropping items, incontinence, and slurred speech may lead to self-consciousness, anxiety, and depression. The individual's personal coping mechanisms and the support provided by family, friends, and the community are crucial to the active problem solving required in living with multiple sclerosis (Shuman and Schwartz: 1988). Men who exhibit these symptoms may also benefit from individual or group counseling.

PROFESSIONAL SERVICE PROVIDERS

The unique symptoms of each man with multiple sclerosis require individualized treatment plans. The physical and emotional needs of each individual are best served through a team approach involving medical, allied health, and rehabilitation professionals.

Neurologists, who specialize in diseases and conditions of the brain and central nervous system, conduct neurological examinations and interpret the results of tests such as MRIs to diagnose multiple sclerosis and to rule out other possible conditions. *Physiatrists*, or rehabilitation physicians, design an individual treatment plan for the patient with multiple sclerosis. *Urologists* treat men with sexual dysfunction by performing diagnostic tests to determine the cause of the impotence, prescribing vacuum devices or pharmacologic treatment, or performing surgery.

Physical therapists teach individuals with multiple sclerosis how to perform a range of exercises which help build endurance and strength. Physical therapists also prescribe therapeutic exercises to diminish or eliminate weakness, spasticity, and lack of coordination. Physical therapists provide training in the use of assistive devices such as canes, crutches, and orthoses.

Occupational therapists assess functioning in activities of everyday living and teach simplified techniques of accomplishing them. They may recommend adaptations to the home and work environments. Occupational therapists also suggest adaptive recreation equipment and programs.

Orthotists make and fit assistive devices (orthoses) for improving gait in individuals with multiple sclerosis. Orthotists, physical therapists, or occupational therapists provide instruction in the use of these devices, such as ankle or foot braces.

Rehabilitation nurses provide skilled nursing care; instruct patients and family members in proper patient care; do follow-up upon discharge from a hospital; and make referrals to community services.

Psychologists provide therapy for individuals and families living with multiple sclerosis. Depression and burnout, for example, may be reduced through marital therapy, helping the couple to balance each other's needs.

Social workers offer practical and emotional support to individuals adjusting to a disability or chronic condition and to their families. Social workers provide information about financial and medical benefits, housing, and community resources. They conduct individual, family, or group counseling and may refer individuals to self-help or peer counseling groups.

Rehabilitation counselors help individuals with multiple sclerosis develop a plan that will enable them to continue functioning and working. Some individuals will need assistance in returning to their previous position or retraining to obtain a different type of position. Rehabilitation counselors help make the contacts and placements necessary to attain these goals.

Low vision specialists may be ophthalmologists, optometrists, opticians, or other professionals trained to help individuals with vision loss use their remaining vision to the greatest extent possible with the assistance of optical and nonoptical aids.

WHERE TO FIND SERVICES

Neurologists work in private practices, acute care hospitals, and specialty clinics. Neurologists and other members of the multidisciplinary team may also work in transitional or independent living programs and in rehabilitation hospitals. In addition to medical services, MS Comprehensive Care Centers provide services such as physical and occupational therapy, counseling, and patient and family education. A list of these centers is available from the National Multiple Sclerosis Society (see "ORGANIZATIONS" section below). Individuals who have mobility problems and difficulty traveling to professional service providers' offices often may obtain services in their homes from physical and occupational therapists. Low vision services are often available in ophthalmologists' or optometrists' offices, in private or public agencies that serve individuals who are visually impaired or blind, or in independent practices.

ENVIRONMENTAL ADAPTATIONS

Individuals with multiple sclerosis use a combination of environmental adaptations and assistive devices to make everyday routines easier. When making plans for living arrangements or for travel, individuals with multiple sclerosis must consider a variety of alternatives in the event that their functional abilities deteriorate. For instance, in purchasing a home, it is wise to determine if there is room for a wheelchair ramp or a chair lift.

Some individuals with gait problems use a cane, crutches, walker, wheelchair, scooter, or a combination of these mobility aids. An individual who usually uses a cane or crutches may prefer to use a wheelchair or scooter when traveling long distances.

Heat and humidity affect many individuals with multiple sclerosis. Air conditioning helps to reduce fatigue and weakness. Physicians, rehabilitation counselors, or tax advisers may provide advice on whether the purchase of an air conditioner is a tax deductible expense. A referral to a low vision rehabilitation center offers individuals with vision problems the

180

opportunity to improve visual function with low vision aids. An eye patch may reduce double vision. Prisms, mounted on the eyeglasses lens, will expand the visual field of the eye that is not patched. Sunglasses reduce glare and improve contrast for individuals with optic neuritis. Nonoptical aids such as large print, tape recorders, and high contrast markings are also useful.

Bathtub rails, elevated toilet seats, and grab bars are useful bathroom safety devices. A stall shower is safer and easier to use than a combination tub/shower. A shower chair or tub seat provides additional safety.

Special controls installed on cars with automatic transmissions enable many individuals with multiple sclerosis to continue driving. The gas and brake pedals are operated by hand. These attachments do not interfere with the foot pedals used by other family members. Rehabilitation hospitals and centers offer driver evaluation services such as clinical testing and observation to determine an individual's need for adaptive equipment or training. Major automobile manufacturers offer reimbursement for adaptive equipment installed on new vehicles. (See Chapter 2, "ORGANIZATIONS" section, beginning on p. 75 for a listing of programs that offer adaptive equipment for automobiles.)

Some individuals use assistive devices for dressing, including elastic shoelaces, velcro closures, and buttoning aids. National mail order companies offer clothes that open in front and have reinforced seams, elastic waistbands, and buttons sewn with elastic thread. Formerly these items were limited to leisure and hospital wear, but manufacturers are now designing suits, outerwear, and dressy items for working men who have disabilities. Foam hair rollers, water pipe foam insulation, or layers of tape are used to build up the handles of items as varied as toothbrushes, pens, pencils, eating utensils, paint brushes, and tools. Many mail order catalogues offer a wide selection of assistive devices for individuals with disabilities and chronic conditions (see Chapter 2, "Coping with Daily Activities," p. 71 for sources of these devices).

Remote controls turn on and off lights and televisions and open and close garage doors. Voice dialer telephones permit the storage of frequently called telephone numbers and automatic dialing. A speaker phone allows individuals with poor motor control or tremors to carry on a telephone conversation comfortably.

Individuals with multiple sclerosis can save time and energy by reorganizing the kitchen and changing food preparation routines. Many individuals learn valuable tips and techniques from peers in multiple sclerosis support groups or from occupational therapists.

References

Betts, Christopher D.
1996 "Pathophysiology of Male Sexual Dysfunction in Multiple Sclerosis" Sexuality and Disability 14:1:41-55
Calvano, Margaret
1991 Facts & Issues New York, NY: National Multiple Sclerosis Society
1989 Facts & Issues New York, NY: National Multiple Sclerosis Society
Frames, Robin
1992 Sexual Dysfunction: Dare We Discuss It? New York, NY: National Multiple Sclerosis Society

Frankel, Debra
1994 <u>Living with MS</u> New York, NY: National Multiple Sclerosis Society

Goodkin, Donald E.
1994 "Interferon Beta-Ib" <u>The Lancet</u> 344:8929:1057

Holland, Nancy
1996 "For Urinary Problems: Get A Diagnosis First!" <u>Inside MS</u> New York, NY: National Multiple Sclerosis Society 14:1:19-20

Kalb, Rosalind et al.
1997 "Multiple Sclerosis: The Questions You Have, The Answers You Need, 1997 Update" <u>Multiple Sclerosis Quarterly Report</u> 16:3

Kalb, Rosalind (ed.)
1996 <u>Multiple Sclerosis: The Questions You Have, The Answers You Need</u> New York, NY: Demos Vermande

Lechtenberg, Richard
1995 <u>Multiple Sclerosis Fact Book</u> Philadelphia, PA: F.A. Davis Company

Mahler, M.E.
1992 "Behavioral Manifestations Associated with Multiple Sclerosis" <u>Psychiatric Clinics of North America</u> 15(June)2:425-438

Minden, Sarah L. and Debra Frankel
1989 <u>PLAINTALK: A Booklet About Multiple Sclerosis for Family Members</u> New York, NY: National Multiple Sclerosis Society

Nadig, Perry W.
1994 "Vacuum Constriction Devices in Patients with Neurogenic Impotence" <u>Sexuality and Disability</u> 12:1:99-105

National Center for Health Statistics, Collins, John G.
1988 "Prevalence of Selected Chronic Conditions, United States, 1983-85" <u>Advance Data From Vital and Health Statistics</u> No. 155 DHHS Pub. No (PHS) 88-1250. Public Health Service Hyattsville, MD

National Institute of Neurological Disorders and Stroke
1990 <u>Multiple Sclerosis: 1990 Research Program</u> Bethesda, MD: National Institutes of Health

National Multiple Sclerosis Society
1998 <u>National Multiple Sclerosis Society Disease Management Consensus Statement</u> New York, NY: National Multiple Sclerosis Society

1995 "Expansion of Treatment IND Program for Copolymer 1 (Copaxone)" <u>Research & Medical Programs Department News</u> January 6

Opsomer, Reinier J.
1996 "Management of Male Sexual Dysfunction in Multiple Sclerosis" <u>Sexuality and Disability</u> 14:1:57-63

Rao, S. M. et al.
1991 "Cognitive Dysfunction in Multiple Sclerosis II. Impact on Employment and Social Functioning" <u>Neurology</u> 41(May)5:692-696

Rodgers, Jennifer and Peter Calder
1990 "Marital Adjustment: A Valuable Resource for the Emotional Health of Individuals with Multiple Sclerosis" Rehabilitation Counseling Bulletin 34(September)1:24-32

Scheinberg, Labe
1983 "Signs, Symptoms, and Course of MS" pp. 35-43 in Labe C. Scheinberg (ed.) Multiple Sclerosis: A Guide for Patients and Their Families New York, NY: Raven Press

Scheinberg, Labe and Charles R. Smith
1989 Rehabilitation of Patients with Multiple Sclerosis New York, NY: National Multiple Sclerosis Society

Segal, Julia
1991 "Counselling People with Multiple Sclerosis and Their Families" pp.147-160 in Hilton Davis and Lesley Fallowfield (eds.) Counselling and Communication in Health Care London: John Wiley and Sons

Shuman, Robert and Janice Schwartz
1988 Understanding Multiple Sclerosis Riverside, NJ: MacMillan Publishing Company

Smith, Charles R. and Labe Scheinberg
1990 "Symptomatic Treatment and Rehabilitation in Multiple Sclerosis" pp. 327-350 in Stuart D. Cook (ed.) Handbook of Multiple Sclerosis New York, NY: Marcel Dekker, Inc.
1985 "Clinical Features of Multiple Sclerosis" Seminars in Neurology 5(June)2:85-93

Sullivan, Michael J., L. Krista Edgley, and Eric Dehoux
1990 "A Survey of Multiple Sclerosis Part 1: Perceived Cognitive Problems and Compensatory Strategy Use" Canadian Journal of Rehabilitation 4:2:99-105

Vermote, R. and J. Peuskens
1996 "Sexual and Micturition Problems in Multiple Sclerosis Patients: Psychological Issues" Sexuality and Disability 14:1:73-82

Warren, S., K. G. Warren, and R. Cockrill
1991 "Emotional Stress and Coping in Multiple Sclerosis Exacerbations" Journal of Psychosomatic Research 35:1:37-47

White, David M., Marci L. Catanzaro, and George H. Kraft
1991 "An Approach to the Psychological Aspects of Multiple Sclerosis: A Coping Guide for Healthcare Providers and Families" Journal of Neurological Rehabilitation 7:2:43-52

ORGANIZATIONS

Avonex Support Line
(800) 456-2255   http://www.avonex.com

Provides information on Avonex, a drug used in treating relapsing forms of multiple sclerosis, distribution options, insurance reimbursement counseling, and/or training for self-administration of the drug. Phone lines open Monday through Friday, 8:30 a.m. to 8:00 p.m., Eastern Standard Time. Publishes quarterly newsletter, "The Alliance Exchange;" free. Also available on the web site.

Betaseron Foundation
4828 Parkway Plaza Boulevard, Suite 220
Charlotte, NC 28217-1969
(800) 948-5777   FAX (704) 357-0036
http://www.betaseronfoundation.org

Provides Betaseron to qualified underinsured patients. Requirements include a confirmed diagnosis of multiple sclerosis, prescription for Betaseron, inadequate medical insurance, and a Social Security number. Patient financial contribution is required (up to $50.00 per month). Uninsured patients will be referred to Berlex, the manufacturer of Betaseron, for assistance [(800) 788-1467].

MS Pathways
Betaseron
PO Box 52171
Phoenix, AZ 85072-2171
(800) 788-1467   http://www.betaseron.com

Sponsored by Berlex, the manufacturer of Betaseron, this program provides information on Betaseron, a drug used in treating relapsing-remitting multiple sclerosis, self-administration training, insurance reimbursement, community support groups, and online services. Publishes quarterly newsletter, "MessageS," free. Also available on the web site.

National Association for Continence (NAFC)
PO Box 8310
Spartanburg, SC 29305-8310
(800) 252-3337   (864) 579-7900   FAX (864) 579-7902
http://www.nafc.org

An information clearinghouse that answers questions if self-addressed stamped envelope is enclosed with letter. Membership, $20.00, includes a quarterly newsletter, "Quality Care," a "Resource Guide: Products and Services for Continence" (nonmembers, $13.00), and a continence referral service. Free publications list.

National Institute of Neurological Disorders and Stroke (NINDS)
Building 31, Room 8A06
31 Center Drive, MSC 2540
Bethesda, MD 20892-2540
(800) 352-9424   (301) 496-5751   FAX (301) 402-2186
http://www.ninds.nih.gov

A federal agency which conducts basic and clinical research on the causes and treatment of multiple sclerosis.

National Multiple Sclerosis Society
733 Third Avenue
New York, NY 10017-3288
(212) 986-3240   FAX (212) 986-7981
(800) 344-4867 Information Resource Center and Library
e-mail: Nat@nmss.org   http://www.nmss.org

Provides professional and public education and information and referral; supports research. Offers counseling services, physician referrals, advocacy, discount prescription and health care products program, and assistance in obtaining adaptive equipment. Regional affiliates throughout the U.S. Information Resource Center and Library answers telephone inquiries from 11:00 a.m. to 5:00 p.m. E.S.T., Monday through Thursday. Membership, $20.00, includes large print magazine, "Inside MS," published three times per year. Individuals with multiple sclerosis may receive a courtesy membership if they are unable to pay.

Shared Solutions
Teva Marion Partners
2800 Rock Creek Parkway
Kansas City, MO 64117-2551
(800) 887-8100   http://www.tevamarionpartners.com

This program, sponsored by the manufacturer of Copaxone, provides information about the drug, which is used to reduce the frequency of relapses in the relapsing-remitting form of multiple sclerosis, treatment reimbursement programs, and local resources. The web site provides an online medication diary, chat rooms, and advice from professionals.

Simon Foundation for Continence
PO Box 835
Wilmette, IL 60091
(800) 237-4666   (847) 864-3913   FAX (847) 864-9758

Provides information and assistance to people who are incontinent. Organizes self-help groups. Membership, individuals, $15.00; professionals, $35.00; includes quarterly newsletter, "The Informer."

ADA and People with MS
by Laura Cooper and Nancy Law with Jane Sarnoff
National Multiple Sclerosis Society
733 Third Avenue
New York, NY 10017-3288
(212) 986-3240   FAX (212) 986-7981
(800) 344-4867 Information Resource Center and Library
e-mail: Nat@nmss.org   http://www.nmss.org

This booklet explains how the Americans with Disabilities Act applies to individuals with multiple sclerosis. Large print. $1.00 plus $2.00 shipping and handling

Aqua Exercise for Multiple Sclerosis
National Multiple Sclerosis Society
733 Third Avenue
New York, NY 10017-3288
(212) 986-3240   FAX (212) 986-7981
(800) 344-4867 Information Resource Center and Library
e-mail: Nat@nmss.org   http://www.nmss.org

This videotape presents exercises for building strength and endurance as well as reducing spasticity. Includes print reference card. 15 minutes. $12.00 plus $2.00 shipping and handling

At Home with MS: Adapting Your Environment
National Multiple Sclerosis Society
733 Third Avenue
New York, NY 10017-3288
(212) 986-3240   FAX (212) 986-7981
(800) 344-4867 Information Resource Center and Library
e-mail: Nat@nmss.org   http://www.nmss.org

This booklet suggests modifications that can be made to the home to compensate for mobility or visual impairment. $1.00 plus $2.00 shipping and handling

Clinical Trials in MS: Searching for New Therapies
National Multiple Sclerosis Society
733 Third Avenue
New York, NY 10017-3288
(212) 986-3240   FAX (212) 986-7981
(800) 344-4867 Information Resource Center and Library
e-mail: Nat@nmss.org   http://www.nmss.org

This videotape describes the clinical trials used to evaluate new drugs and discusses the role of participants. 20 minutes. $20.00 plus $2.00 shipping and handling

dirty details, the days and nights of a well spouse
by Marion Deutsche Cohen
Temple University Press
1601 North Broad Street
Philadelphia, PA 19122
(800) 447-1656   FAX (215) 204-4719
e-mail: tempress@astro.ocis.temple.edu
http://www.temple.edu/tempress

A frank, personal account, written by a woman whose husband has multiple sclerosis, this book describes her caregiving experiences. Hardcover, $49.95; softcover, $18.95; plus $4.00 shipping and handling.

Employment Issues and Multiple Sclerosis
by Philip D. Rumrill
Demos Vermande
386 Park Avenue South, Suite 201
New York, NY 10016
(800) 532-8663   (212) 683-0072   FAX (212) 683-0118

This book discuss how employment may be affected by multiple sclerosis. Includes information about vocational rehabilitation, job placement and retention, the Americans with Disabilities Act, and other legal issues. $29.95 plus $4.00 shipping and handling

Enabling Romance: A Guide to Love, Sex, and Relationships for the Disabled
by Ken Kroll and Erica Levy Klein
Woodbine House
6510 Bells Mill Road
Bethesda, MD 20817
(800) 843-7323   FAX (301) 897-5838
e-mail: info@woodbinehouse.com   http://www.woodbinehouse.com

Written by a man who has a disability and his wife who does not, this book provides examples of how people with a variety of disabilities have established fulfilling relationships. $15.95 plus $4.50 shipping and handling

Frank Talk
by JoAnn LeMaistre
Alpine Guild
PO Box 4848
Dillon, CO 80435
(800) 869-9559   FAX (970) 262-9378

In this videotape, individuals with multiple sclerosis share their concerns about living with chronic illness and discuss coping strategies. 30 minutes. $39.95

Intermittent Self-Catheterization
Media Services
Sacred Heart Medical Center
PO Box 2555
Spokane, WA 99220-2555
(509) 458-5236   FAX (509) 626-4475
http://www.spokanehealth.org/shmc/mediaservices

This videotape demonstrates the use of sterile techniques for intermittent catheterization and shows the necessary supplies and procedures. 8 minutes. Available in English and Spanish. Purchase, individual, $19.95; institution, $99.00; rental for one week, $45.00 (may be applied toward purchase); plus $5.00 shipping and handling. Accompanying booklet, "Clean Intermittent Self-Catheterization," available in English and Spanish; $.50.

Knowledge is Power
National Multiple Sclerosis Society
733 Third Avenue
New York, NY 10017-3288
(212) 986-3240   FAX (212) 986-7981
(800) 344-4867 Information Resource Center and Library
e-mail: Nat@nmss.org   http://www.nmss.org

This home study course provides information about multiple sclerosis including a medical overview, emotional aspects, legal issues, fatigue, sexuality, job accommodation under the Americans with Disabilities Act, family issues, and more. Once individuals are registered for the program, one article per week is mailed to them. Free

Living Well with MS: A Guide for Patient, Caregiver, and Family
by David L. Carroll and Jon Dudley Dorman
Harper Collins Publishers
PO Box 588
Scranton, PA 18512
(800) 331-3761   http://www.harpercollins.com

In addition to information on multiple sclerosis and its diagnosis, prognosis, and treatment, this book discusses emotional and sexual functioning. $13.00 plus $2.75 shipping and handling

Living with Low Vision: A Resource Guide for People with Sight Loss
Resources for Rehabilitation
33 Bedford Street, Suite 19A
Lexington, MA 02420
(781) 862-6455   FAX (781) 861-7517
e-mail: info@rfr.org   http://www.rfr.org

A large print (18 point bold type) comprehensive directory that helps people with sight loss locate the services that they need to remain independent. Chapters describe products that enable people to keep reading, working, and carrying out their daily activities. Information about resources on the Internet is included. $44.95 plus $5.00 shipping and handling (See order form on last page of this book.)

Living with Multiple Sclerosis: A New Handbook for Families
by Robert Shuman and Janice Schwartz
MacMillan Publishing Company
201 West 103rd Street
Indianapolis, IN 46290
(800) 428-5331   FAX (800) 882-8583
http://www.superlibrary.com

In this book, two psychologists discuss the role of the family with a member who has multiple sclerosis. Includes chapters on adolescents with multiple sclerosis, employment, and research. Uses real life experiences to suggest coping strategies and adaptations. $12.95 plus $3.50 shipping and handling

Living with Multiple Sclerosis: A Wellness Approach
by George H. Kraft and Marci Catanzaro
Demos Vermande
386 Park Avenue South, Suite 201
New York, NY 10016
(800) 532-8663   (212) 683-0072   FAX (212) 683-0118

This book suggest strategies for everyday living with multiple sclerosis. Includes information on diet, nutrition, and exercise. $15.95 plus $4.00 shipping and handling

Mainstay: For the Well Spouse of the Chronically Ill
by Maggie Strong
Bradford Books
160 Main Street
Northampton, MA 01060-3134
(413) 584-4597   http://gcim.com/mainstay

Written by a woman whose husband was diagnosed with multiple sclerosis at age 46, this book provides her personal account and others' stories, practical suggestions, and advice from health care professionals. $15.00 plus $3.00 shipping and handling

Managing Incontinence
by Cheryle B. Gartley (ed.)
Simon Foundation for Continence
PO Box 835
Wilmette, IL 60091
(800) 237-4666   (847) 864-3913   FAX (847) 864-9758

This book provides medical advice, information on products, interviews with individuals who are incontinent, and advice on sexuality. $11.95

Moving with Multiple Sclerosis: An Exercise Manual for People with Multiple Sclerosis
by Iris Kimberg
National Multiple Sclerosis Society
733 Third Avenue
New York, NY 10017-3288
(212) 986-3240   FAX (212) 986-7981
(800) 344-4867 Information Resource Center and Library
e-mail: Nat@nmss.org   http://www.nmss.org

This booklet describes four types of exercises designed to relieve some multiple sclerosis symptoms. Includes passive range of motion and stretching, active and active restrictive, coordination and balance, and exercises to reduce spasticity. Numerous illustrations guide the individual and helper through each exercise sequence. Large print. $3.00 plus $2.00 shipping and handling

Multiple Sclerosis: A Guide for Families
by Rosalind C. Kalb (ed.)
Demos Vermande
386 Park Avenue South, Suite 201
New York, NY 10016
(800) 532-8663   (212) 683-0072   FAX (212) 683-0118

This book discusses issues such as caregiving, adults with MS and their parents, cognitive problems, financial planning, sexuality, and reproduction. Includes bibliography and resources. $24.95 plus $4.00 shipping and handling

Multiple Sclerosis: A Guide for the Newly Diagnosed
by Nancy Holland, T. Jock Murray, and Stephen Reingold
Demos Vermande
386 Park Avenue South, Suite 201
New York, NY 10016
(800) 532-8663   (212) 683-0072   FAX (212) 683-0118

This book provides information about multiple sclerosis and medical treatments as well as its effect on the individual and the family. $21.95 plus $4.00 shipping and handling

Multiple Sclerosis: A Personal Exploration
by Alexander Burnfield
Demos Vermande
386 Park Avenue South, Suite 201
New York, NY 10016
(800) 532-8663   (212) 683-0072   FAX (212) 683-0118

Written by a physician who has multiple sclerosis, this book discusses many of the psycho-social aspects of the condition, including grief, self-pity, guilt, anger, and resentment and their effects on marriage and the family. $16.95 plus $4.00 shipping and handling

Multiple Sclerosis: A Self-Care Guide to Wellness
by Nancy Holland and June Halper
PVA Distribution Center
PO Box 753
Waldorf, MD 20604-0753
(888) 860-7244   (301) 932-7834   FAX (301) 843-0159
http://www.pva.org

This book discusses how MS affects the lives of both those with the disease and those who provide care, emphasizing strategies to promote independence, well-being, and productivity. $9.00

Multiple Sclerosis Fact Book
by Richard Lechtenberg
F.A. Davis Company
404-420 North 2nd Street
Philadelphia, PA 19123
(800) 323-3555   FAX (215) 440-3016
e-mail: orders@fadavis.com   http://www.fadavis.com

Written for the lay person, this book describes up-to-date diagnostic tests and therapies and provides practical ideas for coping with multiple sclerosis. $21.95

Multiple Sclerosis Quarterly Report
Demos Vermande
386 Park Avenue South, Suite 201
New York, NY 10016
(800) 532-8663   (212) 683-0072   FAX (212) 683-0118

This newsletter reports advances in the diagnosis and treatment of multiple sclerosis. $19.50

Multiple Sclerosis: The Questions You Have, The Answers You Need
by Rosalind Kalb (ed.)
Demos Vermande
386 Park Avenue South, Suite 201
New York, NY 10016
(800) 532-8663   (212) 683-0072   FAX (212) 683-0118

Written by professionals who care for individuals with multiple sclerosis, this book provides information about living with the condition and answers questions most commonly asked. Topics include neurology, treatment, employment, legal issues, physical and occupational therapy, psychosocial issues, sexuality, and reproductive health. $39.95 plus $4.00 shipping and handling

The Other Victim - Caregivers Share Their Coping Strategies
by Alan Drattell
Seven Locks Press
PO Box 25689
Santa Ana, CA 92799
(800) 354-5348   e-mail: sevenlocks@aol.com

This book is a collection of personal accounts of nine caregivers of individuals with multiple sclerosis. Also includes a resource list of organizations and suggestions for coping. $17.95 plus $4.00 shipping and handling

PLAINTALK: A Booklet about Multiple Sclerosis for Family Members
by Sarah L. Minden and Debra Frankel
National Multiple Sclerosis Society
733 Third Avenue
New York, NY 10017-3288
(212) 986-3240   FAX (212) 986-7981
(800) 344-4867 Information Resource Center and Library
e-mail: Nat@nmss.org   http://www.nmss.org

This booklet simulates a support group meeting for families of individuals with multiple sclerosis. Discusses diagnosis, everyday living, talking with children, and the well parent. Large print. $1.00 plus $2.00 shipping and handling

Providing Services for People with Vision Loss
by Susan L. Greenblatt (ed.)
Resources for Rehabilitation
33 Bedford Street, Suite 19A
Lexington, MA 02420
(781) 862-6455   FAX (781) 861-7517
e-mail: info@rfr.org   http://www.rfr.org

This anthology discusses how health and rehabilitation professionals can work together to provide coordinated care for individuals who have experienced vision loss. Also available on audiocassette. $19.95 plus $5.00 shipping and handling (See order form on last page of this book.)

Real Living with Multiple Sclerosis
Springhouse Corporation
1111 Bethlehem Pike
Springhouse, PA 19477
(800) 783-4903   http://www.springnet.com

This monthly publication provides information about research and medical treatment as well as support through personal experiences and tips for everyday living with multiple sclerosis. $49.00

Rehabilitation Resource Manual: VISION
Resources for Rehabilitation
33 Bedford Street, Suite 19A
Lexington, MA 02420
(781) 862-6455   FAX (781) 861-7517
e-mail: info@rfr.org   http://www.rfr.org

This desk reference helps service providers make effective referrals for individuals with vision loss. Provides information on understanding responses to vision loss and describes optical and nonoptical aids. Chapters on services and products for special population groups and by eye conditions and diseases. $39.95 plus $5.00 shipping and handling (See order form on last page of this book.)

Reproductive Issues for Persons with Physical Disabilities
by Florence P. Haseltine, Sandra S. Cole, and David B. Gray (eds.)
Brookes Publishing Company
PO Box 10624
Baltimore, MD 21285-0624
(800) 638-3775   FAX (410) 337-8539
e-mail: custserv@pbrookes.com   http://www.pbrookes.com

This book provides an overview of sexuality, disability, and reproductive issues across the lifespan for individuals with disabilities including multiple sclerosis.   Includes academic articles as well as personal narratives written by individuals with disabilities. $34.95

Someone You Know Has MS: A Book for Families $1.00
by Cyrisse Jaffee, Debra Frankel, Barbara LaRoche, and Patricia Dick
When a Parent Has MS: A Teenager's Guide $1.00
by Pamela Cavallo with Martha Jablow
National Multiple Sclerosis Society
733 Third Avenue
New York, NY 10017-3288
(212) 986-3240   FAX (212) 986-7981
(800) 344-4867 Information Resource Center and Library
e-mail: Nat@nmss.org   http://www.nmss.org

These two booklets, one written for children age 6-12 and the other for teenagers, help youngsters understand their parent's condition and discuss the youngsters' concerns and fears. Large print.   Add $2.00 shipping and handling

Symptom Management in Multiple Sclerosis
by Randall T. Shapiro
Demos Vermande
386 Park Avenue South, Suite 201
New York, NY 10016
(800) 532-8663   (212) 683-0072   FAX (212) 683-0118

A multidisciplinary guide for health care professionals and individuals with multiple sclerosis which suggests management strategies for treating multiple sclerosis and minimizing and controlling its symptoms. $19.95 plus $4.00 shipping and handling

Taking Care: A Guide for Well Partners
by Nancy J. Holland with Jane Sarnoff
National Multiple Sclerosis Society
733 Third Avenue
New York, NY 10017-3288
(212) 986-3240   FAX (212) 986-7981
(800) 344-4867 Information Resource Center and Library
e-mail: Nat@nmss.org   http://www.nmss.org

This booklet discusses how to balance the needs of both partners and how to ask for and receive help. Large print. $1.00 plus $2.00 shipping and handling

Talking Books for People with Physical Disabilities
National Library Service for the Blind and Physically Handicapped (NLS)
1291 Taylor Street, NW
Washington, DC 20542
(800) 424-8567 or 8572 (Reference Section)
(800) 424-9100 (to receive application)
(202) 707-5100   (202) 707-0744 (TT)   FAX (202) 707-0712
e-mail: nls@loc.gov   http://www.loc.gov/nls

This brochure describes a free program which provides books and magazines recorded on discs and audiocassettes for individuals with multiple sclerosis and other disabling conditions. Application forms are available from the NLS, public libraries, or local affiliates of the National Multiple Sclerosis Society. A health professional must certify that the individual is unable to hold a book or turn pages; has blurred or double vision; extreme weakness or excessive fatigue; or other physical limitations which prevent the individual from reading standard print.

Therapeutic Claims in Multiple Sclerosis: A Guide to Treatments
by William A. Sibley
Demos Vermande
386 Park Avenue South, Suite 201
New York, NY 10016
(800) 532-8663   (212) 683-0072   FAX (212) 683-0118

In addition to basic information about the symptoms and diagnosis of multiple sclerosis, this book describes the most frequently used therapies and their effectiveness. An opinion statement, made by the International Federation of Multiple Sclerosis Societies, accompanies each listing. $24.95 plus $4.00 shipping and handling

Understanding Bladder Problems in Multiple Sclerosis
by Nancy J. Holland and Michele G. Madonna
Understanding Bowel Problems in MS
by Nancy J. Holland and Robin Frames
National Multiple Sclerosis Society
733 Third Avenue
New York, NY 10017-3288
(212) 986-3240   FAX (212) 986-7981
(800) 344-4867 Information Resource Center and Library
e-mail: Nat@nmss.org   http://www.nmss.org

These booklets describe how multiple sclerosis affects the urinary and digestive tracts; how to control symptoms; and how to manage bladder and bowel dysfunction. Large print. $1.00 each plus $2.00 shipping and handling

Vignettes: Stories of Life with MS
by John K. Wolf
Academy Press
PO Box 757
Rutland, VT 05702
(800) 356-3002   FAX (802) 773-6892

This collection of essays, poems, and stories is written by and about individuals with multiple sclerosis. $24.95

Wheelchairs: Your Options and Rights Guide to Obtaining Wheelchairs from the Department of Veterans Affairs
PVA Distribution Center
PO Box 753
Waldorf, MD 20604-0753
(888) 860-7244   (301) 932-7834   FAX (301) 843-0159
http://www.pva.org

This booklet provides information on eligibility criteria, lists the types of wheelchairs available, and describes DVA procedures. Available in English and Spanish. Free

You Are Not Your Illness
by Linda Noble Topf
Simon and Schuster
200 Old Tappan Road
Old Tappan, NJ 07675
(800) 223-2336   FAX (800) 445-6991
e-mail: ss cust serv@prenhall.com http://www.simonsays.com

This book describes the author's personal perspectives on living with multiple sclerosis and provides a step-by-step process for dealing with loss and maintaining feelings of self-worth. $12.00

Chapter 8

PROSTATE CONDITIONS

Many men who encounter urinary problems as they grow older attribute these problems to the normal aging process. However, frequent or painful urination, urgency, or the need to get up at night to urinate may be signs of prostate disease. The quality of a man's life may be greatly affected by an inflamed or enlarged prostate that causes urinary problems. Cancer of the prostate is life-threatening.

The prostate, a gland about the size of a walnut, is located in front of the rectum and below the bladder. It surrounds the urethra which carries urine from the bladder through the penis out of the body. The prostate supplies fluid that becomes part of semen along with sperm and is ejaculated from the penis.

Prostate conditions accounted for more than 25% of all visits to urologists in 1989-90 (Woodwell: 1992). Benign prostatic hyperplasia (BPH) was the most frequent primary diagnosis (13% of visits). Prostate cancer (7%) and prostatitis (5.4%) were other principal diagnoses.

The American Urological Association recommends that men over age 50 have an annual prostate examination, which includes a digital rectal examination (DRE) and a prostate-specific antigen (PSA) blood test (Prostate Health Council: 1991a). In a DRE, the physician examines the prostate by inserting a gloved and lubricated finger into the rectum. The physician can determine by touch whether the prostate is enlarged or if there are any irregularities in texture. The DRE is used to detect two prostate conditions, benign prostatic hyperplasia, an enlargement of the prostate, and prostate cancer. Although benign prostatic hyperplasia is not cancer, individuals may have both BPH and prostate cancer.

PROSTATITIS

Prostatitis is a term used to describe several conditions that cause inflammation of the prostate gland. Although most prostate conditions affect men later in life, prostatitis can occur in younger men. Symptoms include chills and fever; lower back, joint, or muscle pain; urinary problems such as difficulty in urinating, a frequent urge to urinate, burning or pain when urinating, or pus or blood in the urine; prostate tenderness or swelling; and painful ejaculation. Risk factors for prostatitis include recent use of a urinary catheter, urinary infections, rectal intercourse, an enlarged prostate due to aging, and abnormalities in the urinary tract. Prostatitis is not contagious.

Acute and *chronic bacterial prostatitis* are associated with urinary tract infections and are most commonly seen in elderly men (Cunha et al.: 1991). A bacterial localization test should be performed to confirm prostatic infections (Walsh and Worthington: 1995). In this test, a three-glass urine collection method is used to analyze urine and prostatic fluid (Prostate Health Council: 1991b). First, two urine samples are collected separately: the first ounce from the urethra, the second from the bladder (midstream flow). After nearly emptying the bladder, the physician massages the prostate and collects the prostatic fluid on a laboratory slide. This procedure is called *prostate stripping* or *prostate massage*. The remainder of the urine in the bladder is then collected in a third container. The results of this test will help determine treatment. Acute bacterial prostatitis is the least common form of the condition. Its symptoms, such as fever and flu-like symptoms, flare up suddenly but respond well to treatment with antibiotics. An initial high dose of an antibiotic such as ciprofloxacin is recommended to avoid chronic recurrence (Walsh and Worthington: 1995). *Chronic bacterial prostatitis* is more difficult to treat, since the antibiotics used to clear the urinary tract infection do not diffuse well in prostatic tissue.

Individuals with *chronic nonbacterial prostatitis*, the most common form of prostatitis, test negatively for infection and have no history of urinary tract infections. Since this condition is not caused by bacteria, it is not responsive to antibiotic treatment. Despite this fact, however, according to a recent study, nearly 50% of men who were diagnosed with prostatitis with genitourinary symptoms received prescriptions for antibiotics (Collins et al.: 1998). Some men find relief through the use of sitz baths and muscle relaxers.

BENIGN PROSTATIC HYPERPLASIA

Benign prostatic hyperplasia (BPH), or an enlarged prostate gland, is a condition that affects more than half of men over age 60 and nearly 90% by age 85, although not all men experience the symptoms of BPH or require treatment (McConnell et al.: 1994). It is the most common benign tumor in men. As a man ages, the glandular tissue in the prostate grows and the smooth muscle tissue tightens, squeezing the urethra, often causing problems in urinating. These problems may include frequent urination, weak urinary stream, urgency, inability to empty the bladder completely, difficulty starting the urinary stream, dribbling, incontinence, and the need to get up at night to urinate. BPH increases a man's risk of developing urinary tract infections when he is unable to empty his bladder completely. This in turn may lead to acute or chronic bacterial prostatitis. BPH is diagnosed through a combination of the medical history, DRE, urinalysis, blood tests, and general physical examination. Since BPH may be detected as part of routine care, in the absence of symptoms, not all cases require treatment. The individual may opt for "watchful waiting," undergoing periodic checkups but choosing to delay medical or surgical treatment. Some men find that restricting liquids before bedtime and limiting use of decongestants may reduce the need for frequent urination (Prostate Health Council: 1996).

However, if symptoms interfere with activities of daily living or if the individual's urinary tract is affected, there are a variety of treatment options, including medications, surgery, and balloon dilation. Surgery remains the most common treatment for BPH, since it relieves symptoms and its risks and benefits are well known. There are three types of prostatic surgery. *Transurethral resection of the prostate* (TURP) reduces pressure on the urethra. An instrument called a resectoscope is inserted through the penis into the urethra and some of the tissue inside the enlarged prostate is removed. A catheter is necessary for several days after surgery, and antibiotics may be given to prevent infection. In a recent five year study of men with moderate symptoms of BPH who were randomized for either watchful waiting or TURP, the men who underwent surgery had fewer genitourinary symptoms than those in the untreated group (Flanigan et al.: 1998).

Transurethral incision of the prostate (TUIP) is used in men whose prostate is not as severely enlarged. One or two small cuts are made from the neck of the bladder into the prostate, relieving pressure on the urethra and reducing problems in urination. In an ***open prostatectomy***, an inside part of the greatly enlarged prostate is removed through an incision made in the lower abdomen. Since a man can have both BPH and prostate cancer, tissue removed during surgery will be examined for the presence of cancer cells.

The Agency for Health Care Policy and Research (1994) reports that the chance of an improvement in BPH symptoms is 75 to 96% with each of the three procedures. TURP has a 5 to 31% chance of complications such as infection, bleeding, and temporary inability to urinate. If the prostate tissue grows back or scar tissue blocks the urinary tract, additional surgery may be required. A common problem after surgical treatment is retrograde ejaculation, in which semen flows back into the bladder instead of out through the penis, causing a dry ejaculation. This will affect a man's fertility but does not cause impotence, and orgasm may still be achieved. TUIP is more likely than TURP to preserve normal ejaculation and is better suited to a younger man whose prostate is less enlarged and who wishes to remain fertile (Walsh and Worthington: 1995).

In 1996, the Food and Drug Administration approved the use of lasers in the surgical treatment of BPH (National Institute of Diabetes and Digestive and Kidney Diseases: 1998). Using a cystoscope, the physician passes the laser fiber through the urethra into the prostate gland. The tissue which is obstructing the prostate is vaporized in 30 to 60 second bursts of energy. Men must be hospitalized for this type of surgery. There is less blood loss in laser surgery than in TURP and a shorter recovery period; however, the long term effectiveness is unknown.

After surgery, it is recommended that men drink up to eight cups of water a day to help flush out the bladder; prevent constipation with a balanced diet; and refrain from heavy lifting and driving or operating heavy machinery (National Institute of Diabetes and Digestive and Kidney Diseases: 1998).

Drugs known as ***alpha blockers*** relax the muscle tissue in the prostate and the neck of the bladder, improving the man's urinary symptoms. In recent years, the Food and Drug Administration approved terazosin (Hytrin), doxazosin (Cardura), and tamsulosin (Flomax) for use in treating BPH. Symptoms should improve within a few weeks. Possible side effects include headaches, dizziness, fatigue, and feeling lightheaded; some individuals have developed low blood pressure or have difficulty achieving an erection (Prostate Health Council: 1996).

Finasteride (Proscar) lowers the level of testosterone, the major male hormone found in the prostate, thereby shrinking the enlarged prostate and increasing urinary flow. It may take six months or more to note a reduction in symptoms. Side effects may include reduced libido and problems achieving an erection and ejaculating (Agency for Health Care Policy and Research: 1994). Since alpha blocker and finasteride treatments are new, long term benefits and risks are unknown. One recent study to test the effectiveness of terazosin and finasteride alone or together has revealed that terazosin alone is effective, whereas finasteride, alone is not. The combination of the two drugs had no advantage over terazosin alone (Lepor et al.: 1996).

Balloon dilation is a procedure in which a limp balloon is inserted into the urethra, through a catheter in the penis. The balloon is inflated to stretch the urethra where it has been squeezed by the enlarged prostate. Improvement of symptoms is likely to be temporary, and some men experience urinary bleeding or infection. Nonsurgical treatment options for BPH that have been approved by the Food and Drug Administration include two devices that heat and destroy prostate tissue, reducing urinary problems, in a procedure called transurethral microwave thermotherapy (TUMT). The devices send microwaves through a catheter, heating the prostate and destroying tissue; a cooling system protects the urinary tract. The Transurethral Needle Ablation (TUNA) System uses needles to deliver radiofrequency energy directly to the prostate to burn away excess tissue, relieving symptoms and improving urine flow.

In 1996, the Food and Drug Administration approved the use of stents to correct urinary obstructions in men whose symptoms were unrelieved by surgery. The Urolume Endoprosthesis, a spring-like device is inserted into the narrowed area of the urethra and allowed to expand, pushing the prostatic tissue back and widening the urethra (National Institute of Diabetes and Digestive and Kidney Diseases: 1998).

PROSTATE CANCER

Prostate cancer is the second most common cancer in men in the United States, (American Cancer Society: 1998). In 1995, the National Cancer Institute estimated that nearly 250,000 men would be diagnosed with prostate cancer and that about 40,000 would die from it. The greatest risk factor for prostate cancer is age; nearly 75% of prostate cancer diagnoses are in men over the age of 65. African-American men are at highest risk, followed by men who have a father or brother with prostate cancer.

Prostate cancer initially affects the outer part of the prostate, spreading to the inner portion as the tumor grows. The symptoms of prostate cancer are very similar to those experienced by men with benign prostatic hyperplasia (BPH) but are caused by the growth of a malignant tumor. Symptoms such as difficulty with urination may not occur until the tumor is large enough to press on the urethra. Since prostate cancer is most curable in early stages, it is important that men undergo a DRE during annual physical examinations. If abnormalities are detected, additional tests will help determine whether or not cancer is present.

Although it is normal to find small amounts of PSA in the blood, levels tend to rise in men over age 60. Conditions other than prostate cancer may cause a rise in the PSA level. Both prostatitis and benign prostatic hyperplasia can raise the PSA two or three times the normal rate (American Cancer Society: 1995). It may take several weeks following prostate surgery for PSA levels to return to normal. Although there is no benchmark PSA level that indicates a positive cancer diagnosis, an elevation in PSA level can point to the presence of a tumor. Unfortunately, high or low levels can be misleading. False-negative and false-positive PSA tests have led to questions about the reliability of PSA testing as a tool to detect curable prostate cancer (Prostate Health Council: 1995). It should also be noted that finasteride (Proscar) lowers PSA levels in men who are being treated for benign prostatic hyperplasia (BPH). Therefore, PSA testing in these men may not be helpful in detecting prostate cancer (Prostate Health Council: 1995). If an initial PSA test is positive, it is wise to have the test repeated, in combination with a DRE. In the American Cancer Society's National Prostate Cancer Detection Project, about 30% of the cancer diagnoses were made in men whose PSA score level was lower than "normal" range; their cancer was diagnosed because DRE and ultrasound examinations were conducted in addition to the PSA test (Mettlin: 1997).

There is a great deal of controversy over the usefulness of the diagnostic tests now available to detect the presence of prostate cancer. Despite the current lack of evidence that prostate cancer screening reduces mortality (Collins and Barry: 1996), the American Urological Association recommends that men over age 50 have an annual prostate examination, which includes a DRE and a PSA blood test (Prostate Health Council: 1991). The American Cancer Society previously recommended that a PSA blood test be performed for men annually after the age of 50 and after age 40 for men in high risk groups, African-American men and men with a family history of prostate cancer; in 1997, however, it revised its guidelines. It now recommends that men over age 50 discuss the need for PSA testing and DRE with their health care providers. Men in high risk groups are advised to consider DREs and PSA testing before the age of 50 (American Cancer Society: 1997). The American College of Physicians recommends that its members inform men about the benefits and risks of screening, diagnosis, and treatment; listen to the individual's concerns; and make joint decisions on whether to screen or not (Rose: 1997). In a survey of primary care physicians, only a quarter of the subjects conducted PSA testing about half the time as a part of routine care (Collins et al.: 1997).

In a recent study, men who were considering PSA screening viewed a videotape that discussed PSA screening, its uncertainties, treatment for prostate cancer, and treatment complications. The men who viewed the videotape were less likely to proceed with PSA testing than men who had not viewed the videotape (Flood et al.: 1996).

The editors of <u>JAMA</u> (Journal of the American Medical Association) questioned the use of the PSA:

> Because many of the tumors detected by PSA would never become apparent clinically, it is not clear that the costs of detection and treatment, and the unpleasant adverse effects of treatment, are balanced by real benefit to the patient (Chabner et al.: 1997, p. 1475)

A transrectal ultrasound, another diagnostic tool, enables the physician to visualize the entire prostate. A probe, inserted into the rectum, transmits sound waves that bounce off the prostate and create a picture of it on a computer screen. The ultrasound procedure guides a needle that is used to remove prostatic tissue for biopsy. The needle may be inserted through the rectum into the prostate or into the perineum, the area between the scrotum and the anus. A biopsy is the only test that confirms the diagnosis of prostate cancer.

After a diagnosis of cancer is made, the physician will use a staging system to determine the site and location of the disease. This information is used in planning treatment. Stage A is the term used to describe symptomless prostate cancer found during surgery, usually for BPH. These tumors are so small or located so deep in the prostate that they are not found in a DRE. A firm or hard area confined to the prostate but large enough to be felt during a rectal examination is called stage B. In stage C, the tumor has spread throughout the prostate and into the seminal vesicles, which are located just behind the bladder. In Stage D, cancer

202

has spread (metastasized) to the lymph nodes and other parts of the body such as the bones, lungs, or liver (National Cancer Institute: 1996). Another staging system is the international TNM scale in which Tumor size (T), the extent of spread to the lymph Nodes (N), and the extent the cancer has spread or Metastasized (M) to other parts of the body is used to provide specific information about cancer stages (American Cancer Society: 1996).

In addition to staging, cancer cells are graded to determine how aggressive the tumor is. Grading measures how similar cancer cells are to normal cells. The more similar they are, the less aggressive the tumor. The Gleason system is the most common grading system. It ranges from a low score of 2 to a high score of 10. A Gleason score of 2 to 4 indicates that the cancer cells are less aggressive and usually slower to progress. An intermediate score is 5 to 7; a score of 8 to 10 predicts that the cancer cells are more likely to be aggressive (American Cancer Society: 1996).

Treatment options vary depending on the individual's tumor stage, age, and his overall health. The individual should seek advice from a number of sources in order to take an active part in making a decision about treatment. Sexual function and continence are frequently affected during treatment. Urologists, radiation oncologists, and other specialists may have biases for treatment based on their particular specialty. Individuals should contact national health organizations such as the American Cancer Society and the National Cancer Institute for information on cancer treatments, clinical trials, and community services. If possible, they should speak with others who have prostate cancer, possibly at support group meetings (described in "ORGANIZATIONS" section).

Some individuals may choose to do nothing. An elderly man with stage A disease, who is asymptomatic but has another serious health condition, may opt for *watchful waiting*, being closely monitored by the physician but delaying surgical or medical treatment.

Individuals whose tumors are confined to the prostate may choose to undergo a *radical prostatectomy*. This procedure is performed through a midline incision, from navel to pubic bone, or through the perineum. The entire prostate, the section of urethra that passes through it, and some of the surrounding tissue are removed from their position below the bladder. Pelvic lymph nodes may also be removed. The neck of the bladder is sutured to the remaining section of the urethra, and a catheter is inserted through the penis into the bladder to drain the urine while the wound heals. The catheter will remain in place for about 21 days following surgery. In the past, virtually all men who had this surgery became impotent. A nerve sparing technique is now used to preserve the nerves going to the penis so that potency may be maintained, although it may take 12 to 18 months for potency to return (Marks: 1995). A study of 600 men following radical prostatectomy indicated that post-operative sexual function in those over age 50 was better when both neurovascular bundles were preserved than if only one bundle was preserved (Quinlan et al.: 1991).

Incontinence is a common side effect of prostatectomy. The urinary sphincter muscle that controls urine outflow located below the prostate and the nerves that control it may be damaged when the prostate is removed. In overflow incontinence, the bladder retains urine after voiding and leaks involuntarily. Stress incontinence occurs when pressure to the bladder increases, usually during coughing, sneezing, exercise, and, sometimes, merely when rising from a chair or bed. Men with urge incontinence lose urine as soon as they feel the need to go to the bathroom. Some men find that incontinence is relieved with bladder training and pelvic muscle exercises. In bladder training, individuals learn to control the urge to urinate. They may also use a technique called prompted voiding or urinating on a schedule. Pelvic muscle exercises, also called Kegel exercises, strengthen pelvic muscles to hold back urine flow. During recuperation from surgery, incontinence products such as absorbent undergarments or pads may be used to manage incontinence. Men who continue to have severe incontinence may undergo urodynamic testing to evaluate bladder and sphincter function. The physician may suggest the use of a condom catheter or indwelling catheter, a penis clamp, or the surgical implantation of an artificial urinary sphincter.

The experiences of a writer who underwent surgery for prostate cancer provide an informative source for men who are contemplating surgery themselves. Korda (1996) was embarrassed to ask his doctor about a second opinion regarding treatment for prostate cancer; he worried that the physician would think that he did not trust him. When Korda consulted with a second urologist and showed him articles about patients' survival rates, the urologist became very angry. As in the case of Korda's physicians, urologists, radiation oncologists, and other specialists are likely to have biases for treatment based on their particular specialty; urologists recommend surgery, oncologists suggest radiation therapy. Different physicians gave Korda differing opinions as to the best course of treatment, yet he felt pressured to make a fast decision.

Physicians often downplay the need for post-surgical care. Although Korda's physician told him that he would not need nursing care at home after prostate surgery, he found that he did need nursing care. His community home health agency gave him a list of practical supplies that he would require, such as waterproof pads, surgical dressings, and incontinence products, and provided a home health aide for personal care.

The first national randomized controlled trial comparing watchful waiting with radical prostatectomy in men with prostate cancer will not report its results until 2008 (Agency for Health Care Policy and Research: 1997). Yet the results of a survey of urologists conducted by Plawker (1997) reveal that the majority of the survey respondents performed radical prostatectomies on men even if their age suggested that they would receive little benefit. Indicators such as PSA scores and Gleason staging were disregarded by the respondents. The findings of this study suggest that men should be especially wary when a surgeon recommends surgery for prostate cancer.

Another treatment option is *external radiation therapy*, in which a beam of radiation is aimed at the prostate in order to destroy cancer cells. Treatment is provided on an outpatient basis and usually extends six to eight weeks. External radiation may cause damage to rectal tissue. *Internal radiation therapy*, also called *interstitial brachytherapy*, is administered through radioactive seeds surgically implanted in the prostate, guided by transrectal ultrasound and computed tomography (CT) imaging. These seeds contain radioisotopes that emit rays for about three months. Rectal complications are rare, because the radiation is administered directly to the tumor. Many cancer centers use external radiation therapy rather than internal therapy to avoid the risks of surgery. The major side effects of either type of radiation therapy are fatigue, diarrhea, and painful urination, symptoms that appear during the latter part of treatment and improve over time. In addition, the nerves around the prostate and the arteries that carry blood to the penis are damaged by the radiation, leading to problems in achieving an erection. Forty to fifty percent of those treated with radiation therapy become impotent

(National Cancer Institute: 1995). Men with symptoms of rectal bleeding and fecal discharge may have radiation proctitis, caused by damage to the tissue that lines the rectum. This condition is more likely in men with other health complications such as diabetes, high blood pressure, heart disease, or peripheral vascular disease (Bank: 1996). Laser treatment is used to reduce the bleeding of rectal tissues, and a high fiber diet is recommended to improve stool formation.

When cancer has spread beyond the prostate to the lymph nodes or other parts of the body, *hormone therapy* is used to decrease the amount of testosterone, the male hormone that fuels the growth of the cancer cells. The testicles, a major source of testosterone, may be removed in a surgical procedure, called an orchiectomy. The side effects of this surgery are impotence and hot flashes. A nonsurgical alternative is an injection of drugs called luteinizing hormone releasing hormone analogs (LHRH) that shut down the production of testosterone. The injection can be given once a month or every three months. LHRH analogs can also cause hot flashes and impotence. An anti-androgen drug that blocks the action of testosterone in the adrenal gland may be used in conjunction with an LHRH analog. Its side effects include nausea, vomiting, diarrhea, hot flashes, and impotence. The female hormone, estrogen, is also used to suppress the supply of testosterone, although it can lead to cardiovascular problems such as blood clots and stroke.

Chemotherapy is used to reduce pain and slow tumor growth in individuals with advanced prostate cancer, but it has not been found to be effective in achieving remission or stopping the spread of the disease (McDougal: 1996). Anti-cancer drugs are administered by injection or taken orally. Since these drugs flow throughout the body, the dosage and frequency must be monitored carefully to avoid damage to healthy cells. Chemotherapy treatments may be given in the hospital, physician's office, or at home. Many individuals experience side effects such as nausea, vomiting, anemia, hair loss, susceptibility to infection, and sores in the mouth.

For men who have stage A or B prostate cancer, surgery and radiation therapy seem to be equally effective (National Cancer Institute: 1993b). Individuals with stage C usually receive radiation therapy or a combination of radiation and hormone therapy.

Clinical trials are underway to examine new treatments for prostate cancer. To learn more about these trials, individuals should contact the National Cancer Institute's Cancer Information Service (see "ORGANIZATIONS" section below). PDQ, the Institute's computerized database, provides information about clinical trials on the Internet, through e-mail, and by telephone request to the Cancer Information Center (see "ORGANIZATIONS," below).

SEXUAL FUNCTIONING

Radiation therapy or chemotherapy drugs used to treat prostate cancer can affect the man's fertility, reducing the number and mobility of sperm and causing abnormalities. It is wise for a couple to discuss birth control methods because of the effects of chemotherapy drugs on chromosomes (National Cancer Institute: 1993a). A man's fertility is also affected by radical prostatectomy, because semen is not produced when the prostate gland and seminal vesicles are removed. In transurethral resection of the prostate (TURP), used in treating benign prostatic hyperplasia (BPH), retrograde ejaculation forces the semen back into the bladder rather than out through the penis. Men who wish to father a child should consider sperm banking before undergoing these treatments.

Erectile dysfunction is a major side effect of treatment for benign prostatic hyperplasia and prostate cancer. Individuals should obtain information about risks of impotence associated with each form of treatment. Since aging and medical conditions such as diabetes and high blood pressure also affect potency, men who are young, otherwise healthy, and sexually active are more apt to remain potent than older men (McDougal: 1996). Men who choose radiation therapy may develop impotence during the months following treatment due to scarring of the arteries that carry blood to the penis. Individuals whose erections are reduced during chemotherapy usually recover when treatment ends. Hormone therapy may affect both desire and erections. Even if these side effects cannot be avoided, men and their partners should be given realistic expectations for the return of potency and information about treatment for impotence.

Treatments for impotence include injections into the penis, external vacuum pump devices, and penile implants. Injections directly into the base of the penis result in erections that enable men to have intercourse. Vacuum pump devices create a partial vacuum around the penis, drawing blood into the penis and resulting in an erection. The vacuum pump works satisfactorily in most cases, with no serious side effects (Nadig: 1994). Penile implants should be considered only when other treatments have failed. Penile implants may be semi-rigid or inflatable. Possible complications include infection and mechanical malfunction, requiring replacement. If implants must be removed (due to recurrent infection), the man loses the ability to have an erection permanently. It is important to ensure that a man's expectations of a penile implant are realistic. The man should be aware that penile implants do not result in normal erections. His partner should be included in counseling sessions, and both partners should learn about the advantages and disadvantages of each type of implant.

The emotional and physical stress associated with diagnosis and treatment of prostate cancer may affect sexual desire. Changes in appearance, nausea, pain, weakness due to treatment, and depression may interfere with a man's self-image. He may worry that these changes may make him less desirable. The need for physical comfort, tenderness, and affection is often most acute when faced with a grave prognosis. Sexual counseling may prove beneficial to couples in these situations, although pain, fatigue, and the effects of medication may interfere with participation in counseling (Schover and Jensen: 1988). Changes in sexual routines, sensual touching, and experimenting with new positions during intercourse may help couples feel more comfortable in resuming sexual activity.

A single man with cancer may not have the emotional supports that are so important in coping with diagnosis and treatment of the disease. Dating relationships are affected by anxiety, uncertainty, and lowered self-esteem. A man who becomes infertile due to treatment may be reluctant to marry. Men fear rejection by potential lovers due to changes in appearance caused by hormone therapy, chemotherapy, or surgical scars. Incontinence and impotence may make the man with cancer reject the possibility of sexual relationships in both new and long term relationships. Support groups and sexual counseling are helpful in building the self-esteem and confidence necessary to build new relationships and maintain ongoing relationships.

Some centers that specialize in treating individuals with cancer offer sexual rehabilitation programs (Schover: 1995). Sexual dysfunction clinics or programs may be offered by medical schools and some private medical practices. It is wise to look for a program that includes a diverse staff of physicians, psychologists, social workers, and other specialists and that offers services to both sexual partners.

PSYCHOLOGICAL ASPECTS OF PROSTATE CONDITIONS

In addition to the effects of prostate disease on a man and his partner's sexual relationship, diagnosis and treatment affect other aspects of their lives. Individuals with urinary incontinence may fear having an accident in public. They worry about leakage, odor, and others' reactions. They may restrict social activities and withdraw from friends. They may become angry and frustrated at their loss of control of their bodies and may develop symptoms of depression.

Changes in appearance may affect the individual's self-image and interactions with family, friends, and work colleagues. Loss of hair is common in individuals undergoing chemotherapy. They may also lose weight due to loss of appetite, nausea, or diarrhea. Many individuals find it helpful to consult with a nutritionist or dietitian about ways to increase protein and calorie intake during chemotherapy. Eating frequent, small meals may be one solution.

Feelings of vulnerability, loss of independence, and loss of physical strength affect the man's social relationships. He may become isolated due to others' fears and anxieties about the future. Family members may often find that they are taking on additional responsibilities for supporting the household and making important decisions. Role reversal is not an uncommon phenomenon, and even though it may be temporary during the course of treatment, it may be difficult to return to former routines. Children need special attention to help them cope with a parent's illness and the upheaval it causes in the family.

An individual may fear that his cancer history will affect his employment prospects; knowledge of federal laws may prove useful in these situations. Although many cancer survivors may not see themselves as individuals with disabilities, they are protected by the Americans with Disabilities Act. The Family and Medical Leave Act of 1993 requires employers to permit eligible employees 12 workweeks of unpaid leave during a 12 month period. (See Chapter 3, "Laws that Affect Men with Disabilities" for more details on these laws.) Cancer survivors are eligible for vocational rehabilitation services through the Rehabilitation Services Administration (National Institute on Disability and Rehabilitation Research: 1992), although the services have been vastly underutilized. (See Chapter 1, "Men and Disabilities," p. 18 for a description of these services.) Physicians, employers, and cancer information organizations must work with vocational rehabilitation service providers to insure that cancer survivors receive referrals that will help them continue working.

Self-help groups provide emotional support and practical information for individuals coping with prostate disease or the side effects of the treatment. Stress management or relaxation audiotapes use visual imagery and meditation to help individuals cope with stress associated with fear, pain, anxiety, and isolation (Dollinger: 1994).

Primary care physicians are often the first physicians to perform the DRE. They make referrals to specialists such as urologists for further tests and treatment. *Urologists* are physicians who specialize in the medical and surgical treatment of diseases of the urinary and reproductive tracts. They conduct the tests that diagnose the specific condition and perform surgery on the prostate. *Oncologists* are physicians who specialize in the medical and surgical treatment of cancer. A radiation oncologist treats cancer with radiation therapy in order to destroy cancer cells. *Sex therapists* are mental health professionals such as psychiatrists, psychologists, and social workers, who have special training in treating sexual problems. Professional societies such as the American Association of Sex Educators make referrals to sex therapists (see "ORGANIZATIONS" section below).

WHERE TO FIND SERVICES

The National Cancer Institute (NCI) Cancer Centers Program conducts cancer research at basic science, clinical, comprehensive, and consortium cancer centers. Nearly 30 comprehensive cancer centers provide a multidisciplinary approach to research, patient care, and community outreach. A list of these centers is available from the NCI. Some of these centers may have specialists in the treatment of related sexual problems that result from cancer. The National Cancer Institute's Cancer Information Center provides information by telephone and literature. Database services such as Physician Data Query (PDQ), CancerNet, and CANCERLIT provide similar information. (see "ORGANIZATIONS" below).

The American Cancer Society has developed its Man to Man Education and Support Program for men with prostate cancer and their families. The Wellness Community encourages individuals to become active participants in their recovery through educational programs and discussion groups. Impotents Anonymous and I-ANON (for partners) serve men who are impotent as a result of treatment for BPH or prostate cancer. US TOO! is an international support network for men with prostate cancer and benign prostatic hyperplasia, health professionals, and family members. (see "ORGANIZATIONS," below.)

Divisions of the American Cancer Society (ACS) exist in every state. These divisions provide publications, educational programs, support groups for cancer survivors and family members, and referrals to local resources. The national office can provide the address and phone number of local divisions.

Medical social workers or hospital discharge planners help match the individual's needs with resources available in his community. Home care may include skilled nursing services for chemotherapy and other intravenous treatments, physical or occupational therapy services, and home health aides. Meals on Wheels provides nutritious meals to those who are unable to prepare meals themselves or who are alone for long periods of time.

Palliative care, often called hospice care, is provided to individuals who are dying. It focuses on pain relief, psychological and spiritual care and provides support for family members. Hospice workers may provide respite care, staying with the individual while family members take a break from caregiving. They also help the family during the grieving period.

The National Hospice Organization will make local referrals for hospice services (see "ORGANIZATIONS" below).

References

Agency for Health Care Policy and Research
1997 "Debate Continues Over Appropriate Treatment of BPH and Localized Prostate Cancer" Research Activities December Volume 211, pp. 6-8
1994 Treating Your Enlarged Prostate Rockville, MD: Agency for Health Care Policy and Research
American Cancer Society
1998 Facts on Prostate Cancer Atlanta, GA: American Cancer Society
1997 American Cancer Society's New Guidelines for the Early Detection of Prostate Cancer Atlanta, GA: American Cancer Society
1996 After Diagnosis: Prostate Cancer Atlanta, GA: American Cancer Society
1995 The PSA Blood Test and Prostate Cancer Atlanta, GA: American Cancer Society
Bank, Leslie
1996 "Radiation Proctitis--Cause and Treatment" Participate 5:2:3
Chabner, Bruce A. et al.
1997 "Screening Strategies for Cancer: Implications and Results" JAMA 277:18(May 14):1475
Collins, Mary McNaughton and Michael J. Barry
1996 "Controversies in Prostate Cancer Screening" JAMA 276:24(December 25):1976-1979
Collins, Mary McNaughton et al.
1998 "How Common Is Prostatitis? A National Survey of Physician Visits" Journal of Urology 159:(April):1224-1228
1997 "Medical Malpractice Implications of PSA Testing for Early Detection of Prostate Cancer" Journal of Law, Medicine & Ethics 25:4:234-242
Cunha, B. A., J. Marx, and D. Gingrich
1991 "Managing Prostatitis in the Elderly" Geriatrics 46:1(January):60-63
Dollinger, Lenore
1994 "Relaxation and Cancer Recovery" pp. 178-181 in Lenore Dollinger et al. (eds.) Everyone's Guide to Cancer Therapy Toronto, Ontario: Somerville House Books Limited
Flanigan, R. C. et al.
1998 "5-Year Outcome of Surgical Resection and Watchful Waiting for Men With Moderately Symptomatic Benign Prostatic Hyperplasia: A Department of Veterans Affairs Cooperative Study" Journal of Urology 160:(July):12-17
Flood, A. B. et al.
1996 "The Importance of Patient Preference in the Decision to Screen for Prostate Cancer" Journal of General Internal Medicine 11(6):342-9

Korda, Michael

1996 <u>Man to Man: Surviving Prostate Cancer</u> Westminster, MD: Random House

Lepor, Herbert et al.

1996 "The Efficacy of Terazosin, Finasteride, or Both in Benign Prostatic Hyperplasia" <u>New England Journal of Medicine</u> 335:8(August 22):533-39

Marks, Sheldon

1995 <u>Prostate Cancer: A Family Guide to Diagnosis, Treatment and Survival</u> Tucson, AZ: Fisher Books

McConnell, J. D. et al.

1994 <u>Benign Prostatic Hyperplasia: Diagnosis and Treatment Clinical Practice Guideline</u>, Number 8. AHCPR Publication No. 94-0582 Rockville, MD: Agency for Health Care Policy and Research, Public Health Service, U.S. Department of Health and Human Services. February

McDougal, W. Scott

1996 <u>Prostate Disease</u> Westminster, MD: Random House

Mettlin, Curtis

1997 "The American Cancer Society National Prostate Cancer Detection Project and National Patterns of Prostate Cancer Detection and Treatment" <u>CA: A Cancer Journal for Clinicians</u> 47:5:265-273

Nadig, Perry W.

1994 "Vacuum Constriction Devices in Patients with Neurogenic Impotence" <u>Sexuality and Disability</u> 12:1:99-105

National Cancer Institute

1996 <u>PDQ State-of-The Art Cancer Treatment Summary for Patients: Prostate Cancer</u> Washington, DC: National Cancer Institute

1995 <u>Prostate Cancer: Causes, Detection, Prevention, and Treatment</u> Washington, DC: National Cancer Institute

1993a <u>Chemotherapy and You</u> Washington, DC: National Cancer Institute

1993b <u>What You Need to Know About Prostate Cancer</u> Washington, DC: National Cancer Institute

National Institute of Diabetes and Digestive and Kidney Diseases

1998 <u>Prostate Enlargement: Benign Prostatic Hyperplasia</u> Bethesda, MD: National Institute of Diabetes and Digestive and Kidney Diseases

National Institute on Disability and Rehabilitation Research

1992 "Helping People and Saving Money: A Multimethod Analysis of the Employment Experiences of Cancer Survivors" <u>Rehab Brief</u> Arlington, VA: PSI International, Inc.

Plawker, Marc W.

1997 "Current Trends in Prostate Cancer Diagnosis and Staging among United States Urologists" <u>Journal of Urology</u> 158:1853-1858

Prostate Health Council

1996 <u>Treatment Choices for BPH--Enlarged Prostate</u> Baltimore, MD: American Foundation for Urologic Disease, Inc.

1995 <u>Important Information About Prostate-Specific Antigen (PSA)</u> Baltimore, MD: American Foundation for Urologic Disease, Inc.

1991a <u>Prostate Disease: Vital Information for Men Over 40</u> Baltimore, MD: American Foundation for Urologic Disease, Inc.

1991b <u>Prostatitis: Answers to Your Questions</u> Baltimore, MD: American Foundation for Urologic Disease, Inc.

Quinlan, D. M. et al.

1991 "Sexual Function Following Radical Prostatectomy: Influence of Preservation of Neurovascular Bundles" <u>Journal of Urology</u> 145:5(May):998-1002

Rose, Verna L.

1997 "ACP Issues Guidelines on the Early Detection of Prostate Cancer and Screening for Prostate Cancer" <u>American Family Physician</u> 56:6(October 15):1674

Schover, Leslie

1995 <u>Sexuality and Cancer</u> Atlanta, GA: American Cancer Society

Schover, Leslie and Soren Buus Jensen

1988 <u>Sexuality and Chronic Illness: A Comprehensive Approach</u> New York, NY: Guilford Press

Walsh, Patrick C. and Janet Farrar Worthington

1995 <u>The Prostate: A Guide for Men and the Women Who Love Them</u> Baltimore, MD: Johns Hopkins University Press

Woodwell, D. A.

1992 "Office Visits to Urologists 1989-90 National Ambulatory Medical Care Survey" <u>Advance Data from Vital and Health Statistics</u> No 234, DHHS Pub. No. (PHS) 93-1250. Hyattsville, MD: National Center for Health Statistics

ORGANIZATIONS

American Cancer Society (ACS)
1599 Clifton Road
Atlanta, GA 30026
(800) 227-2345   http://www.cancer.org

This national voluntary health organization funds research and provides education, advocacy, and services to individuals with cancer, their families, and professionals. Produces many publications on prostate cancer including "For Men Only: What You Should Know About Prostate Cancer," "The PSA Blood Test and Prostate Cancer," and "Facts On Prostate Cancer." Also publishes self-help guides such as "Radiation Therapy and You," "Chemotherapy and You," "Questions and Answers About Pain Control," and "Facing Forward: A Guide for Cancer Survivors." All publications are free.

American Foundation for Urologic Disease (AFUD)
1128 North Charles Street
Baltimore, MD 21201
(800) 242-2383   (410) 468-1800   FAX (410) 468-1808
e-mail: admin@afud.org   http://www.afud.org

Supports research, education, and patient support services, including the Prostate Cancer Support Network. Sponsors annual low cost or free prostate cancer screenings. Membership, $35.00, includes subscription to quarterly newsletter, "FAMILY Urology."

American Prostate Society
1340 Charwood Road
Hanover, MD 21076
(410) 859-3735   FAX (410) 850-0818
e-mail: cgerard@www.ameripros.org
http://www.ameripros.org

Provides education about prostate diseases and treatment. Quarterly newsletter, "Update," free. Membership is free.

Cancer Care, Inc.
1180 Avenue of the Americas
New York, NY 10036
National Toll-free Counseling Line (800) 813-4673
(212) 302-2400   e-mail: info@cancercare.org
http://www.cancercare.org

The national toll-free counseling line offers psychological support to individuals with cancer and their families. Social workers also provide information and referral to community resources, educational materials, guidelines for doctor-patient communication, and telephone support groups. Direct services, such as financial assistance to help with costs of home care and transportation, are provided in New York, New Jersey, Connecticut, and San Diego and Imperial counties, California only. All services are free.

Cancer Information Center, National Cancer Institute (NCI)
31 Center Drive, MSC 2580
Building 31, Room 10A16
Bethesda, MD 20892-2580
(800) 422-6237   FAX (301) 330-7968   http://www.nci.nih.gov

Provides information on many types of cancer, treatment, resource organizations, and publications, including "Publications for Cancer Patients and the Public" and "Materials for Community Outreach Programs and Health Professionals." Both are free. Spanish-speaking staff members available.

CanSurmount
American Cancer Society
1599 Clifton Road
Atlanta, GA 30026
(800) 227-2345   http://www.cancer.org

This peer-visitor rehabilitation program for cancer patients and family members provides one-to-one emotional support and information about services and resources. Requires physician referral. Call toll-free number to request information about this program in local areas.

Impotence Information Center
Incontinence Information Center
Prostate Information Center
PO Box 9
Minneapolis, MN 55440
(800) 843-4315   http://www.ammedsys.com

These information centers are sponsored by American Medical Systems, Inc., a subsidiary of Pfizer, Inc. They provide free information and physician referrals. Pfizer is the manufacturer of Viagra.

Impotence World Institute (IWA)
PO Box 410
Bowie, MD 20718-0410
(800) 669-1603   (301) 262-2400   FAX (301) 262-6825
e-mail: IWABOWIE@aol.com   http://www.impotenceworld.org

This organization provides information about the causes and treatment of impotence, makes physician referrals, and offers support programs including Impotents Anonymous (IA) and I-ANON (for partners). Membership, $25.00, includes quarterly newsletter, "Impotence Worldwide," and discounts on fact sheets, audiocassettes, videotapes, and books.

Man to Man: Prostate Cancer Education and Support Program
American Cancer Society (ACS)
1599 Clifton Road
Atlanta, GA 30026
(800) 227-2345   http://www.cancer.org

This program provides practical information and emotional support to men who have been diagnosed with prostate cancer and their families. Call toll-free number to request information about this program in local areas.

National Association for Continence (NAFC)
PO Box 8310
Spartanburg, SC 29305-8310
(800) 252-3337   (864) 579-7900   FAX (864) 579-7902
http://www.nafc.org

An information clearinghouse for consumers, family members, and medical professionals. Will answer individual questions if self-addressed stamped envelope is enclosed with letter. Membership, $20.00, includes a quarterly newsletter, "Quality Care," a "Resource Guide: Products and Services for Continence" (nonmembers, $13.00), discount on publications, and a continence referral service. Free publications list.

National Cancer Data Base
http://www.facs.org

Reports on oncology outcomes at 1600 hospitals in 50 states. Annotated bibliographies and cancer statistics may be downloaded from web site.

National Cancer Institute (NCI)
Physician Data Query (PDQ)
CancerNet
CANCERLIT
31 Center Drive MSC 2580
Building 31, Room 10A16
Bethesda, MD 20892-2580
(800) 422-6237   FAX (301) 330-7968
e-mail: cancernet@icicc.nci.nih.gov
http://www.nci.nih.gov   CancerFax (800) 624-2511   FAX (301) 402-5874

The National Cancer Institute supports basic and clinical research investigations into the causes, prevention, and cure for cancer. The PDQ database provides up-to-date information on cancer prevention, screening, treatments, and care. PDQ is available on the Internet through CancerNet, which also contains fact sheets and publications, CancerNet news, and CANCERLIT abstracts and citations. CancerFax provides access by fax machine to information statements from the PDQ Database, CANCERLIT citations and abstracts, and fact sheets on cancer topics. Most information is also available in Spanish.

National Coalition for Cancer Survivorship (NCCS)
1010 Wayne Avenue, Suite 505
Silver Spring, MD 20910
(301) 650-8868   FAX (301) 565-9670
e-mail: info@cansearch.org   http://www.cansearch.org

This grassroots network advocates on behalf of individuals with any type of cancer to improve the quality of their lives. Special interests are health care delivery, employment rights, and insurance coverage. Sponsors NCCS Town Hall meetings in local communities for cancer survivors, healthcare professionals, and community leaders. Membership, individuals, $35.00; physicians, $100.00; organizations, fees vary by organization budget; includes quarterly newsletter, "NCCS Networker," and discounts on publications.

National Hospice Organization (NHO)
1901 North Moore Street, Suite 901
Arlington, VA 22209
(800) 658-8898   (703) 243-5900   FAX (703) 525-5762
http://www.nho.org

A group that advocates for the rights of terminally ill patients and promotes hospice. Provides informational and educational materials and referrals. The web site enables users to locate hospices in their geographical area. For referral to a hospice, call NHO's toll-free Hospice Helpline at (800) 658-8898.

National Kidney and Urologic Diseases Information Clearinghouse (NKUDIC)
3 Information Way
Bethesda, MD 20892-3580
(301) 654-4415   FAX (301) 907-8906
e-mail: nddic@info.niddk.nih.gov   http://www.niddk.nih.gov

Responds to requests from the public and professionals about impotence and prostate conditions. Maintains a publications database. Free list of publications.

National Prostate Cancer Coalition (NPCC)
1156 15th Street, NW, Suite 905
Washington, DC 20005
(202) 463-9455   FAX (202) 463-9456   e-mail: info@4npcc.org
http://www.4npcc.org

This advocacy organization lobbies for funding for prostate cancer research.

PACCT-PCOG (Patient Advocates for Advanced Cancer Treatments-Prostate Cancer Oncology Group)
1143 Parmelee, NW
Grand Rapids, MI 49504-3844
(616) 453-1477   FAX (616) 453-1846
e-mail: PCA@PCAPAACTINC.com
http://www.osz.com/paact

This patient advocacy organization provides information about detection, diagnosis, and treatment options. Offers recorded information service accessible by touch-tone phone; (616) 453-1351; free. Membership, $50.00, includes quarterly newsletter, "Cancer Communication." Newsletter also available on the web site.

Simon Foundation for Continence
PO Box 835
Wilmette, IL 60091
(800) 237-4666   (847) 864-3913   FAX (847) 864-9758

Provides information and assistance to people who are incontinent. Organizes self-help groups. Membership, individuals, $15.00; professionals, $35.00; includes quarterly newsletter, "The Informer."

US TOO! International, Inc.
930 North York Road, Suite 50
Hinsdale, IL 60521-2993
(800) 808-7866   (630) 323-1002   FAX (630) 323-1003
e-mail: ustoo@ustoo.com   http://www.ustoo.com

This international support network of chapters links prostate cancer and BPH survivors, families, and health care professionals. Membership, $25.00, includes quarterly newsletter, "The US TOO Prostate Cancer Communicator."

The Wellness Community
10921 Reed Hartman Highway, Suite 215
Cincinnati, OH 45242
(513) 794-1116   FAX (513) 794-1822
http://www.brugold.com

Provides free psychological, social, and educational support services for adults with cancer, their families, and friends as an adjunct to medical treatment. The "Wellness Community Physician/Patient Statement" may be downloaded from the web site.

After Diagnosis: Prostate Cancer
American Cancer Society
1599 Clifton Road
Atlanta, GA 30026
(800) 227-2345   http://www.cancer.org

This booklet discusses the diagnosis of prostate cancer, staging and grading of tumors, and treatment options such as surgery, radiation, and hormone therapy and their side effects. Includes glossary and resource guide. Free

Answers to Your Questions About Urinary Incontinence
Bladder Health Council
American Foundation for Urologic Disease (AFUD)
1128 North Charles Street
Baltimore, MD 21201
(800) 242-2383   (410) 468-1800   FAX (410) 468-1808
e-mail: admin@afud.org   http://www.afud.org

This booklet discusses the causes and types of urinary incontinence. Includes a bladder diary to be used to record episodes of incontinence. Free

Before, During, and After Your Radical Prostatectomy
American Foundation for Urologic Disease (AFUD)
1128 North Charles Street
Baltimore, MD 21201-5559
(800) 242-2383   (410) 468-1800   FAX (410) 468-1808
e-mail: admin@afud.org   http://www.afud.org

This booklet discusses pre-operative tests, surgical details, pain control, and post-operative care. Free. Also available on the web site.

A Cancer Survivor's Almanac: Charting Your Journey
by Barbara Hoffman (ed.)
National Coalition for Cancer Survivorship (NCCS)
1010 Wayne Avenue, Suite 505
Silver Spring, MD 20910
(301) 650-8868   FAX (301) 565-9670
e-mail: info@cansearch.org   http://www.cansearch.org

This book provides practical information on topics ranging from cancer diagnosis and treatment, health insurance, and finding doctors and hospitals to communicating with family and friends, peer support programs, and personal advocacy. Includes resource list. $18.95 plus $4.00 shipping and handling

Cancer Tests You Should Know About: A Guide for People 65 and Over
National Cancer Institute Cancer Information Center
31 Center Drive MSC 2580
Building 31, Room 10A16
Bethesda, MD 20892-2580
(800) 422-6237   FAX (301) 330-7968
e-mail: cancernet@icicc.nci.nih.gov
http://www.nci.nih.gov   CancerFax (800) 624-2511   FAX (301) 402-5874

This brochure describes diagnostic tests for cancers found in older men such as prostate, colon and rectum, and skin cancer. A fold-out checklist helps individuals keep track of when the tests are done. Free

Enlarged Prostate: BPH and Male Urinary Problems
Prostate Health Council
American Foundation for Urologic Disease (AFUD)
1128 North Charles Street
Baltimore, MD 21201
(800) 242-2383   (410) 468-1800   FAX (410) 468-1808
e-mail: admin@afud.org   http://www.afud.org

This booklet describes the symptoms, diagnosis, and surgical and nonsurgical treatments for benign prostatic hyperplasia. Free. Also available on the web site.

Everyone's Guide to Cancer Therapy
by Malin Dollinger, Ernest H. Rosenbaum, and Greg Cable
Andrews and McMeel
PO Box 419242
Kansas City, MO 64141
(800) 642-6480

This book describes the diagnosis, treatment, and daily management of common cancers, including prostate cancer. Includes chapters on treatment options, supportive care, sexuality, improving quality of life, and new advances in research, diagnosis, and treatment. Provides a glossary of medical terms, and lists of anticancer drugs and their side effects, cancer associations and support groups, comprehensive cancer care centers, clinical trials sites, and suggested reading. Hardcover, $29.95; softcover, $21.95; plus $2.50 shipping and handling.

For Women Who Care: Information on Prostate Disease to Share With the Men in Your Life
Prostate Health Council
American Foundation for Urologic Disease (AFUD)
1128 North Charles Street
Baltimore, MD 21201
(800) 242-2383   (410) 468-1800   FAX (410) 468-1808
e-mail: admin@afud.org   http://www.afud.org

This booklet provides basic facts about the prostate, prostate examination, prostate conditions, and diseases. Free. Also available on the web site.

Harvard Men's Health Watch
PO Box 420235
Palm Coast, FL 32142-0235
(800) 829-5921
http://www.countway.harvard.edu/publications/Health_Publications

This monthly newsletter reports on men's health issues, including prostate conditions, screening, diagnosis, and treatments. $24.00

Important Information About Prostate-Specific Antigen (PSA)
Prostate Health Council
American Foundation for Urologic Disease (AFUD)
1128 North Charles Street
Baltimore, MD 21201
(800) 242-2383   (410) 468-1800   FAX (410) 468-1808
e-mail: admin@afud.org   http://www.afud.org

This booklet discusses testing for the prostate-specific antigen (PSA) found in blood. Free. Also available on the web site.

Impotence: A Matter Most Delicate
Focus International
1160 East Jericho Turnpike, Suite 15
Huntington, NY 11743
(800) 843-0305   (516) 549-5320   FAX (516) 549-2066
e-mail: Sex_Help@focusint.com   http://www.hip.com/focus

This videotape describes treatments for impotence, including drugs, implants, and prostheses. 26 minutes. $29.95 plus $6.00 shipping and handling

It Takes Two: A Couple's Guide to Erectile Dysfunction
Sexual Function Health Council
American Foundation for Urologic Disease (AFUD)
1128 North Charles Street
Baltimore, MD 21201
(800) 242-2383   (410) 468-1800   FAX (410) 468-1808
e-mail: admin@afud.org   http://www.afud.org

This brochure discusses the causes and treatment of erectile dysfunction (impotence) and its effect on relationships. Available in English and Spanish. Free. Also available on the web site.

Lifelines: A Guide to Life with Prostate Cancer
TAP Pharmaceuticals, Inc.
2355 Waukegan Road
Deerfield, IL 60015
(800) 621-1020

This videotape discusses the stages of prostate cancer, diagnosis and treatment, and strategies for coping. Includes a list of questions to ask the physician and a resources list of organizations and publications. Single copy, free.

Man to Man: Surviving Prostate Cancer
by Michael Korda
Random House, Order Department
400 Hahn Road, PO Box 100
Westminster, MD 21157
(800) 793-2665   http://www.randomhouse.com

Written by a prostate cancer survivor, this book describes the author's experiences receiving his diagnosis and choosing surgical treatment, undergoing radical prostatectomy, and coping with side effects such as incontinence and impotence. $12.00 plus $3.00 shipping and handling

The Prostate: A Guide for Men and the Women Who Love Them
by Patrick C. Walsh and Janet Farrar Worthington
Johns Hopkins University Press
2715 North Charles Street
Baltimore, MD 21218
(800) 537-5487   FAX (410) 516-6998
http://muse.jhu.edu/press

Written by a urologist and a science writer, this book discusses prostate cancer, benign prostatic hyperplasia, and prostatitis. Describes diagnosis, treatments, and side effects, such as impotence. Includes a glossary. Hardcover, $39.95; softcover, $15.95; plus $4.00 shipping and handling

The Prostate Book
by Stephen N. Rous
W. W. Norton & Company
800 Keystone Industrial Park
Scranton, PA 18512
(800) 223-2588   (717) 346-2029   FAX (800) 458-6515
http://www.wwnorton.com

Written by a urologist, this book describes the anatomy and function of the prostate as well as diagnosis and treatment of prostatitis, BPH, and prostate cancer. Complications and side effects of treatment are also discussed. Includes a glossary. Hardcover, $22.95; softcover, $13.00; plus $4.00 shipping and handling

Prostate Cancer: A Non-Surgical Perspective
by Kent Wallner
Pathways Book Service
PO Box 89
Gilsum, NH 03448
(800) 345-6665   e-mail: pbs@top.monad.net

This book, written by a radiation oncologist, describes and compares treatment options, listing side effects and complications. Includes chapter on impotence. Large print. $15.95 plus $4.00 shipping and handling

Prostate Cancer Resource Guide
American Foundation for Urologic Disease (AFUD)
1128 North Charles Street
Baltimore, MD 21201-5559
(800) 242-2383   (410) 468-1800   FAX (410) 468-1808
e-mail: admin@afud.org   http://www.afud.org

This booklet discusses treatment choices and lists prostate cancer support groups, resource organizations, and publications. Includes prostate cancer bibliography. $8.00 Also available on the web site at no charge.

Prostate Cancer: What You Should Know
by Michael Lancaster
Coffey Communications, Inc.
1505 Business One Circle
Walla Walla, WA 99362
(800) 952-9089   (509) 525-0101   FAX (509) 525-0281
e-mail: coffey@coffeycomm.com   http://www.life-and-health.com

This booklet discusses prostate cancer risk factors, screening, diagnosis and staging, and treatment. $1.25 plus 7% shipping and handling (minimum order, $5.00).

Prostate Disease
by W. Scott McDougal with P.J. Skerrett
Times Books
Random House, Order Department
400 Hahn Road, PO Box 100
Westminster, MD 21157
(800) 793-2665   http://www.randomhouse.com

Written by a urologist, this book discusses diagnosis and treatment of prostatitis, benign prostatic hyperplasia, and prostate cancer. Includes chapters on surgery, radiation therapy, hormone therapy, "watchful waiting," coping with incontinence and impotence, and living with prostate cancer. Also includes resource list. $14.00

Prostate Disease: Vital Information for Men Over 40
Prostate Health Council
American Foundation for Urologic Disease (AFUD)
1128 North Charles Street
Baltimore, MD 21201-5559
(800) 242-2383   (410) 468-1800   FAX (410) 468-1808
e-mail: admin@afud.org   http://www.afud.org

This booklet provides information about symptoms and diagnosis of prostate conditions such as benign prostatic hyperplasia, prostatitis, and prostate cancer. Available in English and Spanish. Free. Also available on the web site.

Prostate Enlargement: Benign Prostatic Hyperplasia
National Kidney and Urologic Diseases Information Clearinghouse (NKUDIC)
3 Information Way
Bethesda, MD 20892-3580
(301) 654-4415   FAX (301) 907-8906
e-mail: nddic@info.niddk.nih.gov   http://www.niddk.nih.gov

This booklet describes the symptoms, diagnosis, and surgical and nonsurgical treatment of benign prostatic hyperplasia (BPH). Includes a glossary and reading list. Free. Also available on the web site.

Prostate Problems
National Institute on Aging Information Center
PO Box 8057
Gaithersburg, MD 20898-8057
(800) 222-2225   (800) 222-4225 (TT)   (301) 587-2528
e-mail: niainfo@access.digex.com

This brochure describes noncancerous prostate problems such as prostatitis and benign prostatic hyperplasia (BPH) and prostate cancer. Discusses symptoms, diagnosis, and treatment choices. Includes resource list. Free

Prostatitis: Disorders of the Prostate
National Kidney and Urologic Diseases Information Clearinghouse (NKUDIC)
3 Information Way
Bethesda, MD 20892-3580
(301) 654-4415   FAX (301) 907-8906
e-mail: nddic@info.niddk.nih.gov   http://www.niddk.nih.gov

This brochure describes four types of prostatitis. Free. Also available on the web site.

Prostatitis: Answers to Your Questions
Prostate Health Council
American Foundation for Urologic Disease (AFUD)
1128 North Charles Street
Baltimore, MD 21201-5559
(800) 242-2383   (410) 468-1800   FAX (410) 468-1808
e-mail: admin@afud.org   http://www.afud.org

This booklet describes the prostate's function, types of prostatitis, diagnosis, and treatment. Free. Also available on the web site.

Sexuality and Cancer: For the Man Who Has Cancer and His Partner
by Leslie Schover
American Cancer Society (ACS)
1599 Clifton Road
Atlanta, GA 30026
(800) 227-2345   http://www.cancer.org

This booklet discusses the effects of cancer treatment on male sexuality, suggests strategies for dealing with sexual problems, and describes sources for professional help and additional publications. American Cancer Society service programs are listed, including self-help support groups. Free

Sexuality and Fertility After Cancer
by Leslie Schover
John Wiley and Sons
1 John Wiley Drive
Somerset, NJ 08875
(800) 225-5945   (908) 469-4400   FAX (908) 302-2300
http://www.wiley.com

This book answers common questions about sexuality and fertility asked by cancer survivors, their partners, and families. Topics include men's sexual health, erectile dysfunction, and prostate cancer. Includes resource list. $15.95 plus $2.50 shipping and handling

Surgical and Nonsurgical Treatments for Benign Prostatic Hyperplasia
National Kidney and Urologic Diseases Information Clearinghouse
3 Information Way
Bethesda, MD 20892-3580
(301) 654-4415   FAX (301) 907-8906
e-mail: nddic@info.niddk.nih.gov   http://www.niddk.nih.gov

This information packet contains reprints from medical journals which describe treatment for BPH. Free

Teamwork: The Cancer Patient's Guide to Talking with Your Doctor
by Elizabeth J. Clark (ed.)
National Coalition for Cancer Survivorship (NCCS)
1010 Wayne Avenue, Suite 505
Silver Spring, MD 20910
(301) 650-8868   FAX (301) 565-9670
e-mail: info@cansearch.org   http://www.cansearch.org

This publication provides practical suggestions to help people with cancer communicate with their doctors. Based on the experience of individuals with cancer, it includes questions that they should ask and information the doctor should get from them. Available in English and Spanish. Free plus $1.00 shipping and handling

Treating Your Enlarged Prostate
AHCPR Publications Clearinghouse
PO Box 8547
Silver Spring, MD 20907
(800) 358-9295   e-mail: info@ahcpr.gov   http://www.ahcpr.gov

This booklet describes benign prostatic hyperplasia (BPH), its symptoms, diagnosis, treatment choices, and the benefits, risks, and side effects of these treatments. Available in English and Spanish. Free

Treatment Choices for BPH
Prostate Health Council
American Foundation for Urologic Disease (AFUD)
1128 North Charles Street
Baltimore, MD 21201-5559
(800) 242-2383   (410) 468-1800   FAX (410) 468-1808
e-mail: admin@afud.org   http://www.afud.org

This booklet discusses the benefits and risks of treatment options for BPH: watchful waiting, drug treatment, and surgery. Free. Also available on the web site.

Understanding Incontinence: A Patient's Guide
Agency for Health Care Policy and Research (AHCPR)
Publications Clearinghouse
PO Box 8547
Silver Spring, MD 20907
(800) 358-9295   e-mail: info@ahcpr.gov   http://www.ahcpr.gov

This booklet describes the causes, types, and diagnosis of urinary incontinence and discusses the benefits and risks of treatment. Includes a sample bladder function record. Free

Urinary Incontinence
National Institute on Aging Information Center
PO Box 8057
Gaithersburg, MD 20898-8057
(800) 222-2225   (800) 222-4225 (TT)   (301) 587-2528
e-mail: niainfo@access.digex.com

This brochure discusses the types, treatment, and management of urinary incontinence. Large print, free.

What Cancer Survivors Need to Know About Health Insurance
by Kimberly J. Calder and Karen Pollitz
National Coalition for Cancer Survivorship (NCCS)
1010 Wayne Avenue, 5th Floor
Silver Spring, MD 20910
(301) 650-8868   FAX (301) 565-9670
e-mail: info@cansearch.org   http://www.cansearch.org

This booklet discusses the basics of health insurance and gives cancer survivors tips for purchasing health insurance. Suggests strategies for submitting claims and handling rejected claims. Includes worksheets and glossary. $1.25 plus $5.00 shipping and handling

What You Need To Know About Prostate Cancer
National Cancer Institute Cancer Information Center
31 Center Drive MSC 2580
Building 31, Room 10A16
Bethesda, MD 20892-2580
(800) 422-6237   FAX (301) 330-7968
e-mail: cancernet@icicc.nci.nih.gov
http://www.nci.nih.gov   CancerFax (800) 624-2511   FAX (301) 402-5874

This booklet, written for patients and their families, discusses symptoms, diagnosis, staging, treatment methods and side effects, and follow-up care associated with prostate cancer. A list of medical terms and resources is also included. Free

Working It Out: Your Employment Rights as a Cancer Survivor
by Barbara Hoffman (ed.)
National Coalition for Cancer Survivorship (NCCS)
1010 Wayne Avenue, 5th Floor
Silver Spring, MD 20910
(301) 650-8868   FAX (301) 565-9670
e-mail: info@cansearch.org   http://www.cansearch.org

This booklet describes laws that prohibit employment discrimination, suggests strategies to avoid discrimination, and how individuals can advocate for their legal rights. $1.25 plus $5.00 shipping and handling

Wrongful Death
by Sandra M. Gilbert
W. W. Norton & Company
800 Keystone Industrial Park
Scranton, PA 18512
(800) 223-2588   (717) 346-2029   FAX (800) 458-6515
http://www.wwnorton.com

Written by a woman whose husband died after routine prostate surgery, this book examines her shock and grief and the decision to sue the hospital for medical negligence. Hardcover, $22.50; softcover, $13.00; plus $3.50 shipping and handling.

Your Choice for Treating Prostate Cancer
TAP Pharmaceuticals, Inc.
2355 Waukegan Road
Deerfield, IL 60015
(800) 621-1020

This videotape describes palliative hormone treatment for advanced prostate cancer. Single copy, free.

Chapter 9

SPINAL CORD INJURY

The spinal cord is responsible for transmitting the brain's electrical impulses that control other organs of the body. Therefore, when the spinal cord is injured, there are effects on many of the body's systems, requiring modifications of activities of everyday living and of the home and workplace environments.

Tumors and diseases such as *poliomyelitis*, *arthritis*, *spina bifida*, and *multiple sclerosis* may cause spinal cord injuries; however, spinal cord injuries occur most frequently as a result of *accidents*. Young males who have been in an automobile accident account for the greatest proportion of spinal cord injuries. Because it is often the case that individuals with spinal cord injury were extremely physically active prior to their injury, the effects of the injury may seem overwhelming to them at first. However, rehabilitation opportunities and the development of a wide variety of special assistive devices have enabled thousands of individuals with spinal cord injuries to live productive lives and to continue to participate in many recreational activities, albeit in modified forms.

It has been estimated that there are about 200,000 living Americans who have experienced spinal cord injuries, the majority of whom were injured during or after World War II. The annual incidence of accidents that cause spinal cord injury where the injured individual survives is between 30 and 35 per million population or approximately eight to ten thousand per year (Young et al.: 1982). Prior to World War II and the development of penicillin and of sulfa drugs that prevented death from urinary tract infections, it was unusual for those who had a spinal cord injury to survive (DeVivo et al.: 1987). Today, due to the development of these drugs and improved emergency medical care at the scene of accidents, the vast majority of individuals with spinal cord injuries live for many years.

Studies of patients admitted to the Model Spinal Cord Injury Care Systems (Stover: 1996) have yielded demographic characteristics about the population. Over four-fifths (82.2%) of individuals with spinal cord injuries are males. The average age at onset is 30.7 years, and the most common age at which spinal cord injury occurs is 19, with a third of the injuries occurring between the ages of 17 and 23. Automobile accidents account for 35.9% of spinal cord injuries. Violence as a cause of spinal cord injury has increased in recent years; it now accounts for 29.8% of all spinal cord injuries. Sports accidents (frequently diving accidents) account for 7.4% of all spinal cord injuries and are a major cause of spinal cord injuries among the younger population, while falls are a major cause among the older population.

A study (DeVivo et al.: 1992) investigated the characteristics of individuals who had received treatment for spinal cord injuries at six federally supported model treatment centers between 1973 and 1986. The study found several significant differences between the population who had been injured in the period 1973-77 and those who had been injured in the period 1984-86; the mean age at the time of injury increased over time as did the proportion of individuals who were not white and the proportion with quadriplegia. Although the mean length of stays in hospitals for rehabilitation decreased, the cost of the rehabilitation increased. For those who entered the centers within the first 24 hours of injury, the probability of dying in the first two years following injury decreased by two-thirds. While virtually all of the subjects were discharged to live in the community during the entire study period, only a small percentage of the subjects were employed two years post-injury, ranging from a low of 12.5% in the 1978-80 period to a high of 14.7% for those who had been injured from 1984-86. While a substantial proportion were students and small proportions were either homemakers or retired two years post-injury, over half of the subjects were unemployed throughout the study period.

THE SPINAL CORD

The spine has 33 bony, hollow, interlocking vertebrae including seven cervical or neck vertebrae, 12 thoracic or high back vertebrae, five lumbar or low back vertebrae, five sacral vertebrae near the base of the spine, and four coccygeal vertebrae fused to form the coccyx. The spinal cord, consisting of a narrow bundle of nerve cells and fibers, runs from the base of the brain through the hollow structure of the vertebrae. The brain's communication with the rest of the body is carried out through these nerve fibers.

Paralysis, the loss or impairment of motor function, occurs below the site of the injury or fracture. Not all injuries are complete, meaning that sometimes the individual may retain some sensation or movement below the site of the injury. *Paraplegia,* or paralysis of the legs and often the lower part of the body, occurs when the spinal cord is injured at the thoracic, lumbar, or sacral level of the spine. When injuries are complete, individuals also lose their sense of touch, pain, and temperature in the affected region.

Quadriplegia (or tetraplegia) is paralysis of all four limbs and the part of the body beneath the site of the spinal cord injury. Quadriplegia occurs when the injury to the spinal cord is at the level of the cervical vertebrae or the neck region. The lower the lesion within the cervical area, the greater amount of function that remains. Some individuals with cervical spinal cord injuries retain some function of the shoulders, biceps, upper arms, and the wrists. In general, the higher the site of the injury, the less function the individual retains. Individuals whose injuries are complete and at the chin level require respirators in order to breathe. These individuals require assistance with their everyday activities, although the use of mouthsticks and sip-and-puff mechanisms enables them to operate wheelchairs, computers, and other devices (Trieschmann: 1988).

According to Young and his associates (1982), there is a higher prevalence of quadriplegia (53%) than paraplegia (47%), but the injuries are more likely to be complete in paraplegia (60%) than for quadriplegia (52%).

TREATMENT AND COMPLICATIONS OF SPINAL CORD INJURY

Acute medical care following an accident that has caused spinal cord injury includes x-rays, possible treatment for shock, and immobilization of the patient. Patients are often placed in a Stryker frame, which is used to immobilize the spine and prevent further injury. A catheter to control bladder function is inserted and urine output is monitored. In some cases, surgery may be performed to stabilize or fuse the spine, free nerve roots, or remove bony fragments. Immediately following the injury, swelling and bruising near the site of the fracture may be present, preventing the determination of the extent of neurological damage (Trieschmann: 1988). Patients are positioned and turned frequently in an effort to prevent pressure sores (see below). Other injuries that often accompany spinal cord injury, such as

230

fractures and lung injuries, must also be treated. Pain may also be a major problem in the first weeks following injury.

Preliminary studies on the use of drugs immediately following spinal cord injury have found some positive benefits. Administration of methylprednisolone within eight hours following the injury resulted in the recovery of an average of 20% of the motor and sensory function lost (Hingley: 1993).

Although treatments have been developed for many of the complications of spinal cord injury, it is still necessary to constantly be aware of the development of these complications and to take measures to prevent them. *Pressure sores* or *decubitus ulcers* are lesions on the skin that usually occur over a bony surface and result from lack of motion. Because the individual may have no sensation at the site where the sores begin to develop, they may become deep before they are discovered. In an effort to prevent pressure sores, individuals who are confined to bed immediately following the injury should be moved frequently and great attention should be paid to cleansing the skin regularly. Special flotation pads and sheepskins are sometimes used to relieve pressure and distribute body weight. Because of their restricted mobility, individuals with spinal cord injury must take precautions to prevent pressure sores for the rest of their lives.

Despite the loss of sensation to temperature and touch below the site of the lesion, *pain* and unusual sensations may be a problem for people with spinal cord injuries. According to Trieschmann (1988), until recently it was assumed that pain was not a problem, and little attention was paid to the subject. However, Trieschmann states that many individuals experience a tingling or pins and needles sensation as well as other types of pain, such as shooting or burning sensations.

Transcutaneous electric nerve stimulation (TENS) is a treatment method for pain in which low level electric impulses are delivered to nerve endings under the skin near the source of pain. It is not known why TENS should be effective in relieving pain or if it is really effective.

Loss of bladder and bowel control is another complication of spinal cord injury. One study (Kuhlemeier et al.: 1985) concluded that patients with spinal cord injuries are likely to maintain good renal output ten years after injury. Those individuals who have indwelling catheters are prone to develop bladder infections. When the extent of nerve damage permits, it is preferable to have the individual learn how to control his or her bladder through an individualized training program. When urinary tract infections become symptomatic, they are treated with antibiotics for a period of 7 to 14 days (National Institute on Disability and Rehabilitation Research: 1992). Programs for bowel control enable the individual to empty the bowel on a regular schedule, thereby avoiding gastrointestinal complications such as distention and impaction. Attention to diet and the use of rectal suppositories may also contribute to control of bowel movements.

Spasticity (involuntary jerky motions) is common in individuals with spinal cord injuries. These spasms are caused by random stimulation of the nerves leading to the muscles. Severe spasms may interfere with some activities and in some cases may be strong enough to throw the individual from the bed or chair.

Functional electrical stimulation (FES) is an experimental method that uses electrical stimulation to evoke skeletal muscle responses in areas that do not function normally because injury or disease has cut off the pathway for central nervous system communication from the brain. A functional electrical stimulation system consists of a control unit, a stimulator unit, and electrodes. In some instances, the goal of functional electrical stimulation is to restore movement or function and in other cases to strengthen muscles. A study by Petrofsky (1992) found that subjects with spinal cord injuries who participated in a two year experiment using functional electrical stimulation to exercise muscles had a reduction in the incidence of pressure sores and urinary tract infections. Another experiment (Granat et al.: 1992) that used functional electrical stimulation to restore movement in six subjects with incomplete spinal cord injuries found that all subjects were able to stand and walk using an FES system, but half of the subjects found that the system was not practical for their lifestyles.

A recent technological advance, the Freehand System developed by NeuroControl Corporation (see "ORGANIZATIONS" section below), enables some individuals with quadriplegia to regain control over one hand. The system requires that the individual have some motion in the upper body, so that he or she can use the shoulder to control the system. The Freehand System is a neural prosthesis that involves the surgical implantation of electrodes that send signals to muscles in the hand. Individuals control the processor that sends the signals by moving the shoulder. Using the Freehand System, individuals may be able to carry out activities such as using dining utensils, grooming, and writing.

A number of research projects around the country are working on potential cures for spinal cord injury through nerve regeneration and drug therapy. Other projects have the goal of re-training individuals to walk (Huelskamp: 1998). Devices that use technology similar to the Freehand System are potential aids that will improve bowel and bladder control and enable individuals with paraplegia to walk (Finn: 1998).

SEXUAL FUNCTIONING

Sexual function may be affected in both men and women with spinal cord injuries, although the effects are greater for men. Men with spinal cord injuries who were asked to rank 12 life areas ranked sex life as the fifth most important but as the least satisfactory. Nearly half (49%) of the men had had sexual intercourse in the preceding 12 months, and nearly two-thirds (63%) had concerns about not satisfying a partner, fear of giving or getting a sexually transmitted disease (58%), urinary accidents (53%), and not enough personal satisfaction (53%) (White et al.: 1994). Another study (Romeo et al.: 1993) found that men with either paraplegia or quadriplegia had more negative body image, less sexual experience, and more psychological distress than men without disabilities. The groups were comparable, however, on intensity of sex drive and sexual satisfaction.

The ability of a man with spinal cord injury to have an erection is often impaired, depending upon the level and completeness of the injury. When the injury occurs in the thoracic or cervical vertebrae, the erection reflex remains intact; about 80% of men with this level of injury can obtain an erection by tactile stimulation of the penis. However, the erection is usually short-lived. These injuries also result in a lack of sensation in the genital area. Men with injuries at a high level in the spinal cord who have a reflex erection are incapable of responding normally, resulting in autonomic dysreflexia (rapid rise in blood pressure, sweating, flushing, and pounding headache (Schover and Jensen: 1988).

Men with injuries to the sacral area or below have a much higher rate of erectile dysfunction; only about 30% of men with complete injuries in this area are able to have a full erection, which is the result of psychological stimulation. Men with lesions in this area are more likely to retain sensitivity in the genital area. Men who have incomplete lesions and those whose lesions are below the T10 (10th thoracic vertebra) level and above the S2 (2nd sacral vertebra) area have the best prognosis for full erections (Schover and Jensen: 1988).

Treatments for erectile dysfunction include injections into the penis, external vacuum pump devices, and penile implants. Injections directly into the base of the penis have resulted in satisfactory erections that enable men to have intercourse. The drugs used for this purpose include papaverine, prostaglandin E1, and phentolamine, often used in combination. A recent study of men with spinal cord injuries who used pharmacologic injections found that erections were satisfactory for most of the subjects and side effects were minimal (Lloyd and Brown: 1995).

Vacuum pump devices create a partial vacuum around the penis, drawing blood into the penis and causing an erection. The device consists of a plastic cylinder placed over the penis; a pump which draws air out of the cylinder; and an elastic band placed at the base of the penis to maintain the erection. The vacuum pump does not have any side effects and works satisfactorily in most cases (Nadig: 1994).

Penile implants should be considered only when other treatments have failed. Penile implants may be semi-rigid or inflatable. Possible complications include infections, leaks, and mechanical malfunctions. If they must be removed (due to recurrent infection), it is unlikely that other treatment methods will be successful (Green et al.: 1995).

Prior to scheduling surgery for a penile implant, a man should undergo a psychological evaluation to determine whether the cause of his erectile dysfunction is organic or psychological and to ensure that his expectations of a penile implant are realistic. Penile implants do not result in normal erections, and the man should be aware of this prior to undergoing the surgery. His partner should be included in counseling sessions, and both partners should learn about the advantages and disadvantages of each type of implant.

Each of these methods has disadvantages for men with spinal cord injuries. Both injections and vacuum pump devices require manual dexterity. Men with spinal cord injuries may not be able to utilize these methods on their own, but their partners may learn how to carry out the procedure. Men with spinal cord injuries are more likely than other men to experience infections after penile implantation, primarily because of urinary tract infection, and erosion of the implants (Montague and Lakin: 1994). Because of the various disadvantages of each of these methods, sexual activities that are alternatives to intercourse present a viable option.

Individuals who have spinal cord injuries lose sensation in the parts of their bodies that are below the lesion in their spinal cord; however, they retain sensitivity in parts of the body above the injury and may derive sexual pleasure through physical stimulation. It may take some experimenting for men and their partners to discover the parts of the body that are most sensitive to touch and that produce sexual pleasure with stimulation.

The lack of mobility caused by spinal cord injury changes the role that men play in sexual relationships. Many men traditionally view their role as dominant in sexual activities. The loss of mobility may require a role reversal for men with spinal cord injuries. In some cases, alternatives to sexual intercourse, such as oral sex, must be considered. Although many individuals initially feel that sexual intercourse is the only way to achieve sexual pleasure, after experimenting with alternatives, they often find that their sexual activities are pleasurable and satisfying.

Men who have recently experienced spinal cord injuries may find it difficult to resume a sexual relationship or to begin a relationship with a new partner. As in all sexual relationships, good communication facilitates the process. When men feel comfortable talking to their partners, they can discuss their preferences and ways to experiment with new positions and techniques that were not used prior to their injuries.

Some men fear the embarrassment of bladder and bowel incontinence during sexual relations. It is not necessary for men with indwelling catheters to remove them during sex, although some may feel more comfortable doing so. Men who are on regular bowel programs are advised to empty their bowel prior to sexual activity to avoid the fear of bowel accidents. Urinary tract infections may be passed from the man to his partner; therefore, it is advisable to wash the penis and void prior to sexual relations (Sandowski: 1989).

In cases where attendant care is necessary (usually in cases of quadriplegia), the partner often becomes a caretaker by default when financial resources do not permit hiring an attendant. Yet some men have difficulty conceiving of a sexual relationship if their partner assists with their bladder and bowel control. For other men, their partner's role as personal attendant is viewed as normal and does not create problems in the area of sexual relationships. In those instances where a paid personal attendant helps the man with his bodily functions, it is often necessary for the attendant to prepare and position the man for sexual activity. Since being involved in another person's intimate affairs may cause embarrassment or tension, an open discussion between the attendant and the couple may prove useful. Rehabilitation programs for people with spinal cord injuries should include counseling in the area of sexual functioning. A recent study reveals that two-thirds of men with spinal cord injuries received information about sexuality (White et al.: 1994). However, this study included men in one metropolitan area only and may not be representative of other sections of the country.

FAMILY PLANNING

Most spinal cord injuries in men occur during the time of life in which they plan to father children. Impaired ejaculatory function in most men precludes this possibility unless medical procedures are used. Men with spinal cord injuries have lower sperm counts and poor quality of sperm. However, many of these men may still father children by undergoing electroejaculation. In this procedure, an electric probe is inserted in the rectum, stimulating the prostate and resulting in the production of semen which is collected for artificial insemination. For men who retain sensation in this area, the procedure is done under anesthesia; those whose lesion is high in the spinal cord and have lost sensation do not need anesthesia as they cannot feel the pain. Attempts at pregnancy through electroejaculation and artificial insemination can be very draining physically, emotionally, and financially, as the procedures may need to be repeated a number of times. A successful pregnancy cannot be guaranteed.

234

Planning a family requires special preparations when mobility impairment is involved. Society's attitudes toward parenting with a disability have been negative, although more individuals with disabilities are asserting their legal rights to become parents. In addition, special devices and adaptations are on the market; the necessities for child care vary with the man's level of injury, his special role in raising the children, his home environment, and the amount of assistance he and his wife receive from other family members and paid help. Adaptive devices include special trays that attach to wheelchairs and hold the baby (Through the Looking Glass: 1994). Individuals with spinal cord injuries have noted that their children quickly learn to respond to verbal discipline, become involved in household activities, and develop independence at an early age. As children begin socializing with other children in the neighborhood and at school, they must learn to respond effectively to the taunts they may receive about their father's condition. Some fathers may wish to visit their children's classrooms to explain their condition and to answer questions, so that classmates feel more comfortable and interested in visiting their home.

PSYCHOLOGICAL ASPECTS OF SPINAL CORD INJURY

Men who experience spinal cord injuries have changed in an instant from able-bodied individuals into individuals with severe physical limitations. Many of these men have acquired these injuries because they were extremely physically active in either their occupation or their recreational pursuits. Going from extensive physical activity to extreme limitation in mobility of any kind is likely to cause a loss of self-esteem (Lemon: 1993). The suddenness with which this change takes place and the wide ranging effects are likely to cause great anguish to the individuals as well as to their families and friends. The more severe the disability, the greater the loss of independence. Men with spinal cord injuries have lost the ability to carry out many physical activities, a loss which threatens their sense of masculinity. In many cases, they are unable to continue in their previous occupational roles, and their sexuality is impaired. These impairments and losses are direct attacks on their identities, which are formed largely by traditional masculine values.

It is essential that men with spinal cord injuries receive help with their emotional adjustment, through individual or group counseling from professionals, self-help groups, or role models of other men who have adjusted successfully to spinal cord injuries. However, many men, especially young men, are resistant to receiving psychological counseling. They must be convinced that the need for counseling does not mean that they are "crazy" (Marmer: 1996).

Krause and Crewe (1987) compared survivors of spinal cord injuries and those who had died several years after their injuries on a number of variables that measured adjustment. Those who were better adjusted in terms of vocational and social activity were more likely to survive regardless of their age. Krause and Crewe suggest that the frequent neglect of counseling in social skills and sexual functioning during the rehabilitation process contributes to poor adjustment. A study by Krause (1991) that builds upon the earlier study confirmed the findings that social, psychological, and vocational maladjustment was higher among deceased subjects than among the survivors. A recent study by McColl and Rosenthal (1994) found that emotional support continues to be crucial many years after the injury occurred. In a sample of men age 45 or over who had experienced spinal cord injuries at least 15 years before, emotional support was the only variable that predicted life satisfaction, adjustment to disability, and lack of depression. Other investigations have found relationships between social support and well-being (Rintala et al.: 1992) and employment and self-perception of both physical and psychological adjustment (Krause: 1992).

Some men may never lose the anger or guilt they feel about the circumstances surrounding the accident that caused the injury. In the period immediately following the accident, they may feel overpowered by the many professionals who have begun to make major decisions for them. In many cases, the accident that caused spinal cord injury involved the use of alcohol while driving. These factors, combined with inadequate counseling and the inability to cope with the effects of the injury, may cause some men to abuse alcohol or other drugs. Bozzacco (1990) suggests that all patients in rehabilitation units be assessed for their vulnerability to alcohol and drug abuse. She further suggests that patients become part of the decision-making process for their own treatment and rehabilitation plans as soon as possible and that alcohol and drug treatment programs be an integral part of rehabilitation.

The need to modify the activities of everyday living as well as the physical environment; the impairment of sexual function; and the financial aspects of living with a spinal cord injury may place a great strain on marital and family relationships. In cases where attendant care is necessary, the wife often becomes a caretaker by default when financial resources do not permit hiring an attendant. In these instances, it is not uncommon for the wife and offspring to feel both overburdened and guilty. When an attendant is hired, a stranger becomes part of a family structure that is already strained and may even be involved in preparing the man with a spinal cord injury for sexual relations. Since sexual intimacy is considered to be a private matter, the need for an attendant adds yet another source of tension to the relationship.

Young and his associates (1982) found that four years after spinal cord injury, nearly 16% of the males were divorced. Brown and Giesy (1986) found that 18.1% of males with spinal cord injuries were divorced, separated, or widowed compared to 9.3% of males in the general population. Only 40.7% of the males with spinal cord injuries were married compared to 62.6% in the general population. While the differences between the general population and those with spinal cord injuries was greater for females than for males, marriage is still problematic for men. Three-quarters (76%) of the men blamed their divorce on the injury itself.

DeVivo and his colleagues (1995) found that individuals with spinal cord injuries who married post-injury had higher divorce rates than the general public. Both education and severity of injury were related to divorce rates. Individuals without a college education had higher divorce rates than those with a college education; those with lumbosacral injuries had lower divorce rates than individuals with higher injuries. Divorce rates were higher for men than for women and for African-Americans than for whites.

Other issues that affect marriages where one partner has a spinal cord injury include the spouse's feelings of guilt. A study (Gerhart: 1995) of Britons who had survived spinal cord injuries at least 20 years and their spouses found that spouses often feel guilty about leaving their mate alone and about participating in activities that are not possible for their spouse. Participants indicated that it was important for each spouse to develop his or her own special interests and to adapt activities that they had enjoyed prior to the injury so that both spouses could participate. Furthermore, spouses who were caregivers for their injured mates experienced more depression, physical and emotional stress, fatigue, anger, and resentment than spouses who did not act as caregivers.

Social workers should work with the family where spouses and children feel psychologically, physically, and financially overburdened and socially isolated. Arranging for respite care, financial assistance, and other services may alleviate some of the burden. According to Young and his associates (1982), over half (54%) of all individuals with spinal cord injuries were single when their injury occurred; these individuals may benefit from counseling in order to develop satisfactory relationships and marriage.

PROFESSIONAL SERVICE PROVIDERS

In most cases, the physician in charge serves as the case manager or coordinator for the person with spinal cord injury. The physician in charge may be a *physiatrist* (a specialist trained in rehabilitation medicine); an *orthopedist* (a specialist in treatment of the skeletal system); or a *neurologist* or *neurosurgeon* (a specialist in disorders of the nervous system). All of these physicians receive training in treatment of spinal cord injury. Also on the multidisciplinary team are *urologists*, who specialize in treatment of kidneys, the bladder, the ureter, and the urethra. Urologists treat men with sexual dysfunction by performing surgery on the penis or prescribing vacuum devices or pharmacologic treatment.

Rehabilitation nurses receive special training available at schools throughout the country and may receive certification in this specialty after working two years in a rehabilitation setting (Livingston: 1991). They work closely with the physicians and in some instances may serve as case managers. In inpatient settings, rehabilitation nurses work with other health care and rehabilitation professionals to develop and implement medical and rehabilitation plans for patients. They may act as consultants in planning for discharge and may evaluate the individual's home to ensure that appropriate environmental modifications have been made. They are often the professionals in charge of following up on the individual's needs after discharge from the rehabilitation unit.

Orthotists specialize in the design of braces and other devices that help with mobility, support, and prevention of further injury. They also fit the devices and provide instruction in their use. *Rehabilitation engineers* specialize in the design of devices that enable people with disabilities to function at their maximum level of independence. Their research includes the development of robotic devices and other computer driven devices that serve as substitutes for the function that was lost as a result of injury or disease. In some instances, they may consult on individual cases to adapt wheelchairs or other devices for specific needs.

Physical therapists design exercise programs to maintain and strengthen residual motor function. They also teach transfer skills to and from the bed and how to use wheelchairs and orthotic devices such as canes, braces, and walkers. They develop exercise programs to help individuals who are able to use crutches to build up muscles in their arms and shoulders.

Occupational therapists teach individuals with spinal cord injuries how to re-learn the activities of daily living. Included are eating, dressing, grooming, and the use of "high tech" devices that contribute to increased independence.

Psychologists provide individual or group counseling to people with spinal cord injuries and to their family members. They may also provide special help in the area of sexual functioning. *Social workers* help to make the arrangements that enable individuals to return to the community. They also ensure that individuals with spinal cord injuries receive the financial assistance that they are entitled to. Social workers may also provide counseling for individuals and their families.

Rehabilitation counselors help individuals with spinal cord injuries develop a plan that will enable them to continue functioning and working. Many individuals with spinal cord injuries will need assistance in returning to their previous position or retraining to obtain a different type of position. Rehabilitation counselors help make the contacts and placements necessary to attain these goals.

Employment after spinal cord injury is more likely for people who have higher education and who work in office jobs that do not require physical effort. Individuals who were employed in office or clerical work prior to their spinal cord injuries are most likely to be able to perform the same type of work, with or without modifications in the office environment. Individuals whose work involved physical skills will in most instances need to be trained to carry out the requirements of more sedentary occupations.

WHERE TO FIND SERVICES

The federal government sponsors the "Model System of Spinal Cord Injury Care" in order to provide coordinated comprehensive care and to conduct research related to spinal cord injury. Administered by the National Institute on Disability and Rehabilitation Research (NIDRR) within the U.S. Department of Education, this model system encompasses treatment centers throughout the country that participate in research and data collection efforts. The major components of the model system include early access to care through rapid, effective transportation; an acute level one traumatology setting; a comprehensive acute rehabilitation program; psychosocial and vocational services that begin in the hospital and continue through discharge; and follow-up to ascertain that medical and psychosocial needs are met once patients have re-entered the community (Thomas: 1990).

Another federal system that offers special treatment for individuals with spinal cord injuries is the U.S. Department of Veteran Affairs (VA). Spinal cord units are located at a number of VA Medical Centers across the country. The National Institutes of Health also funds model research and treatment centers at several facilities.

Many rehabilitation hospitals have spinal cord injury units. One of the advantage of obtaining treatment in these settings is that other patients serve as role models. Some acute care hospitals also have rehabilitation units, and outpatient rehabilitation facilities offer services to people with spinal cord injuries. Many long term care facilities provide services to people with spinal cord injuries. The Commission on Accreditation of Rehabilitation Facilities (CARF) provides accreditation for these facilities (see "ORGANIZATIONS" section below). Independent living centers offer services and referrals to people with spinal cord injuries.

MODIFICATIONS IN EVERYDAY LIVING

In order to remain living in the community, many individuals with spinal cord injuries, especially those with quadriplegia, require personal assistance services (PAS). Personal assistance services may be provided by a family member, friend, or a person specifically employed for this purpose. Personal assistants perform tasks that enable the man with a disability to carry out his activities of daily living. Health care providers have observed that personal assistance services contribute not only to the improved physical well-being of individuals with spinal cord injuries and other disabilities, but also to their mental well-being (Nosek: 1993).

The major source of funding for the employment of personal assistants is Medicaid, although other state, local, and federal programs as well as private agencies often contribute. According to Nosek (1991), most individuals with disabilities rely on family members and have had no contacts with formal programs that provide personal assistants. Furthermore, those interested in hiring personal assistants often have difficulty locating qualified individuals. A number of consumer advocacy organizations, research organizations, and the federal government are paying increased attention to the issue of personal assistance services in an attempt to improve the provision of these services.

Most individuals with spinal cord injuries use wheelchairs for mobility. A wide variety of wheelchairs designed for different purposes and different types of impairments is available. Individuals whose injury prohibits them from using manually operated wheelchairs may use battery operated wheelchairs. Sip-and-puff controls, tubes that respond to changes in pressure caused by inhaling and exhaling, enable people with more severe impairments to control the movement of their wheelchairs. Wheelchairs are prescribed by physicians and must accommodate the individual's body size, disability, and functional criteria.

Individuals whose injury has resulted in paraplegia sometimes use braces as an alternative to wheelchairs. One study (Heinemann et al.: 1987) found that only about a quarter of those individuals who had braces continued to use them, while the remainder preferred using wheelchairs. Those who continued to use braces were less likely to have complete lesions than those who stopped using braces. Those who stopped using braces said that they preferred wheelchairs because they were safer, required less energy, and were less likely to fail.

Modification of the home environment requires the installation of ramps; wide doorways with doors that open easily; the removal of thresholds between rooms; and lifts for getting from one level of the home to the other. The kitchen should have accessible appliances, shelves, and working space, and pulls and knobs that are easy to use. The bathroom should be large enough to accommodate a wheelchair; the sink must be at an accessible level; showers should be the roll-in variety with grab bars; and toilets should have grab bars.

Many individuals with paraplegia learn to drive with special hand controls, locks, steering mechanisms, and wheelchair lifts. Major automobile manufacturers offer programs to purchase adapted vehicles with special controls and wheelchair lifts; some individuals may be eligible for reimbursement of the cost of this equipment from the automobile manufacturer (see Chapter 2, "ORGANIZATIONS" section, beginning on p. 71 for a listing of these programs). Parking must be arranged so that there is enough space for entering and exiting the vehicle.

Special feeding devices are available for individuals with quadriplegia who do not have the use of their upper limbs. Devices may be installed that move people around a room. Use of these specialized devices increases the independence of individuals with quadriplegia.

References

Bozzacco, Victoria
1990 "Vulnerability and Alcohol and Substance Abuse in Spinal Cord Injury" Rehabilitation Nursing 15(March-April):2:70-72

Brown, Julia S. and Barbara Giesy
1986 "Marital Status of Persons with Spinal Cord Injury" Social Science and Medicine 3:3:313-322

DeVivo, Michael J. et al.
1995 "Outcomes of Post-Spinal Cord Injury Marriages" Archives of Physical Medicine and Rehabilitation 76(February):130-138

DeVivo, Michael J. et al.
1992 "Trends in Spinal Cord Injury Demographics and Treatment Outcomes Between 1973 and 1986" Archives of Physical Medicine and Rehabilitation 73(May):424-430

DeVivo, Michael J. et al.
1987 "Seven-Year Survival Following Spinal Cord Injury" Archives of Neurology 44(August):872-875

Finn, Robert
1998 "Neural Prosthetics Come of Age as Research Continues" FES Update 8:1(Summer):1-2

Gerhart, Kenneth A.
1995 "Marriage to a Spinal Cord Injury Survivor" Spinal Cord Injury Life Fall 24-27

Granat, M. et al.
1992 "The Use of Functional Electrical Stimulation to Assist Gait in Patients with Incomplete Spinal Cord Injury" Disability and Rehabilitation 14(2):93-97

Green, Bruce G. et al.
1995 "Complications of Penile Implants in Spinal Cord Injured Patients" Topics in Spinal Cord Injury Rehabilitation 1:2(Fall):44-52

Heinemann, Allen W. et al.
1987 "Mobility for Persons with Spinal Cord Injury: An Evaluation of Two Systems" Archives of Physical Medicine and Rehabilitation 68(February):90-93

Hingley, Audrey T.
1993 "Spinal Cord Injuries: Science Meets Challenge" FDA Consumer July/August:15-19

Huelskamp, Scott
1998 "When Will We Cure Spinal Cord Injuries?" Advance for Occupational Therapy Practitioners 14:31(August 3):28-30

Krause, James S.

1992 "Adjustment to Life after Spinal Cord Injury: A Comparison among Three Participant Groups Based on Employment Status" <u>Rehabilitation Counseling Bulletin</u> 35(June)4:218-229

1991 "Survival Following Spinal Cord Injury: A Fifteen-Year Prospective Study" <u>Rehabilitation Psychology</u> 36:2:89-98

Krause, James S. and Nancy M. Crewe

1987 "Prediction of Long-Term Survival of Persons with Spinal Cord Injury: An 11-Year Prospective Study" <u>Rehabilitation Psychology</u> 32:4:205-213

Kuhlemeier, K. V., L. K. Lloyd, and S. L. Stover

1985 "Urological Neurology and Urodynamics" <u>Journal of Urology</u> 134(September):510-513

Lennon, Marilyn

1993 "Sexual Counseling and Spinal Cord Injury" <u>Sexuality and Disability</u> 11:1:73-97

Livingston, Carolyn

1991 "Opportunities in Rehabilitation Nursing" <u>American Journal of Nursing</u> 91 (February):2:90-95

Lloyd, L. Keith and Jane Brown

1995 "Management of Erectile Dysfunction in Spinal Cord Injury with Intracavernous Pharmacotherapy" <u>Topics in Spinal Cord Injury Rehabilitation</u> 1:2(Fall):53-61

Marmer, Loretta

1996 "Model Treatment Systems for SCI Target Quality of Life" <u>Advance for Occupational Therapists</u> 12:26(July 1):13, 46

McColl, M. A. and C. Rosenthal

1994 "A Model of Resource Needs of Aging Spinal Cord Injured Men" <u>Paraplegia</u> 32:261-70

Montague, Drogo K. and Milton M. Lakin

1994 "Penile Prosthesis Implantation in Men with Neurogenic Impotence" <u>Sexuality and Disability</u> 12:1:95-98

Nadig, Perry W.

1994 "Vacuum Constriction Devices in Patients with Neurogenic Impotence" <u>Sexuality and Disability</u> 12:1:99-105

National Institute on Disability and Rehabilitation Research

1992 <u>The Prevention and Management of Urinary Tract Infection among People with Spinal Cord Injuries</u> Washington, DC: U.S. Department of Education

Nosek, Margaret A.

1993 "Personal Assistance: Its Effect on the Long-Term Health of a Rehabilitation Hospital Population" <u>Archives of Physical Medicine and Rehabilitation</u> 74(February):127-132

1991 "Personal Assistance Services: A Review of the Literature and Analysis of Policy Implications" <u>Journal of Disability Policy Studies</u> 2(2):1-17

Petrofsky, Jerrold S.

1992 "Functional Electrical Stimulation, a Two-Year Study," <u>Journal of Rehabilitation</u> July/August/September 29-34

Rintala, Diana H. et al.
1992 "Social Support and the Well-Being of Persons with Spinal Cord Injury Living in the Community" Rehabilitation Psychology 37:3:155-163

Romeo, Allen J., Richard Wanlass, and Silverio Arenas
1993 "A Profile of Psychosexual Function in Males Following Spinal Cord Injury" Sexuality and Disability 11:4(Winter):269-276

Sandowski, Carol L.
1989 Sexual Concerns When Illness or Disability Strikes Springfield, IL: Charles C. Thomas Publishers

Schover, Leslie R. and Soren Buus Jensen
1988 Sexuality and Chronic Illness New York, NY: Guilford Press

Stover, Samuel L.
1996 "Facts, Figures, and Trends on Spinal Cord Injury" American Rehabilitation Autumn

Thomas, J. Paul
1990 "Definition of the Model System of Spinal Cord Injury Care" pp. 7-9 in David F. Apple and Lesley M. Hudson (eds.) Spinal Cord Injury: The Model Atlanta, GA: Spinal Cord Injury Care System, Sheperd Center for the Treatment of Spinal Injuries

Through the Looking Glass
1994 "Adaptive Parenting Equipment" Parenting with a Disability 3(January)1:4

Trieschmann, Roberta B.
1988 Spinal Cord Injuries: Psychological, Social and Vocational Rehabilitation New York, NY: Demos Publications

White, Mary Joe et al.
1994 "A Comparison of the Sexual Concerns of Men and Women with Spinal Cord Injuries" Rehabilitation Nursing Research Summer

Young, John S. et al.
1982 Spinal Cord Injury Statistics Phoenix, AZ: Good Samaritan Medical Center

ORGANIZATIONS

American Association of Spinal Cord Injury Nurses (AASCIN)
75-20 Astoria Boulevard
Jackson Heights, NY 11370-1177
(718) 803-3782   FAX (718) 803-0414   e-mail: info@epva.org
http://www.epva.org/AASCIN/aascin.html

A professional membership organization that encourages and improves nursing care of individuals with spinal cord injuries and sponsors research. Membership, $75.00, includes quarterly journal, "SCI Nursing."

American Paralysis Association (APA)
500 Morris Avenue
Springfield, NJ 07081
(800) 225-0292   (973) 379-2690   FAX (973) 912-9433
http://www.apacure.com

Supports research to find a cure for paralysis caused by spinal cord injury and other central nervous system disorders. Publishes "Walking Tomorrow," a newsletter about the organization's activities, and "Progress in Research," a newsletter about spinal cord injury research. Various levels of membership fees.

American Paraplegia Society
75-20 Astoria Boulevard
Jackson Heights, NY 11370-1177
(718) 803-3782   FAX (718) 803-0414
http://www.epva.org/APS.html

A professional membership organization for physicians, scientists, and allied health care professionals. Holds an annual meeting for the presentation of scientific research related to spinal cord injury. Membership, $100.00, includes quarterly journal, "Journal of Spinal Cord Medicine."

American Spinal Injury Association (ASIA)
Rehabilitation Institute of Chicago
345 East Superior, Room 1436
Chicago, IL 60611
(312) 908-1242   FAX (312) 503-0869
e-mail: mkaplan@asia-spinalinjury.org
http://www.asia-spinalinjury.org

A professional membership organization for health care providers dedicated to improving the care of individuals with spinal cord injury through research, education, and development of regional spinal cord injury care systems. Holds an annual meeting with presentation of scientific papers. Membership, physicians, $200.00; nonphysicians, $50.00; includes newsletter "ASIA Bulletin."

Commission on Accreditation of Rehabilitation Facilities (CARF)
4891 East Grant Road
Tucson, AZ 85712
(520) 325-1044 (V/TT)   FAX (520) 318-1129   http://www.carf.org

Conducts site evaluations and accredits organizations that provide rehabilitation. Publishes the "Directory of Accredited Organizations," $60.00 plus $5.50 shipping and handling.

Craig Hospital Aging with Spinal Cord Injury
Craig Hospital
3425 South Clarkson
Englewood, CO 80110
(303) 789-8202   FAX (303) 789-8441
http://www.craighospital.org

A federally funded center that studies the physiological and psychological effects of changes brought about by aging on individuals with spinal cord injuries. Produces consumer information brochures in English and Spanish.

Functional Electrical Stimulation Information Center
11000 Cedar Avenue, Suite 230
Cleveland, OH 44106-3052
(800) 666-2353   (216) 231-3257 (V/TT)   FAX (216) 231-3258
e-mail: fesinfo@po.cwru.edu   http://feswww.fes.cwru.edu

Affiliated with the Rehabilitation Engineering Center at Case Western Reserve University, the center provides information to consumers and professionals about functional electrical stimulation. Publishes quarterly newsletter, "FES Update," in standard print and on audiocassette; free. Free publications list.

National Association for Continence (NAFC)
PO Box 8310
Spartanburg, SC 29305-8310
(800) 252-3337   (864) 579-7900   FAX (864) 579-7902
http://www.nafc.org

An information clearinghouse for consumers, family members, and medical professionals. Will answer individual questions if self-addressed stamped envelope is enclosed with letter. Membership, $20.00, includes a quarterly newsletter, "Quality Care," a "Resource Guide:

Products and Services for Continence" (nonmembers, $13.00), discount on publications, and a continence referral service. Free publications list.

National Association on Alcohol, Drugs, and Disability, Inc. (NAADD)
2165 Bunker Hill Drive
San Mateo, CA 94402-3801
(650) 578-8047   FAX (650) 286-9205
e-mail: jdem@aimnet.com   http://www.naadd.org

Promotes awareness and education about substance abuse in individuals with disabilities. Membership, individuals, $15.00; agencies, $25.00; organizations, $100.00.

National Institute of Neurological Disorders and Stroke (NINDS)
Building 31, Room 8A06
31 Center Drive, MSC 2540
Bethesda, MD 20892-2540
(800) 352-9424   (301) 496-5751   FAX (301) 402-2186
http://www.ninds.nih.gov

A federal agency that sponsors basic and clinical research to understand, prevent, and cure paralysis. Supports a national program of Spinal Cord Injury Research Centers. The Neural Prosthetic Program offers bibliographies of publications from research projects supported by the program (http://www.ninds.nih.gov/npp).

National Institute on Disability and Rehabilitation Research (NIDRR)
U.S. Department of Education
400 Maryland Avenue, SW
Washington, DC 20202
(202) 205-8134   (202) 205-8198 (TT)   FAX (202) 205-8515
http://www.ed.gov/OSERS/offices/NIDRR

A federal agency that supports research into various aspects of disability and rehabilitation, including demographic analyses, social science research, and the development of assistive devices. Supports a nationwide system of model spinal cord injury centers.

National Spinal Cord Injury Association (NSCIA)
8300 Colesville Road, Suite 551
Silver Spring, MD 20910
(800) 962-9629   (301) 588-6959   FAX (301) 588-9414
e-mail: nscia2@aol.com   http://www.spinalcord.org

A membership organization with chapters throughout the U.S. Disseminates information to people with spinal cord injuries and to their families; provides counseling; and advocates for the removal of barriers to independent living. Participates in the development of standards of care for regional spinal cord injury care. NSCIA will perform a customized database search; call for details. Holds annual meeting and educational seminars. Membership, individuals with a disability or family members, $25.00; allied health professionals, $50.00; attorneys or physicians, $100.00; organizations, $250.00 to $1000.00; includes quarterly magazine, "SCI Life" (nonmember price, $30.00), fact sheets, and discounts on other publications, medical products, and pharmaceutical supplies.

National Spinal Cord Injury Hotline
2200 Kernan Drive
Baltimore, MD 21207
(800) 526-3456   (410) 448-6623   FAX (410) 448-6627
e-mail: scihotline@aol.com   http://www.scihotline.org

A 24 hour hotline that answers questions, solves individual problems, and makes referrals to professional service providers and peers with spinal cord injuries.

NeuroControl
1945 East 97th Street
Cleveland, OH 44106
(888) 333-4918   (216) 231-6812   FAX (216) 231-2305
http://www.neurocontrol.com

Developed and markets the Freehand System, a system that is surgically implanted and enables some individuals with quadriplegia to regain control over one hand. The company is also developing the NeuroControl VOCARE Bladder System to restore bladder control to individuals with spinal cord injuries.

Paralysis Society of America (PSA)
515 King Street, Suite 420
Alexandria, VA 22314-3317
(888) 772-1711   (703) 684-2660   FAX (703) 684-6048
e-mail: info@psa.org   http://www.psa.org

This organization serves individuals of any age who have experienced paralysis caused by a spinal cord injury or disease. Promotes quality health care, research and education, civil rights, and independence. Membership, $10.00.

Paralyzed Veterans of America (PVA)
801 18th Street, NW
Washington, DC 20006
(800) 424-8200   (800) 795-4327 (TT)   (202) 872-1300
FAX (202) 785-4452   e-mail: info@pva.org   http://www.pva.org

A membership organization for veterans with spinal cord injury. Advocates and lobbies for the rights of paralyzed veterans and sponsors research. Membership fees are set by state chapters. The national office refers callers to the nearest chapter. The PVA Spinal Cord Injury Education and Training Foundation accepts applications to fund continuing education, post-professional specialty training, and patient/client and family education. The PVA Spinal Cord Research Foundation accepts applications to fund basic and clinical research, the design of assistive devices, and conferences that foster interaction among scientists and health care providers. Some publications are available on the web site.

Rehabilitation Research and Training Center in Community Integration for Individuals with Spinal Cord Injury
Baylor College of Medicine
1333 Moursund
Houston, TX 77030
(713) 797-5940   FAX (713) 797-5982

A federally funded center that conducts research and training on the health needs, psychological adjustment, and community integration of individuals with spinal cord injuries. Its training component, The Institute for Rehabilitation Research [TIRR), (713) 797-5945], produces a variety of audiocassettes, videotapes, and publications for professionals, people with disabilities, and family members. Some materials have been translated into Spanish. TIRR will conduct special searches of its database on spinal cord injury (See National Database of Educational Resources on Spinal Cord Injury listed in "PUBLICATIONS AND TAPES" section below). Free publications list.

Rehabilitation Research and Training Center in Prevention and Treatment of Secondary Complications of Spinal Cord Injury
Spain Rehabilitation Center
University of Alabama at Birmingham
1717 Sixth Avenue South, Room 506
Birmingham, AL 35233
(205) 934-3450   (205) 934-4642 (TT)   FAX (205) 975-4691
e-mail: Lindsey@sun.rehabm.uab.edu
http://www.spinalcord.uab.edu

A federally funded center that conducts research and holds educational conferences for people with spinal cord injuries, their families, and professionals. The National Spinal Cord Injury Statistical Center collects data from spinal cord injury centers throughout the country. Produces a variety of audio-visual materials and books for professional care providers and consumers, as well as a series of information sheets. A list of articles documenting some of the center's research findings is also available. Information sheets are available on the web site. Newsletter, "Pushin' On," is published twice a year; free.

Simon Foundation for Continence
PO Box 835
Wilmette, IL 60091
(800) 237-4666   (847) 864-3913   FAX (847) 864-9758

Provides information and assistance to people who are incontinent. Organizes self-help groups. Membership, individuals, $15.00; professionals, $35.00; includes quarterly newsletter, "The Informer."

Substance Abuse Resources & Disability Issues (SARDI)
Rehabilitation Research and Training Center on Drugs and Disability
Wright State University
Dayton, OH 45401-0927
(937) 259-1384
http://www.med.wright.edu/som/sardi

A federally funded research center that investigates the relationship between drug use and disabilities. Free newsletter.

Vocational Rehabilitation Services
Veterans Benefits Administration
Department of Veterans Affairs (VA)
810 Vermont Avenue, NW
Washington, DC 20420
(202) 273-5400   (800) 827-1000 (connects with regional office)
FAX (202) 273-7485   http://www.va.gov

Provides education and rehabilitation assistance and independent living services to veterans with service related disabilities through offices located in every state as well as regional centers, medical centers, and insurance centers. Medical services are provided at VA Medical Centers, Outpatient Clinics, Domiciliaries, and Nursing Homes.

Aging with Spinal Cord Injury
by Gale G. Whiteneck et al.
Demos Vermande
386 Park Avenue South, Suite 201
New York, NY 10016
(800) 532-8663   (212) 683-0072   FAX (212) 683-0118

This book is an anthology of articles by a multidisciplinary group of experts in the field of spinal cord injury. Topics include research in the area of aging with a spinal cord injury, physiological and psychological aspects of the aging process, and societal perspectives. $99.95 plus $4.00 shipping and handling

Alcohol, Disabilities, and Rehabilitation
by Susan A. Storti
Singular Publishing Group
401 West A Street, Suite 325
San Diego, CA 92101
(800) 521-8545   FAX (800) 774-8398
e-mail: singpub@mail.cerfnet.com   http://www.singpub.com

This book discusses alcohol abuse in individuals with disabilities and chronic conditions. Includes treatment and rehabilitation strategies. $34.95 plus $6.00 shipping and handling

The Challenged Life: Spinal Cord Injury
Rehabilitation Institute of Chicago
Education and Training Center
345 East Superior Street, Suite 1641
Chicago, IL 60611
(312) 908-2859   FAX (312) 9008-4451   e-mail: ric-lrc@nwu.edu
http://www.rehabchicago.org

A videotape in which a young man with a spinal cord injury discusses his feelings and his need to relearn how to carry out functional activities. The staff members who treated him discuss the function of the spinal cord, mobility skills, and social skills that individuals with spinal cord injuries need to learn. 22 minutes. $75.00 plus $3.00 shipping and handling

A Change in Perspective
Video Management Services
115 Newfield Avenue
Raritan Center
Edison, NJ 08818-6292
(800) 867-5432   FAX (732) 225-7555

Produced by the Eastern Paralyzed Veterans Association [EPVA, (718) 803-3782], this videotape shows five individuals with spinal cord injury during the course of their everyday life. 30 minutes. $39.95 plus $4.95 shipping and handling

A Consumer's Guide to Home Adaptation
Adaptive Environments Center
374 Congress Street, Suite 301
Boston, MA 02210
(800) 949-4232 (V/TT)   (617) 695-1225 (V/TT)   FAX (617) 482-8099
e-mail: adaptive@adaptenv.org   http://www.adaptenv.org

A workbook that enables people with mobility impairments to plan the modifications necessary to adapt their homes. Includes descriptions of widening doorways, lowering countertops, etc. $12.00

Don't Worry, He Won't Get Far on Foot
by John Callahan
Random House, Order Department
400 Hahn Road
Westminster, MD 21157
(800) 793-2665   http://www.randomhouse.com

Written by a nationally known cartoonist who experienced a spinal cord injury as a result of an accident caused by drinking and driving, this witty autobiographical account provides details of his rehabilitation and his life after his accident, including his return to sobriety. $12.00 plus $3.00 shipping and handling

Enabling Romance: A Guide to Love, Sex, and Relationships for the Disabled
by Ken Kroll and Erica Levy Klein
Woodbine House
6510 Bells Mill Road
Bethesda, MD 20817
(800) 843-7323   FAX (301) 897-5838
e-mail: info@woodbinehouse.com   http://www.woodbinehouse.com

Written by a man who has a disability and his wife who does not, this book provides examples of how people with a variety of disabilities have established fulfilling relationships. $15.95 plus $4.50 shipping and handling

Family Adjustment in Spinal Cord Injury
Spain Rehabilitation Center
University of Alabama at Birmingham
1717 Sixth Avenue South, Room 506
Birmingham, AL 35233
(205) 934-3283   (205) 934-4642 (TT)   FAX (205) 934-2709
e-mail: Lindsey@sun.rehabm.uab.edu
http://www.spinalcord.uab.edu

This booklet provides support for family members, discussing their concerns and feelings. $2.00

Family Challenges: Parenting with a Disability
Aquarius Health Care Videos
5 Powderhouse Lane
PO Box 1159
Sherborn, MA 01770
(508) 651-2963   FAX (508) 650-4216
e-mail: aqvideos@tiac.net   http://www.aquariusproductions.com

In this videotape, the children and spouses of parents with disabilities describe their relationships and coping strategies. Includes two fathers, one with a spinal cord injury and one with a neuromuscular disease. 25 minutes. $195.00 plus $9.00 shipping and handling

FES Resource Guide for Persons with Spinal Cord Injury or Multiple Sclerosis
by J.O. Teeter, C. Kantor, and D.L. Brown
University Bookstore, Case Western Reserve University
10900 Euclid Avenue
Cleveland, OH 44106-7102
(213) 368-1656   (216) 368-5205

This guide describes the applications of functional electrical stimulation (FES); lists clinical and research programs; and provides information about professional organizations and manufacturers. Includes glossary. $13.35 plus $2.00 shipping and handling

A Guide to Wheelchair Selection: How to Use the ANSI/RESNA Wheelchair Standards to Buy a Wheelchair
PVA Distribution Center
PO Box 753
Waldorf, MD 20604-0753
(888) 860-7244   (301) 932-7834   FAX (301) 843-0159
http://www.pva.org

This book enables wheelchair users to make informed choices when purchasing a wheelchair. $12.00 plus $5.00 shipping and handling

Intermittent Self-Catheterization
Media Services
Sacred Heart Medical Center
PO Box 2555
Spokane, WA 99220-2555
(509) 458-5236   FAX (509) 626-4475
http://www.spokanehealth.org/shmc/mediaservices

This videotape demonstrates the use of sterile techniques for intermittent catheterization and shows the necessary supplies and procedures. 8 minutes. Available in English and Spanish. Purchase, individual, $19.95; institution, $99.00; rental for one week, $45.00 (may be applied toward purchase); plus $5.00 shipping and handling. Accompanying booklet, "Clean Intermittent Self-Catheterization," available in English and Spanish; $.50.

Journal of Rehabilitation Research and Development (JRRD)
Scientific and Technical Publications Section
Rehabilitation Research and Development Service
103 South Gay Street, 5th floor
Baltimore, MD 21202
(410) 962-1800   FAX (410) 962-9670   e-mail: pubs@vard.org
http://www.vard.org

A quarterly publication of scientific and engineering articles related to spinal cord injury, prosthetics and orthotics, sensory aids, and gerontology. Includes abstracts of literature, book reviews, and calendar of events. A special issue on choosing a wheelchair system appeared as Clinical Supplement # 2 to the March, 1990 edition. Free

Journal of Spinal Cord Medicine
American Paraplegia Society
75-20 Astoria Boulevard
Jackson Heights, NY 11370-1177
(718) 803-3782   FAX (718) 803-0414
http://www.epva.org/APS.html

A quarterly journal that covers a wide range of topics related to treatment of the physical and psychological aspects of spinal cord injury. Free

Just What Can You Do?
Multi-Focus
1525 Franklin Street
San Francisco, Ca 94109
(800) 821-0514   (415) 673-5100

A discussion among four individuals with spinal cord injury, this videotape includes information about sexuality, marriage, incontinence, attitudes, and personal experiences. 23 minutes. Purchase, videotape, $220.00; 16mm film, $450.00; rental of either format, $60.00.

Keep Fit While You Sit
Twin Peaks Press
PO Box 129
Vancouver, WA 98666-0129
(800) 637-2256 (Order Line only)   (360) 694-2462   FAX (360) 696-3210
e-mail: 73743.2634@compuserve.com

This videotape demonstrates aerobic exercises for the arms, torso, neck, and shoulders for individuals who have no use of their lower body. 45 minutes. $29.95 plus $6.00 shipping and handling

Living with Spinal Cord Injury
by Barry Corbet
Fanlight Productions
47 Halifax Street
Boston, MA 02130
(800) 937-4113   (617) 524-0980   FAX (617) 524-8838
e-mail: fanlight@fanlight.com   http://www.fanlight.com

A series of three videotapes produced by an individual who has experienced spinal cord injury himself. "Changes" is about the consequences of spinal cord injury and the process of rehabilitation. "Outside" emphasizes the life-long aspect of rehabilitation for people with spinal cord injuries. "Survivors" interviews 23 men and women who have lived at least 24 years with spinal cord injuries. Purchase of single videotape, $99.00; rental for one day, $50.00; rental for one week, $100.00; $9.00 shipping and handling. Purchase of series, $200.00; call for shipping and handling.

Managing Incontinence
by Cheryle B. Gartley (ed.)
Simon Foundation for Continence
PO Box 835
Wilmette, IL 60091
(800) 237-4666   (847) 864-3913   FAX (847) 864-9758

This book provides medical advice, information on products, interviews with individuals who are incontinent, and advice on sexuality. $11.95

Moving Violations: War Zones, Wheelchairs, and Declarations of Independence
by John Hockenberry
Time-Warner Trade Publishing
Attn: Order Department
3 Center Plaza
Boston, MA 02108
(800) 759-0190   FAX (800) 286-9471   (617) 227-0730

Written by a television reporter who became a paraplegic at the age of 19 as a result of an automobile accident, this book describes his adjustment to disability, rehabilitation, jobs in radio and television, and the stories of other family members with disabilities. Hardcover, $24.45; softcover, $14.45.

National Database of Educational Resources on Spinal Cord Injury
The Institute for Rehabilitation and Research (TIRR)
Division of Education, B 107
1333 Moursund
Houston, TX 77030
(800) 732-8124   (713) 797-5944   (713) 797-5970 (TT)
FAX (713) 797-5982   e-mail: mgordon@bcm.tmc.edu

This database of publications, audiocassettes, and videotapes on spinal cord injury covers topics such as environmental modifications and accessibility, adaptive equipment and aids, vocational management, and recreation and leisure. Printouts for up to two subject areas are free. Complete database of both audio-visual materials and unpublished written materials, $55.00 plus $5.00 shipping and handling.

No Barriers: The Mark Wellman Story
Aquarius Health Care Videos
5 Powderhouse Lane
PO Box 1159
Sherborn, MA 01770
(508) 651-2963   FAX (508) 650-4216
e-mail: aqvideos@tiac.net   http://www.aquariusproductions.com

This videotape follows Mark Wellman, who is paraplegic, as he climbs mountains in Yosemite National Park. 48 minutes. $90.00 plus $9.00 shipping and handling

Partners in Independence: The Personal Care Attendant's Role in Pressure Sore Prevention
The Institute for Rehabilitation and Research (TIRR)
Division of Education, B 107
1333 Moursund
Houston, TX 77030
(800) 732-8124   (713) 797-5945   (713) 797-5790 (TT)
FAX (713) 797-5982   e-mail: lherson@bcm.tmc.edu

A videotape that teaches how to detect skin problems and how to prevent them. Available in English and Spanish. 12 minutes. Consumers, $30.00; professionals, $85.00; plus $7.50 shipping and handling.

PN/Paraplegia News
2111 East Highland Avenue, Suite 180
Phoenix, AZ 85016
(888) 888-2201   (602) 224-0500   FAX (602) 224-0507
e-mail: pvapub@aol.com   http://www.pva.org

A monthly magazine sponsored by the Paralyzed Veterans of America. Features information for paralyzed veterans and civilians, articles about everyday living, new legislation, employment, and research. $23.00

Reproductive Issues for Persons with Physical Disabilities
by Florence P. Haseltine, Sandra S. Cole, and David B. Gray (eds.)
Brookes Publishing Company
PO Box 10624
Baltimore, MD 21285-0624
(800) 638-3775   FAX (410) 337-8539
e-mail: custserv@pbrookes.com   http://www.pbrookes.com

This book provides an overview of sexuality, disability, and reproductive issues across the lifespan for individuals with disabilities including spinal cord injuries. Includes academic articles as well as personal narratives written by individuals with disabilities. $34.95

Sexuality After Spinal Cord Injury: Answers to Your Questions
by Stanley H. Ducharme and Kathleen M. Gill
Brookes Publishing Company
PO Box 10624
Baltimore, MD 21285-0624
(800) 638-3775   FAX (410) 337-8539
e-mail: custserv@pbrookes.com   http://www.pbrookes.com

This book discusses both physical and emotional aspects of sexuality, including anatomy, self-esteem, sexually transmitted diseases, fertility, and parenting after spinal cord injury. $22.95

Sexuality in Males with SCI
Spain Rehabilitation Center
University of Alabama at Birmingham
1717 Sixth Avenue South, Room 506
Birmingham, AL 35233
(205) 934-3283   (205) 934-4642 (TT)   FAX (205) 934-2709
e-mail: Lindsey@sun.rehabm.uab.edu
http://www.spinalcord.uab.edu

This information sheet describes changes in sexual functioning due to spinal cord injury and discusses sexual aids and relationships and the role of counseling. Free; send self-addressed stamped envelope.

Sexuality Reborn
New Jersey Spinal Cord Injury System
Kessler Institute for Rehabilitation
1199 Pleasant Valley Way
West Orange, NJ 07052
(800) 435-8866   (973) 243-6977   FAX (973) 243-6963
e-mail: rehab@kessler-rehab.com   http://www.kessler-rehab.com

A videotape in which four couples discuss the physical and emotional aspects of spinal cord injury upon their sex lives, including dating, bowel and bladder control, sexual response, and sexual activity. 48 minutes. $39.95 plus $8.00 shipping and handling

Spinal Cord Injury: A Manual for Healthy Living
The Institute for Rehabilitation and Research (TIRR)
Division of Education, B 107
1333 Moursund
Houston, TX 77030
(800) 732-8124   (713) 797-5945   (713) 797-5790 (TT)
FAX (713) 797-5982   e-mail: lherson@bcm.tmc.edu

This manual provides information on how to prevent complications associated with spinal cord injury. Includes information on skin care, sexuality, exercises, equipment, and more. Available in English and Spanish. $60.00 plus $7.50 shipping and handling

Spinal Cord Injury Home Care Manual
Rehabilitation Educational Fund, Attn: Ellie Farzamian
Santa Clara Valley Medical Center
751 South Bascom Avenue
San Jose, CA 95128
(408) 885-2000   FAX (408) 885-2001

Provides people with spinal cord injuries, their families, and professionals with information about physical care, independent living, psychosocial issues, attendant care, and supplies. $120.00

Spinal Network
by Sam Maddox
Miramar Communications
PO Box 8987
Malibu, CA 90265
(800) 543-4116   (310) 317-4522   FAX (310) 317-9644

This book describes the medical aspects of spinal cord injury and the wide variety of effects on functioning. Presents biographical accounts of people who have lived with spinal cord injuries. Discusses issues of everyday living, including recreation and sports, travel, and legal and financial concerns. $39.95 plus $7.50 shipping and handling. "New Mobility" is a monthly magazine with updated information and articles on similar topics. $27.95

Sports 'N Spokes
2111 East Highland Avenue, Suite 180
Phoenix, AZ 85016-9611
(888) 888-2201   (602) 224-0500   FAX (602) 224-0507
e-mail: snsmagazine@aol.com   http://www.pva.org

A bimonthly magazine that features articles about sports activities for people who use wheelchairs. $21.00

Substance Abuse in Rehabilitation Facilities - No Problem? Think Again...
The Institute for Rehabilitation and Research (TIRR)
Division of Education, B 107
1333 Moursund
Houston, TX 77030
(800) 732-8124   (713) 797-5945   (713) 797-5790 (TT)
FAX (713) 797-5982   e-mail: lherson@bcm.tmc.edu

In this videotape, a psychiatrist moderates a discussion by a panel of individuals with spinal cord injuries who experienced substance abuse while in rehabilitation. The role of the institution staff is also discussed. 38 minutes. $89.95 plus $7.50 shipping and handling

<u>Wheelchairs: Your Options and Rights Guide to Obtaining Wheelchairs from the Department</u>
<u>of Veterans Affairs</u>
PVA Distribution Center
PO Box 753
Waldorf, MD 20604-0753
(888) 860-7244   (301) 932-7834   FAX (301) 843-0159
http://www.pva.org

This booklet provides information on eligibility criteria, lists the types of wheelchairs available, and describes DVA procedures. Available in English and Spanish. Free

Chapter 10

STROKE

Stroke is a vascular disease which affects the arteries of the central nervous system. The technical term for a stroke is cerebrovascular accident (CVA). Strokes occur when a blood vessel either bursts or becomes clogged with a blood clot. A stroke stops the flow of blood that brings oxygen and nutrients to the brain. When brain cells die, they are not replaceable. The effects of stroke may be slight or severe, temporary or permanent. The behavior of stroke patients will differ, depending upon the portion of the brain that has been injured, the type of injury, the severity of the injury, and how recently the stroke occurred (Fowler and Fordyce: 1989).

Stroke is a major cause of long term disability. In 1993, medical and rehabilitation costs of stroke along with lost productivity cost Americans 30 billion dollars (Matchar and Duncan: 1994).

In the United States, stroke is the third leading cause of death, after heart disease and cancer; however, the death rate from stroke declined by 17.3% from 1985 to 1995. The incidence of stroke in men is about 19% higher than in women (American Heart Association: 1998a).

The southeastern section of the United States has become known as the stroke belt, as death from stroke is higher than the national average for both sexes and all races. People living in this region are more likely to be overweight and have high blood pressure than those in other parts of the country. The highest rate of stroke occurs among African-Americans (National Heart, Lung, and Blood Institute: 1993).

There are an estimated 600,000 new and recurrent episodes of stroke each year in the United States. The incidence of stroke is decreasing, in part due to education about improving blood pressure and cholesterol through modification of diet and exercise as well as warnings about the health hazards of smoking. As the older population increases and as more individuals receive immediate post-stroke medical attention, the number of stroke survivors is increasing (Duncan: 1994). There are about four million stroke survivors in the United States (American Heart Association: 1998a).

Other risk factors for stroke include a prior stroke, diabetes, and heredity. The risk factors associated with heart disease which increase the risk of stroke include smoking, elevated blood cholesterol, and high blood pressure and are all amenable to treatment. High blood pressure, the strongest risk factor for stroke, may be treated with diet and medication. African-Americans have a greater risk of stroke due to a greater incidence of high blood pressure. Physical inactivity, another risk factor, can be changed through an exercise program.

The warning signals which may indicate a stroke include sudden weakness or numbing of the face, arm, or leg on one side of the body; a loss of speech, difficulty speaking, or understanding speech; dimness or loss of vision, particularly in one eye only; unexplained dizziness, unsteadiness, or sudden falls; or transient ischemic attacks (described below). Stroke requires immediate care. The diagnosis of stroke is confirmed through a neurological exam, computed tomography (CT scan), arteriography, digitized intravenous arteriography (DIVA), or ultrasonography.

There are two major types of strokes: *ischemic strokes*, which are caused by a blood clot that results in an insufficient flow of blood to the brain, and *hemorrhagic strokes*, in which a blood vessel breaks and leaks into the brain.

Within each of the two major types of strokes are two types of strokes. *Cerebral thrombosis* and *cerebral embolism* are both ischemic strokes and account for 70 to 80% of all strokes (American Heart Association: 1994a). In the cerebral thrombosis, a blood clot forms in the artery which brings blood to the brain or in a blood vessel in the brain itself. Clots form in arteries which are damaged by atherosclerosis (hardening of the arteries). A cerebral thrombosis usually occurs at night or first thing in the morning, when blood pressure is low.

Individuals may be forewarned of potential cerebral thrombotic strokes by experiencing *transient ischemic attacks* (TIAs), which may occur days, weeks, or even months before a major stroke. In a TIA, a blood clot temporarily clogs an artery, interrupting the flow of blood to a part of the brain. Symptoms, such as a loss of mobility in a hand or foot, vertigo, vision or hearing loss, occur rapidly and usually last a short time (24 hours or less). Individuals who experience TIAs are 9.5 times more likely to have a stroke than people of the same age and sex who have not had a TIA (American Heart Association: 1994a). The main distinctions between a TIA and a stroke are the TIA's short duration and lack of permanent damage.

In the cerebral embolism, the bloodstream carries a blood clot to the artery leading to the brain or into the brain itself. These clots arise from diseased areas of the heart.

Cerebral hemorrhage and *subarachnoid hemorrhage* are the two types of hemorrhagic strokes. In a cerebral hemorrhage, a blood vessel within the brain, usually an artery, ruptures. This form of stroke is associated with high blood pressure in 70% of the cases. Subarachnoid hemorrhages occur when a blood vessel on the surface of the brain ruptures and bleeds into the space between the brain and the skull. Subarachnoid hemorrhages may be caused by head injury or burst aneurysms (blood filled pouches that balloon out from weak areas in blood vessels).

About one-fifth to one-quarter of individuals who have had a stroke experience second or third strokes. These sometimes can be prevented with surgery and drugs. Surgery may remove built-up plaque in arteries or bypass ruptured blood vessels in the brain. A study sponsored by the National Institute of Neurological Disorders and Stroke found that carotid endarterectomy, surgery to remove fatty deposits from the carotid artery, the main artery in the neck, is effective in reducing the chances of future strokes in those individuals with extreme narrowing of their carotid arteries (National Stroke Association: 1991a). However, African-Americans, who are at greater risk for stroke, are less likely to undergo this surgery (Horner et al.: 1995). A national survey of stroke prevention practices reported that carotid endarterectomy is perceived as being performed less frequently by physicians who practice in the stroke belt (Goldstein et al.: 1995).

Several large studies have shown that individuals with symptomatic carotid artery blockage (stenosis) of 70% or more benefit from carotid endarterectomy (American Heart Association: 1998b). The reduction in the risk of stroke in individuals with 50 to 69% blockage was only moderate (Barnett et al,: 1998). Surgery was of no benefit to individuals who had less than 50% stenosis. Drug therapy with anticoagulants such as heparin, warfarin, or aspirin may prevent new clots from forming or prevent existing clots from becoming larger.

The effects and complications of ischemic stroke are minimized by early treatment with tissue plasminogen activator (tPA), a drug that dissolves the clot that reduces blood flow to the brain. Antiplatelet therapy (platelets are small structures in the blood concerned with blood coagulation and the contraction of blood clots) has recently been touted as a preventative measure for those who have already experienced a stroke or a stroke precursor, such as a TIA. Both ticlopidine hydrochloride and aspirin appear to be effective in preventing thrombotic strokes in individuals who have had minor strokes or TIAs and have undergone carotid endarterectomy (Easton: 1995). Although ticlopidine hydrochloride is recommended for individuals who cannot tolerate aspirin, it too has side effects. Because ticlopidine may cause neutropenia, a deficiency in the blood, complete blood counts should be taken every two weeks during the first three months of therapy. In addition, possible side effects include skin rash and diarrhea (Atkinson: 1995). Ticlopidine is most effective in the first year following stroke, when the probability of recurrence is also greatest (Biller et al.: 1994).

According to Baldwin and Vacek (1989), careful monitoring of any drug therapy is especially important in older individuals due to variable drug absorption rates, interactions of drugs, metabolism, and excretion. The stroke survivor who participates in the management of hypertension by using a blood pressure monitor and recording readings in a daily diary provides valuable information to the physician who can adjust medications, if necessary. Self-monitoring also gives stroke survivors a sense of control over one risk factor for secondary stroke (Ozer: 1992).

Balloon angiography and stenting, common procedures in the treatment of coronary artery disease, are now being investigated in clinical trials as possible techniques to keep carotid arteries open and avoid restenosis (Cleveland Clinic: 1998).

EFFECTS OF STROKE

About four million people in the United States live with varying degrees of disability caused by stroke (American Heart Association: 1998a). The effects of stroke are more severe for individuals age 65 or over; they experience twice the disability and four times the limitations in activities of daily living as those age 45 to 64 (Evans et al.: 1994).

Paralysis or weakness on one side of the body is usually the most visible sign of stroke. When one side of the body is affected, there is an injury to the opposite side of the brain. For example, paralysis on the right side of the body, or right hemiplegia, means that there is an injury to the left side of the brain. The man who has a right hemiplegia is apt to have *aphasia*, which affects the ability to express thoughts and understand what is said or written by others. In expressive aphasia, speech is slow and labored, and words connecting nouns and verbs are often missing; the individual is aware of his difficulties. In receptive aphasia, the man has difficulty understanding speech and in monitoring his own conversation; he is often unaware of these difficulties. Global aphasia consists of both expressive and receptive aphasia (Zezima: 1994). Individuals with aphasia often have a weakness in the right arm and leg. Vision may also be affected, and in some instances, seizures may occur. *Dysarthria* is the term used to describe the speech problems that occur when muscles in the tongue, palate, and lips are affected. Speech may be slowed, slurred, or distorted.

Loss of spatial-perceptual skills is often the result of a stroke affecting the right side of the brain and producing left hemiplegia. The ability to judge size, distance, rate of movement, and position is affected. Individuals may have trouble steering a wheelchair through a doorway, may confuse left and right, miss buttons, or lose their place when reading.

Many individuals who have had a stroke lose some of their visual field; individuals with right hemiplegia lose right field vision in both eyes, individuals with left hemiplegia lose left visual fields in both eyes. Although many individuals learn to turn their heads to compensate, some do not. This failure to compensate is called *neglect*. Neglect can also affect all the senses on one side of the body; individuals may not recognize their own left or right arms and legs as part of their bodies. They act as though they were selectively ignoring all that happens on the impaired side.

In many individuals, the loss of function of upper extremities may be more of a problem than loss of lower extremity function. Range of motion, or the extent to which a joint can be extended and flexed, may be maintained through the use of a sling, support pillow, armboard, or medication, but it is important to use only the adaptive equipment which is actually needed.

Changes in individuals' behavior may also be attributable to stroke. The term *quality control* is used to describe the ability to guide and check one's own behavior, sometimes known as social judgment. Individuals may become aggressive or uncommunicative, may neglect personal hygiene, or swear inappropriately. Gentle coaching, appropriate feedback, and simple memory cues may help individuals with these memory defects.

Memory problems occur with almost any injury to the brain and can have language and spatial-perceptual components. *Retention span* is a term used to describe the amount of information which can be retained, used, or acted upon. Short retention spans are characteristic after a stroke. Using short, concise phrases, and brief, simple messages may avoid confusing these individuals. After a stroke, individuals have difficulty with new learning, even though they are able to recall information from the past quite well. *Generalization*, or applying learning from one situation to another, may also be affected. Individuals with generalization problems are very sensitive to changes in their environment and may not be able to transfer skills learned in the rehabilitation program setting to the home. Rehabilitation services provided in the home may ameliorate this problem. For these individuals, it is important to discuss changes in routine and establish new routines as quickly as possible.

STROKE REHABILITATION

The key factor in stroke rehabilitation is that it must start as soon as possible. According to one source, rehabilitation should be instituted within 48 hours of hospital admission (Gibson and Caplan: 1984). Most spontaneous recovery occurs within the first four to six months after the stroke.

> To a large degree, successful rehabilitation depends on the extent
> of brain damage, the person's attitude, the rehabilitation team's
> skill, and the cooperation of family and friends (American Heart
> Association: 1994a, 28).

The purpose of stroke rehabilitation is to reduce dependence; improve physical activity; and enable the stroke survivor to be as independent and productive as possible within the limitations caused by the stroke. The standard goals of stroke rehabilitation include prevention of complications; compensation for physical and intellectual losses; minimizing social and economic loss; and maximizing independence. Early stroke care includes maintaining range of motion in the joints; preventing pressure sores; sensory stimulation; and getting out of bed as soon as possible. Over 70% of stroke survivors can become independent in activities of daily living if they receive appropriate rehabilitation (National Stroke Association: 1991b).

In evaluating an individual who has had a stroke, the rehabilitation team takes into account the following characteristics: functional ability before the stroke; the social situation and the options for a return to the community; ability to cooperate with nurses and therapists; capacity to learn new material; age; and bowel and bladder (in)continence (Gibson and Caplan: 1984). Recent government guidelines recommend that the person undergo rehabilitation as long as there is evidence of progress (Gresham et al.: 1995).

Medicare and other insurance coverage place a limit on the length of time an individual who has had a stroke may spend in an acute hospital, unless there are complications. Since most individuals will benefit from rehabilitation services, they may be discharged to a hospital rehabilitation unit or to a rehabilitation hospital. Individuals who cannot afford stroke rehabilitation services may be eligible for special funding which provides treatment at rehabilitation facilities for people with brain injuries.

The rehabilitation team is also involved in discharge planning, evaluating what the individual and the family can do for themselves; what assistance must be supplied; and what resources are available through community agencies.

SEXUAL FUNCTIONING

The man who has had a stroke has experienced sudden and dramatic changes in his body, and they may lead to a fear of failure in sexual performance (Sandowski: 1989) as well as a fear of the consequences of sexual activity (Stewart: 1979). Changes in self-image, role reversal, and attitudes of partners also disrupt sexual relationships. The physical and behavioral losses of stroke described above may affect sexual functioning as well. Men who have had healthy sexual relationships prior to stroke are more likely to regain sexual functioning after having a stroke (Finger: 1993).

Ageism may account for the lack of attention paid in stroke rehabilitation programs to sexual dysfunction. Other factors include personal attitudes, lack of training, and discomfort in discussing sexual issues among staff members at these programs and the families of the stroke survivor. Although there may be psychological as well as physical causes of impotence following a stroke, damage to the left side of the brain is more likely to cause impotence (Sandowski: 1989). Other medical conditions such as diabetes, hardening of the arteries, and high blood pressure may be responsible for erectile dysfunction. Changing the dosage or timing of medications for hypertension, which often cause sexual dysfunction, can reduce side effects. External vacuum pump devices and injections into the penis may produce satisfactory erections. Vacuum pump devices carry little risk, while drugs used for penile injections have cardiovascular side effects. A man with significant motor function loss will need his partner's help to use these methods of achieving an erection. An auto injector is an option for men with limited dexterity.

The partner of a man whose vision is affected by stroke should try to remain in his visual field. If weakness affects an arm or leg, it is important to try various positions for intercourse. A stroke survivor with reduced sensation or lack of sensation on one side of his body should lie on that side, using the unaffected arm and hand to caress his partner. Men with spasticity may find that antispasmodic medications improve sexual functioning. Aphasia interferes with the ability to communicate. Couples will need to develop their own verbal or nonverbal communication methods.

Sexual counseling should be a part of stroke rehabilitation and should be available to both the stroke survivor and his partner.

PSYCHOLOGICAL ASPECTS OF STROKE

A stroke that causes physical weakness and dependency may be viewed as a direct assault on a man's sense of masculinity. In addition to the physical and mental impairments caused by a stroke, the loss of a job, reduced financial resources, and the loss of independence may cause men to lose self-esteem and become depressed. Although post-stroke depression is very common, it is often overlooked by health care providers (Rusin: 1990). Because men are often reluctant to admit that they need psychological help, their wives are often left to seek assistance and convince the men to accept it. Depression may interfere with motivation for rehabilitation and delay improved functioning; it is important that all individuals who have experienced a stroke be screened for depression. Often, what appears to be depression is actually the result of the brain injury caused by the stroke (organic emotional lability) and characterized by little or no obvious relationship between emotions and what is happening around the individual.

Post-stroke depression may include anxiety, loss of energy, weight and appetite loss, and sleep disturbances. Neurological features of stroke such as verbal and nonverbal communication problems, emotional control, and visual and auditory losses may affect the clinical assessment of depression. The health care professionals on the stroke rehabilitation team work together to determine the extent of post-stroke depression. A neuropsychological assessment should include tests of attention span, memory, language, perceptual abilities, and cognitive functions, such as problem solving and abstract thinking.

For some men, post-stroke depression is reduced as physical recovery progresses. Individual or group counseling, as part of the rehabilitation program or after discharge from the hospital, may enable men to adapt emotionally to their physical condition (Schwartz and Speed: 1989). Volunteer visitation programs enable stroke survivors and family members to talk with other stroke survivors. Talking to other male stroke survivors may encourage men to express their own fears, feelings of dependency, and sexual problems. Men who derive comfort from this type of peer counseling may find self-help groups such as stroke clubs beneficial. Attendance at a day activity program contributes to continuation and maintenance of skills developed through rehabilitation and offers opportunities for socializing. Antidepressant drugs may also be prescribed after careful consideration of any associated medical conditions and risk of side effects.

The family plays a crucial role in rehabilitation of a stroke patient. The stroke survivor's wife may become depressed due to feelings of guilt and fear. Other symptoms apparent in caregivers include inability to sleep, social withdrawal, and marital problems. One study found that caregivers' stress increased over time, although the caregivers had not sought help for themselves (Mcnamara et al.: 1990). A spouse may become over-protective and worry about another stroke once the individual is discharged from the rehabilitation hospital. Conferences with the spouse and other family members may help to alleviate these concerns and also put the individual who has had a stroke at ease. Obtaining information about the effects of stroke and attendance at support groups for caregivers may help to alleviate some of the stress that is inevitable. A caring and able spouse or other caregiver, a supportive family, and an understanding of stroke and its consequences are important parts of a coordinated approach to care.

PROFESSIONAL SERVICE PROVIDERS

A rehabilitation evaluation involves the coordinated efforts of the neurologist, physiatrist, nurse, physical and occupational therapists, speech and language pathologist, audiologist, social worker, and psychologist. Recent guidelines published by the federal government suggest that one member of the rehabilitation team be the coordinator of services, establish a baseline evaluation, and keep track of the person's progress (Gresham et al.:1995).

Neurologists are physicians who specialize in diagnosing and treating disorders of the brain and central nervous system. *Physiatrists*, physicians who specialize in rehabilitation medicine, often act as case managers or team leaders, coordinating medical and rehabilitation services, working with the patient and the family, and arranging additional health care services, if necessary.

Physical therapists help the individual to strengthen muscles and to improve balance and coordination. Mechanical aids such as braces, walkers, crutches, or canes are often used.

Rehabilitation nurses provide day-to-day care of the patient who has had a stroke; report to the rehabilitation team on the progress of the patient; withdraw help as the patient recovers the ability to perform everyday activities in order to promote independence; and offer support to the patient's family in the hospital, outpatient clinic, and during home care visits.

Occupational therapists help the individual to improve hand-eye coordination and to develop skills for everyday activities, such as washing, dressing, homemaking, and recreation. Many assistive devices, such as reaching tools, built-up kitchen utensils, and writing aids are suggested by the occupational therapist. Shorter hospital stays have led to the development of home treatment programs involving stroke survivors and their families; these treatment programs are often managed by occupational therapists.

Speech and language pathologists aid in the recovery or maintenance of speech or language function. After an assessment, speech and language pathologists design and implement a program to treat the individual's language difficulties. Often the test results obtained by speech and language pathologists will help the medical staff in caring for the individual with aphasia. These services are offered both in the hospital and on an out-patient basis.

Audiologists identify and evaluate hearing impairment; determine the need for hearing rehabilitation; decide whether or not a hearing aid will be beneficial; and select and fit the appropriate aid.

Social workers meet with the individual and the family to help plan the individual's rehabilitation after release from the acute care hospital and rehabilitation programs. Social workers may also help individuals and their families with the emotional effects of stroke.

Psychologists assess cognitive deficits and emotional reactions to stroke and provide supportive counseling.

WHERE TO FIND SERVICES

According to the National Stroke Association (no date), there are approximately 75 free-standing rehabilitation hospitals in the United States; many of these have voluntarily sought and received accreditation from the Commission on Accreditation of Rehabilitation Facilities (CARF). Recently, many hospitals have established inpatient rehabilitation units. These rehabilitation hospitals and units provide the services needed by individuals who have had a stroke.

The discharge plan for an individual who has had a stroke should include information about the resources available in the community. Physical therapy, occupational therapy, speech and language therapy, and audiology services may be provided by public and private clinics; local hospitals; home health agencies such as visiting nurse associations; nursing homes; state, federal, and private agencies; Veterans Affairs Medical Centers; and therapists in private practice.

Local offices of organizations such as the American Heart Association and the National Easter Seal Society as well as independent living centers and hospitals may sponsor stroke support groups or clubs to provide emotional and practical support to individuals who have had strokes, their families, and friends. The National Stroke Association defines a stroke support group as one which usually meets in a hospital or long term care facility and is led by a rehabilitation professional. Stroke clubs are primarily social groups run by stroke survivors without professional direction.

ASSISTIVE DEVICES AND TECHNIQUES

Individuals who have had a stroke often learn new techniques to do familiar activities. Residual paralysis or weakness, perceptual problems, vision loss, and difficulty in movement or coordination often require that the individual slow down, plan ahead, and use assistive devices to accomplish daily living activities. Special equipment may be used to give support, prevent deformity, or replace lost abilities. Some devices are readily available in medical supply stores and through mail order catalogues (See Chapter 2, "Coping with Daily Activities," p. 71 for sources of these devices), while others require a prescription from a health care professional.

In the bathroom, for example, nonskid tape should be placed on the bottom of the tub, and shower and grab bars should be installed. A hand-held shower head, soap-on-a-rope, and long-handled bath brushes will assist with bathing. A shower seat or chair with nonskid suction cups on its legs may help the individual feel more comfortable and safe.

When dressing, the individual should put the weaker arm or leg into the garment first, pull the clothing into place, and then insert the stronger arm or leg. In undressing, the opposite order should be followed. Dressing aids such as button hooks, elastic shoe laces, or zipper pulls and clothing with velcro fasteners, elastic waistbands, or snaps will help the individual dress more easily. In the kitchen, jar openers, long-handled tongs, utensils with built-up handles, and other assistive devices will make it easier for the individual to resume homemaking activities.

Adaptations of the physical environment are sometimes required to meet the individual's limitations. Simple adaptations include removing scatter rugs or shag carpets; raising chair seats with double cushions; or rearranging shelves for easy reach. Other adaptations include removing architectural barriers such as thresholds; installing ramps and handrails; and widening doorways.

Individuals who have had a stroke may use mobility aids such as four-legged walkers, canes, braces, and railings that help them to regain independent mobility to the greatest extent possible. Individuals who wish to drive should be evaluated by professionals who are expert in training for drivers with physical disabilities. Some rehabilitation hospitals or centers offer these training courses.

References

American Heart Association
1998a 1998 Heart and Stroke Statistical Update Dallas, TX: American Heart Association
1998b Guidelines for Carotid Endarterectomy Dallas, TX: American Heart Association
1994a Heart and Stroke Facts Dallas, TX: American Heart Association
1994b Heart and Stroke Facts: 1995 Statistical Supplement Dallas, TX: American Heart Association
Atkinson, Richard P.
1995 "Practical Information on the Administration of Antiplatelet Therapy" Reducing the Odds of Stroke (A special report of Postgraduate Medicine) (February):36-39
Baldwin, Thomas and James Vacek
1989 "Use of Cardiovascular Drugs in the Elderly" Postgraduate Medicine 85(April):319-330
Barnett, Henry J. M. et al.
1998 "Benefit of Carotid Endarterectomy in Patients with Symptomatic Moderate or Severe Stenosis" New England Journal of Medicine 339:20(November):425
Biller, Jose et al.
1994 Consensus and Controversy: Medical and Surgical Options for Stroke Prevention New York, NY: Phase Five Communications

Cleveland Clinic
1998 "New Technique to Prevent Stroke" The Cleveland Clinic Heart Advisor Cleveland, OH: Cleveland Clinic

Duncan, Pamela W.
1994 "Stroke Disability" Physical Therapy 74:399-407

Easton, J. Donald
1995 "Preventing Stroke: An Overview of Medical and Surgical Options" Reducing the Odds of Stroke (A special report of Postgraduate Medicine) (February):7-13

Evans, R. L. et al.
1994 "Stroke: A Family Dilemma" Disability and Rehabilitation 16:3:110-118

Finger, William W.
1993 "Prevention, Assessment and Treatment of Sexual Dysfunction Following Stroke" Sexuality and Disability 11:1:39-56

Fowler, Roy S. and W. E. Fordyce
1989 Stroke: Why Do They Behave That Way? Dallas, TX: American Heart Association

Gibson, Charles J. and Bruce M. Caplan
1984 "Rehabilitation of the Patient with Stroke" pp. 145-159 in T. Franklin Williams (ed.) Rehabilitation in the Aging New York, NY: Raven Press

Goldstein, L. B. et al.
1995 "U.S. National Survey of Physician Practices for the Secondary and Tertiary Prevention of Ischemic Stroke" Stroke 26:(September):1607-1625

Gresham, G. E. et al.
1995 Post-Stroke Rehabilitation: Assessment, Referral, and Patient Management Clinical Practice Guideline, No. 16 Rockville, MD: U.S. Department of Health and Human Services, Public Health Service, Agency for Health Care Policy and Research. AHCPR Pub. No. 95-0663

Horner, R. D., E. Z. Oddone, and D. B. Matchar
1995 "Theories Explaining Racial Differences in the Utilization of Diagnostic and Therapeutic Procedures for Cerebrovascular Disease" The Milbank Quarterly 73(3):443-462

Matchar, David B. and Pamela W. Duncan
1994 "Cost of Stroke" Stroke Clinical Updates 5(September):3

Mcnamara, Susan E. et al.
1990 "Caregiver Strain: Need for Late Poststroke Intervention" Rehabilitation Psychology 35:2:71-78

National Heart, Lung, and Blood Institute
1993 "National High Blood Pressure Education Program: Update on the Stroke Belt Projects" Heart Memo (Fall):7

National Stroke Association
1991a "Carotid Endarterectomy - Stroke Prevention Surgery More Effective Than Previously Thought" Be Stroke Smart 8:1(Spring):2-3
1991b "Rehabilitation After Stroke" STROKE CLINICAL UPDATE 1:6(March):21-24
No date Resources for Stroke Treatment and Rehabilitation

Ozer, Mark N.
1992 "Prevention of Secondary Stroke" <u>Be Stroke Smart</u> 9:1(Winter):5 National Stroke Association

Rusin, Michael J.
1990 "Stroke Rehabilitation: A Geropsychological Perspective" <u>Archives of Physical Medicine and Rehabilitation</u> 71(October):914-922

Sandowski, Carol L.
1989 <u>Sexual Concerns When Illness or Disability Strikes</u> Springfield, IL: Charles C. Thomas Publishers

Schwartz, Joseph A. and Nancy Speed
1989 "Depression and Stroke" <u>Rehabilitation Report</u> 5(March-April):1-3

Stewart, W. F. R.
1979 <u>The Sexual Side of Handicap</u> Cambridge, England: Woodhead-Faulkner Limited

Zezima, Michele and Michael
1994 "Louder Than Words: Treating Aphasia and Agnosia" <u>Advance/Rehabilitation</u> 3 (September)8:27-28

ORGANIZATIONS

American Heart Association
7272 Greenville Avenue
Dallas, TX 75231-4596
(800) 242-8721   (214) 373-6300   FAX (214) 706-1341
http://www.americanheart.org

Promotes research and education and publishes professional and public education brochures. Local affiliates. Membership fees vary.

American Speech-Language-Hearing Association (ASHA)
10801 Rockville Pike
Rockville, MD 20852
(800) 498-2071   (301) 897-5700   (301) 897-0157 (TT)
FAX (301) 571-0457   e-mail: irc@asha.org   http://www.asha.org

A professional organization of speech-language pathologists and audiologists. Provides information on communication problems and a free list of certified audiologists and speech therapists for each state. Toll-free HELPLINE offers answers to questions about conditions and services as well as referrals, (800) 638-8255 (V/TT).

Commission on Accreditation of Rehabilitation Facilities (CARF)
4891 East Grant Road
Tucson, AZ 85712
(520) 325-1044 (V/TT)   FAX (520) 318-1129   http://www.carf.org

Conducts site evaluations and accredits organizations that provide rehabilitation. Publishes the "Directory of Accredited Organizations." $60.00 plus $7.00 shipping and handling

National Aphasia Association
156 Fifth Avenue, Suite 707
New York, NY 10010
(800) 922-4622   (212) 255-4329   http://www.aphasia.org

Promotes public awareness, publishes public education brochures, and develops community programs for people with aphasia. Maintains list of health care professionals who will make referrals to local resources. Publishes a variety of inexpensive fact sheets and "Aphasia Community Group Manual," for organizers of local aphasia support groups; $30.00. Membership, $25.00, includes quarterly newsletter.

National Easter Seal Society
230 West Monroe Street, Suite 1800
Chicago, IL 60606
(800) 221-6827   (312) 726-6200   (312) 726-4258 (TT)
FAX (312) 726-1494   http://www.easter-seals.org

Promotes research, education, and rehabilitation for people with physical disabilities and speech and language problems. Sponsors Easter Seal Stroke Clubs for people who have had strokes, their families, and friends.

National Heart, Lung, and Blood Institute (NHLBI)
31 Center Drive, MSC 2480
Bethesda, MD 20892-2480
(301) 496-5166   http://www.nih.gov.

Conducts research and national education programs and issues clinical guidelines on topics such as high blood pressure and high cholesterol. Publications list available, free.

National Heart, Lung, and Blood Institute Information Center
PO Box 30105
Bethesda, MD 20824-0105
(301) 251-1222   FAX (301) 251-1223
http://www.nhlbi.nih/nhlbi

A federal information center which distributes publications about cardiovascular disease. NHLBI Information Line provides recorded messages in English and Spanish about prevention and treatment of high blood pressure; [(800) 575-9355]. Free publications list.

National Hypertension Association
324 East 30th Street
New York, NY 10016
(212) 889-3557   FAX (212) 447-7032

Conducts research, promotes public and professional education, and provides hypertension work-site detection programs. General information packet, free, plus $2.00 shipping and handling. Also available, "Week by Week to a Strong Heart," $8.50; "Lower Your Blood Pressure and Live Longer," $8.50; and "High Blood Pressure & What You Can Do About It," $2.50.

National Institute of Neurological Disorders and Stroke (NINDS)
Building 31, Room 8A06
31 Center Drive, MSC 2540
Bethesda, MD 20892-2540
(800) 352-9424   (301) 496-5751   FAX (301) 402-2186
http://www.ninds.nih.gov

A federal agency that conducts basic and clinical research on the causes, prevention, and treatment of stroke. Publishes pamphlets on stroke and stroke-related conditions. Free

National Institute on Deafness and Other Communication Disorders (NIDCD)
Building 31, Room 3C35
31 Center Drive, MSC 2320
Bethesda, MD 20892-2320
(301) 496-7243   (301) 402-0252 (TT)
FAX (301) 402-0018   http://www.nih.gov/nidcd

A federal agency that funds basic research studies on problems of hearing, balance, voice, language, and speech.

National Institute on Deafness and Other Communication Disorders Information Clearinghouse
1 Communication Avenue
Bethesda, MD 20892-3456
(800) 241-1044   (800) 241-1055 (TT)   FAX (301) 907-8830
e-mail: nidcd@aerie.com   http://www.nih.gov/nidcd

Maintains a database of references and responds to requests for information from the public and professionals on communication disorders including aphasia. Publishes newsletter, "Inside NIDCD Clearinghouse." Free

National Stroke Association
96 Inverness Drive East, Suite I
Englewood, Colorado 80112-5112
(800) 787-6537   (303) 649-9299   (303) 649-0122 (TT)
FAX (303) 649-1328   e-mail: info@stroke.org   http://www.stroke.org

Assists individuals with stroke and educates their families, physicians, and the general public about stroke.   Membership, individuals, $20.00; professionals, $50.00; organizations, $200.00; includes quarterly newsletter, "Be Stroke Smart."

Stroke Connection
American Heart Association
7272 Greenville Avenue
Dallas, TX 75231
(800) 553-6321   e-mail: strokeaha@americanheart.org
http://www.american heart.org

Coordinates a network of more than 800 stroke clubs and groups. Sponsors "Common Threads PenFriends," which matches stroke survivors, caregivers and family members. Publishes "A Stroke of Luck," a free newsletter for survivors and caregivers living with aphasia, and a bimonthly newsletter, "Stroke Connection Magazine," $12.00. A courtesy subscription is available to any stroke survivor unable to pay. Also available on the web site.

American Heart Association Family Guide to Stroke
American Heart Association Fulfillment Center
200 State Road
South Deerfield, MA 01373-0200
(800) 611-6083   FAX (800) 499-6464

This book discusses the causes, diagnosis, and treatment of stroke as well as the rehabilitation process, including lifestyle changes, adapting the home, and coping with residual effects of stroke. $23.00 plus $5.75 shipping and handling

Aphasia, My World Alone
by Helen Harlan Wulf
Wayne State University Press
4809 Woodward Avenue
Detroit, MI 48201-1309
(800) 978-7323   (313) 577-6120   FAX (313) 577-6131

The author shares her experiences in having a stroke and aphasia, with emphasis on speech therapy, family relationships, and the effects of fatigue on recovery. $13.95 plus $3.00 shipping and handling

The Brain At Risk: Understanding and Preventing Stroke
National Stroke Association
96 Inverness Drive East, Suite I
Englewood, Colorado 80112-5112
(800) 787-6537   (303) 649-9299   (303) 649-0122 (TT)
FAX (303) 649-1328   e-mail: info@stroke.org   http://www.stroke.org

This videotape describes risk factors of stroke, warning signs and symptoms, and how a stroke occurs. 19 minutes. $25.00 plus $5.00 shipping and handling

Brain Attacks
Aquarius Health Care Videos
5 Powderhouse Lane
PO Box 1159
Sherborn, MA 01770
(508) 651-2963   FAX (508) 650-4216
e-mail: aqvideos@tiac.net   http://www.aquariusproductions.com

This videotape describes the risk factors, warning signals and treatment available for stroke. Includes personal accounts of stroke survivors. 30 minutes. $195.00 plus $9.00 shipping and handling

Caring for a Person with Aphasia
American Heart Association
7272 Greenville Avenue
Dallas, TX 75231-4596
(800) 242-8721   (214) 373-6300   FAX (214) 706-1341
http://www.americanheart.org

This booklet describes the communication problems associated with aphasia and provides practical tips for improving communication skills. Free

Directory: Information Resources for Human Communication Disorders
National Institute on Deafness and Other Communication Disorders Information Clearinghouse
1 Communication Avenue
Washington, DC 20892-3456
(800) 241-1044   (800) 241-1055 (TT)
e-mail: nidcd@aerie.com   http://www.nih.gov/nidcd

This directory provides a listing and description of professional and consumer organizations related to speech, language, hearing, and balance. Free

How Stroke Affects Behavior
American Heart Association
7272 Greenville Avenue
Dallas, TX 75231-4596
(800) 242-8721   (214) 373-6300   FAX (214) 706-1341
http://www.americanheart.org

This booklet discusses the intellectual, behavioral, and emotional changes which may occur after a stroke and offers guidelines for caregivers. Free

One Hand Can Do the Work of Two
A/V Health Services
PO Box 20271
Roanoke, VA 24018-0028
(540) 725-9288 (Voice and FAX)   e-mail: avhealth4u@aol.com

This videotape shows how someone who has had a cerebral hemorrhage accomplishes household activities with the use of one hand. 20 minutes. $30.00

The One-Handed Way
American Heart Association
7272 Greenville Avenue
Dallas, TX 75231-4596
(800) 242-8721   (214) 373-6300   FAX (214) 706-1341
http://www.americanheart.org

This booklet offers many practical solutions to the challenges experienced by stroke survivors who have the use of just one hand. Free

Pathways: Moving Beyond Stroke and Aphasia
by Susan Adair Ewing and Beth Pfalzgraf
Wayne State University Press
4809 Woodward Avenue
Detroit, MI 48201-1309
(800) 978-7323   (313) 577-6120   FAX (313) 577-6131

In this book, stroke survivors and their families describe methods of coping with disability. $21.95 plus $3.00 shipping and handling.

Portrait of Aphasia
by David R. Knox
Wayne State University Press
4809 Woodward Avenue
Detroit, MI 48201-1309
(800) 978-7323   (313) 577-6120   FAX (313) 577-6131

In this book, the author describes his wife's recovery from a stroke. Includes many helpful suggestions for helping individuals with aphasia regain language skills. $14.95 plus $3.00 shipping and handling

Recovering from a Stroke
American Heart Association
7272 Greenville Avenue
Dallas, TX 75231-4596
(800) 242-8721   (214) 373-6300   FAX (214) 706-1341
http://www.americanheart.org

This booklet suggests how familiar tasks can be performed in new ways and describes financial and legal resources. Free

The Road Ahead: A Stroke Recovery Guide
National Stroke Association
96 Inverness Drive East, Suite I
Englewood, Colorado 80112-5112
(800) 787-6537   (303) 649-9299   (303) 649-0122 (TT)
FAX (303) 649-1328   e-mail: info@stroke.org   http://www.stroke.org

This handbook helps individuals who have had strokes and their families understand the many aspects of recovering from stroke. $14.50 plus $4.00 shipping and handling

Sex After Stroke
American Heart Association
7272 Greenville Avenue
Dallas, TX 75231-4596
(800) 242-8721   (214) 373-6300   FAX (214) 706-1341
http://www.americanheart.org

This booklet provides information for stroke survivors and their partners about intimacy following stroke, describing fears and concerns, sexual positions, and special physical challenges. Free

Sexual Concerns When Illness or Disability Strikes
by Carol L. Sandowski
Charles C. Thomas Publisher
2600 South First Street
Springfield, IL 62794
(800) 258-8980   (217) 789-8980   FAX (217) 789-9130
e-mail: books@ccthomas.com   http://www.ccthomas.com

Written by a social worker who is a certified sex counselor, this book discusses sexuality and self esteem issues that arise with illness or disability, including stroke. $41.95 plus $5.50 shipping and handling

A Stroke Manual for Families
HDI Publishers
PO Box 131401
Houston, TX 77219
(800) 321-7037   In TX, (713) 526-6900   FAX (713) 526-7787

This book offers suggestions for families of stroke survivors. $6.50 plus $2.00 shipping and handling

Stroke Survivors
by William H. Bergquist, Rod McLean and Barbara A. Kobylinski
Jossey-Bass Publishers
350 Sansome Street
San Francisco, CA 94104
(800) 956-7739   (415) 433-1767   FAX (800) 605-2665
http://josseybass.com

This book uses the personal histories of stroke survivors to describe the stroke experience, the recovery and rehabilitation process, and the viewpoints of caregivers. $25.00

Stroke: What Every Person Needs to Know
Coming Back: You're Not Alone
Coming Back: A Gift of Caring
American Heart Association Fulfillment Center
200 State Road
South Deerfield, MA 01373-0200
(800) 611-6083   FAX (800) 499-6464

The first videotape provides general information about stroke, including causes, symptoms, and effects. The second videotape discusses physical, emotional, and lifestyle changes associated with stroke; describes the effects of stroke on the left and right side of the brain; and explains the role of the family, friends, and support groups. The third videotape provides information for caregivers. Each videotape is about 15 minutes in length. $16.00 each; $40.00 for all three; plus $5.75 shipping and handling May also be available through local affiliates' videotape lending libraries; call (800) 242-8721.

Ted's Stroke: The Caregiver's Story
by Ellen Paullin
National Stroke Association
96 Inverness Drive East, Suite I
Englewood, Colorado 80112-5112
(800) 787-6537   (303) 649-9299   (303) 649-0122 (TT)
FAX (303) 649-1328   e-mail: info@stroke.org   http://www.stroke.org

This book describes personal experiences and provides guidance for caregivers of stroke survivors. $14.95 plus $3.00 shipping and handling

Understanding Stroke
by Karen Craddock
Coffey Communications, Inc.
1505 Business One Circle
Walla Walla, WA 99362
(800) 952-9089   (509) 525-0101   FAX (509) 525-0281
e-mail: coffey@coffeycomm.com   http://www.life-and-health.com

This booklet describes the warning signs of stroke, risk factors, diagnosis, treatment, and rehabilitation. A section for families of stroke survivors discusses possible intellectual, behavioral, and emotional changes. $1.25 plus 7% shipping and handling (minimum order, $5.00).

What You Should Know About Stroke
American Heart Association
7272 Greenville Avenue
Dallas, TX 75231-4596
(800) 242-8721   (214) 373-6300   FAX (214) 706-1341
http://www.americanheart.org

This booklet discusses the warning signs and risk factors for stroke, prevention, types of stroke, and rehabilitation. Free

When the Brain Goes Wrong
by Jonathan David and Roberta Cooks
Fanlight Productions
47 Halifax Street
Boston, MA 02130
(800) 937-4113   (617) 524-0980   FAX (617) 524-8838
e-mail: fanlight@fanlight.com   http://www.fanlight.com

A stroke survivor's experience is included in this videotape, which deals with seven types of brain dysfunctions. 47 minutes. Purchase, $195.00; rental for one day, $50.00; rental for one week, $100.00; plus $9.00 shipping and handling.

INDEX TO ORGANIZATIONS

This index contains only those organizations listed under sections titled "ORGANIZA-TIONS." These organizations may also be listed as vendors of publications, tapes, and other products.

PUBLICATIONS FROM RESOURCES FOR REHABILITATION

A Man's Guide to Coping with Disability

Written to fill the void in the literature regarding the special needs of men with disabilities, this book includes information about men's responses to disability, with a special emphasis on the values men place on independence, occupational achievement, and physical activity. Information on finding local services, self-help groups, laws that affect men with disabilities, sports and recreation, and employment is applicable to men with any type of disability or chronic condition. The disabilities that are most prevalent in men or that affect men's special roles in society are included. Chapters on coronary heart disease, diabetes, HIV/AIDS, multiple sclerosis, prostate conditions, spinal cord injury, and stroke include information about the disease or condition, psychological aspects, sexual functioning, where to find services, environmental adaptations, and annotated entries of organizations, publications and tapes, and resources for assistive devices. Includes information about Internet resources.

Second edition   1999   ISBN 0-929718-23-2 $44.95

*"a **unique** reference source." Library Journal*

*"a **unique** purchase for public libraries" Booklist/Reference Books Bulletin*

*"...Thank you for the **high quality** books you provide." A nurse's aide*

A Woman's Guide to Coping with Disability

This book addresses the special needs of women with disabilities and chronic conditions, such as social relationships, sexual functioning, pregnancy, childrearing, caregiving, and employment. Special attention is paid to ways in which women can advocate for their rights with the health care and rehabilitation systems. Written for women in all age categories, the book has chapters on the disabilities that are most prevalent in women or likely to affect the roles and physical functions unique to women. Included are arthritis, diabetes, epilepsy, lupus, multiple sclerosis, osteoporosis, and spinal cord injury. Each chapter also includes information about the condition, service providers, and psychological aspects plus descriptions of organizations, publications and tapes, and special assistive devices.

Second edition 1997   ISBN 0-929718-19-4 $42.95

"...this excellent, empowering resource belongs in all collections." Library Journal

"...crucial information women need to be informed, empowered, and in control of their lives. Excellent self-help information... Highly recommended for public and academic libraries."   Choice

"...a marvelous publication...will help women feel more in control of their lives." A nurse who became disabled

Resources for People with Disabilities and Chronic Conditions

This comprehensive resource guide has chapters on spinal cord injury, low back pain, diabetes, multiple sclerosis, hearing and speech impairments, visual impairment and blindness, and epilepsy. Each chapter includes information about the disease or condition; psychological aspects of the condition; professional service providers; environmental adaptations; assistive devices; and descriptions of organizations, publications, and products. Chapters on rehabilitation services, independent living, self-help, laws that affect people with disabilities (including the ADA), and making everyday living easier. Special information for children is also included. This new edition includes information about special resources on the Internet.

Fourth edition 1999   ISBN 0-929718-22-4 $54.95

"...wide coverage and excellent organization of this encyclopedic guide...recommended..." Choice

"...an excellent guide" Reference Books Bulletin/Booklist

"Sensitive to the tremendous variety of needs and circumstances of living with a disability" American Libraries

"an excellent resource for consumers and professionals..." Journal of the American Paraplegia Society

"...improves the chances of library patrons finding needed services..." American Reference Books Annual

"...an excellent reference that should be in every family physician's office as well as in libraries..."

Journal of the American Board of Family Physicians

Resources for Elders with Disabilities

This book provides information that enables elders, family members and other caregivers, and service providers to locate appropriate services. Published in LARGE PRINT (**18 point bold type**), the book provides information about rehabilitation, laws that affect elders with disabilities, and self-help groups. Each chapter that deals with a specific disability or condition has information on the causes and treatments for the condition; psychological aspects; professional service providers; where to find services; environmental adaptations; and suggestions for making everyday living safer and easier. Chapters on hearing loss, vision loss, Parkinson's disease, stroke, arthritis, osteoporosis, and diabetes also provide information on organizations, publications and tapes, and assistive devices. Throughout the book are practical suggestions to prevent accidents and to facilitate interactions with family members, friends, and service providers. Plus information about aids for everyday living, older workers, falls, travel, and housing.

Third edition 1996   ISBN 0-929718-16-X $48.95

"...especially useful for older readers. Highly recommended." Library Journal
"...a valuable, well organized, easy-to-read reference source." American Reference Books Annual

Making Wise Medical Decisions
How to Get the Information You Need

This book includes a wealth of information about where to go and what to read in order to make informed, rational, medical decisions. It describes a plan for obtaining relevant health information and evaluating the quality of medical tests and procedures, health care providers, and health facilities. Each chapter includes extensive resources to help the reader get started. Chapters include Getting the Information You Need to Make Wise Medical Decisions; Locating Appropriate Health Care; Asking the Right Questions About Medical Tests and Procedures; Protecting Yourself in the Hospital; Medical Benefits and Legal Rights; Drugs; Protecting the Health of Children Who Are Ill; Special Issues Facing Elders; People with Chronic Illnesses and Disabilities and the Health Care System; Making Decisions About Current Medical Controversies; Terminal Illness.

1998   ISBN 0-929718-21-6 $39.95

"It is refreshing to find a source of practical information on how to proceed through the medical maze...this should become a popular resource in any public, hospital, or academic library's consumer health collection."
Library Journal

Living with Low Vision
A Resource Guide for People with Sight Loss

This LARGE PRINT (**18 point bold type**) comprehensive directory helps people with sight loss locate the services, products, and publications that they need to keep reading, working, and enjoying life. Chapters for children and elders plus information on self-help groups, how to keep reading and working, and making everyday living easier. Information on laws that affect people with vision loss, including the ADA, and high tech equipment that promotes independence and employment. Includes information about Internet resources.

Fifth edition 1998   ISBN 0-929718-20-8 $44.95

"no other complete resource guide exists..an invaluable tool for locating services.. for public and academic libraries."   Library Journal
"This volume is a treasure chest of concise, useful information."   OT Week

Meeting the Needs of Employees with Disabilities

A comprehensive resource guide that provides information to help people with disabilities retain or obtain employment. Includes information on government programs and laws, training programs, supported employment, transition from school to work, and environmental adaptations. Chapters on hearing and speech impairments, mobility impairments, visual impairment and blindness describe organizations, adaptive equipment, and services plus suggestions for a safe and friendly workplace.

Second edition 1993   ISBN 0-929718-13-5 $42.95

"...recommended for public libraries and for academic libraries..." Choice

LARGE PRINT PUBLICATIONS

Designed for distribution by professionals, these publications serve as self-help guides for people with disabilities and chronic conditions. They include information on the condition, rehabilitation services, professional service providers, products, and resources that help people with disabilities and chronic conditions to live independently. Titles include "Living with Low Vision," "After a Stroke," and "Living with Diabetes." Printed in 18 point bold type on ivory paper with black ink for maximum contrast. 8 1/2" by 11" Sold in minimum quantities of 25 copies per title. See order form on last page of this book for complete list of titles.

"These are exciting products. We look forward to doing business with you again."
A rehabilitation professional

Rehabilitation Resource Manual: VISION

A desk reference that enables service providers, librarians, and others to make effective referrals. Includes guidelines on starting self-help groups; information on professional research and service organizations; plus chapters on assistive technology; for special populations; and by eye condition/disease. Case vignettes demonstrating multidisciplinary cooperation in providing services to people with vision loss are a new special feature of the Manual.

Fourth edition 1993 ISBN 0-929718-10-0 $39.95

".the best ready-access source available in this field." OT Week
"...should be a part of every eye care professional/service provider library." *Journal of Rehabilitation*

Providing Services for People with Vision Loss
A Multidisciplinary Perspective
Susan L. Greenblatt, Editor

Written by ophthalmologists, rehabilitation professionals, a physician who has experienced vision loss, and a sociologist, this book discusses how various professionals can work together to provide coordinated care for people with vision loss. Chapters include Vision Loss: A Patient's Perspective; Vision Loss: An Ophthalmologist's Perspective; Operating a Low Vision Aids Service; The Need for Coordinated Care; Making Referrals for Rehabilitation Services; Mental Health Services: The Missing Link; Self-Help Groups for People with Sight Loss; and Aids and Techniques that Help People with Vision Loss plus a Glossary. Also available on audiocassette.

1989 ISBN 0-929718-02-X $19.95

"...an excellent guide for professionals" **Journal of Rehabilitation**

Meeting the Needs of People with Vision Loss
A Multidisciplinary Perspective
Susan L. Greenblatt, Editor

Written by rehabilitation professionals, physicians, and a sociologist, this book discusses how to provide appropriate information and how to serve special populations. Chapters include What People with Vision Loss Need to Know; Information and Referral Services for People with Vision Loss; The Role of the Family in the Adjustment to Blindness or Visual Impairment; Diabetes and Vision Loss - Special Considerations; Special Needs of Children and Adolescents; Older Adults with Vision and Hearing Losses; Providing Services to Visually Impaired Elders in Long Term Care Facilities; plus a series of Multidisciplinary Case Studies. Also available on audiocassette.

1991 ISBN 0-929718-07-0 $24.95

"...of use to anyone concerned with improving service delivery to the growing population of people who are visually impaired." **American Journal of Occupational Therapy**

RESOURCES for REHABILITATION →

33 Bedford Street, Suite 19A • Lexington, MA 02420-4460 • (781) 862-6455 • FAX (781) 861-7517
e-mail: orders@rfr.org • http://www.rfr.org
Our Federal Employer Identification Number is 04-2975-007

NAME _____

ORGANIZATION _____

ADDRESS _____

PHONE _____

[ ] Check or signed institutional purchase order enclosed for full amount of order. Purchase orders accepted from government agencies, hospitals, and universities <u>only</u>.

[ ] Mastercard/VISA Card number: _____

Signature: _____Expiration date: _____

ALL ORDERS OF $100.00 OR LESS <u>MUST</u> BE PREPAID.

TITLE	QUANTITY	PRICE	TOTAL
A man's guide to coping with disability	____ X	$44.95	____
A woman's guide to coping with disability	____ X	42.95	____
Resources for people with disabilities and chronic conditions	____ X	54.95	____
Resources for elders with disabilities	____ X	48.95	____
Making wise medical decisions	____ X	39.95	____
Living with low vision: A resource guide	____ X	44.95	____
Providing services for people with vision loss	____ X	19.95	____
[ ] Check here for audiocassette edition			
Meeting the needs of people with vision loss	____ X	24.95	____
[ ] Check here for audiocassette edition			
Rehabilitation resource manual: VISION	____ X	39.95	____
Meeting the needs of employees with disabilities	____ X	42.95	____

<u>MINIMUM PURCHASE OF 25 COPIES PER TITLE FOR THE FOLLOWING PUBLICATIONS</u>
Call for discount on purchases of 100 or more copies of any single title.

TITLE	QUANTITY	PRICE	TOTAL
Living with diabetes	____ X	1.75	____
After a stroke	____ X	1.75	____
Living with low vision	____ X	2.00	____
How to keep reading with vision loss	____ X	1.75	____
Living with diabetic retinopathy	____ X	1.75	____
Living with age-related macular degeneration	____ X	1.25	____
Aids for everyday living with vision loss	____ X	1.25	____
High tech aids for people with vision loss	____ X	1.75	____
Living with arthritis	____ X	1.00	____
Living with hearing loss	____ X	1.00	____

SUB-TOTAL ____

SHIPPING & HANDLING: $50.00 or less, add $5.00; $50.01 to 100.00, add $8.00;
add $4.00 for each additional $100.00 or fraction of $100.00. Alaska, Hawaii,
U.S. territories, and Canada, add $3.00 to shipping and handling charges
Foreign orders must be prepaid in U.S. currency.
Please write for shipping charges.

SHIPPING/HANDLING ____

TOTAL ____